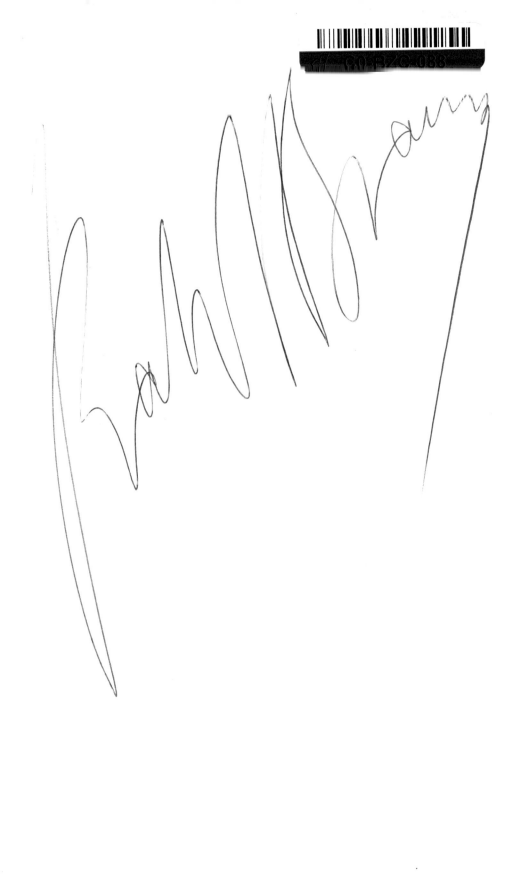

NEW CONCEPTS IN NEUROTRANSMITTER REGULATION

NEW CONCEPTS IN NEUROTRANSMITTER REGULATION

*Proceedings of a Symposium on Drug Abuse and Metabolic Regulation
of Neurotransmitters held in La Jolla, California, in July 1972*

EDITED BY
ARNOLD J. MANDELL

*Department of Psychiatry
School of Medicine
University of California at San Diego
La Jolla, California*

PLENUM PRESS · NEW YORK–LONDON · 1973

First Printing - May 1973
Second Printing - October 1974

Library of Congress Catalog Card Number 73-79222
ISBN 0-306-30737-5

© 1973 Plenum Press, New York
A Division of Plenum Publishing Corporation
227 West 17th Street, New York, N.Y. 10011

United Kingdom edition published by Plenum Press, London
A Division of Plenum Publishing Company, Ltd.
Davis House (4th Floor), 8 Scrubs Lane, Harlesden, London,
NW10 6SE, England

Printed in the United States of America

PREFACE

Historically, the development of biological science has
proceeded from the anatomy to the physiology of particular systems.
Knowledge about neurotransmitters in the brain has evolved from the
discovery of the compounds per se, through the elucidation of their
biosynthetic and degradative pathways, and finally to the current
focus, the regulation of these processes.

Regulation in a biological system implies the capacity to
respond to perturbations. The introduction of standard and speci-
fiable disturbances in a biological system followed by examination
of the mechanisms involved in response, i.e. that dampen and/or
cancel the induced changes, has proved to be a successful way to
elucidate regulatory mechanisms.

Psychotropic drugs have been most useful to students of regulatory mechanisms in that calvarial prisoner, the brain, for they
allow prospective manipulation of variables like dosage and time.
Those of us interested in the biological substrata of behavior are
especially excited that disturbance induced by drugs leaves the
organism intact and behaving, and we can observe behavioral
correlates.

The pharmacological strategy is, of course, not unique to
brain scientists. The relationship between psychotropic drugs
and our emerging knowledge of neurotransmitter regulation is, for
example, akin to the development of anticancer agents in company
with the uncovering of many mysteries of molecular biology.

Working in this field, we are blessed with a very important
impetus to our basic research, namely, relevance. At least two
areas of human suffering justify our continued efforts: psycho-
pathology and the promise of effective treatment thereof with drugs,
and the abuse of and addiction to drugs affecting the central nervous
system. Both areas will benefit ultimately from studies of the
regulation of the biosynthesis and the effects of neurotransmitters.
We see neuropharmacology as the basic science most relevant to
psychiatry, and examples of the best current work in the field
are to be found in these pages.

v

We were delighted that the Center for Studies of Drug Abuse and Narcotics Addiction, and Drs. Bunney, Peterson, Braude, Szara, and Nuite of the National Institute of Mental Health saw fit to aid the private foundation, Friends of Psychiatric Research of San Diego, Inc. in sponsoring a symposium on this important and timely work. We were also very pleased that all the invited guests saw fit to take time from their busy and productive schedules of activity to deliver papers of outstanding quality.

Thanks are also in order to Drs. Suzanne Knapp, Ronald Kuczenski, and David Segal, whose work and effort helped create the local scientific base for the proceedings; to Noelle Cason for immeasurable help in planning and arranging the meeting; and to Linda Bailey and Barbara Blomgren for their assistance with editing and production.

I think we all had a stimulating and delightful time together. I hope a bit of this feeling pervades the book.

                                              Arnold J. Mandell

La Jolla
February, 1973

CONTRIBUTORS

GEORGE K. AGHAJANIAN, Departments of Pharmacology and Psychiatry, School of Medicine, Yale University, New Haven, Conn.

JAMES P. BENNETT, Department of Pharmacology, School of Medicine, The Johns Hopkins University, Baltimore, Maryland

RICHARD BJUR, Department of Pharmacology, School of Medicine, University of Colorado, Denver, Colorado

FLOYD E. BLOOM, Laboratory of Neuropharmacology, National Institute of Mental Health, St. Elizabeth's Hospital, Washington, D.C.

FRANK C. BOVE, Department of Pharmacology, School of Medicine, University of Colorado, Denver, Colorado

BENJAMIN S. BUNNEY, Department of Psychiatry, School of Medicine, Yale University, New Haven, Connecticut

GILLES CLOUTIER, Department of Pharmacology, School of Medicine, University of Colorado, Denver, Colorado

ERMINO COSTA, Laboratory of Preclinical Pharmacology, National Inst. of Mental Health, St. Elizabeth's Hospital, Washington, D.C.

GALE L. CRAVISO, Department of Pharmacology, School of Medicine, New York University, New York, New York

WALLACE DAIRMAN, The Roche Institute of Molecular Biology, Nutley, New Jersey

JACQUES GLOWINSKI, Laboratory of Molecular Biology, College of France, Paris, France

AVRAM GOLDSTEIN, Department of Pharmacology, School of Medicine, Stanford University, Stanford, California

ALESSANDRO GUIDOTTI, Laboratory of Preclinical Pharmacology, Nat'l Inst. of Mental Health, St. Elizabeth's Hosp., Washington, D.C.

MICHEL HAMON, Laboratory of Molecular Biology, College of France, Paris, France

FRANCIS HERY, Laboratory of Molecular Biology, College of France, Paris, France

ING K. HO, Langley Porter Neuropsychiatric Institute, San Francisco, California

BARRY J. HOFFER, Laboratory of Neuropharmacology, National Institute of Mental Health, St. Elizabeth's Hosp., Wash., D.C.

LESLIE L. IVERSEN, Department of Pharmacology, University of Cambridge, England

IRWIN J. KOPIN, Laboratory of Clinical Science, National Institute of Mental Health, Bethesda, Maryland

MICHAEL J. KUHAR, Department of Psychiatry, School of Medicine, Yale University, New Haven, Connecticut

SALOMON Z. LANGER, Institute of Pharmacological Research, Buenos Aires, Argentina

WILLIAM J. LOGAN, Department of Neurology, School of Medicine, The University of Virginia, Charlottesville, Virginia

HORACE H. LOH, The Langley Porter Neuropsychiatric Institute, San Francisco, California

ARNOLD J. MANDELL, Department of Psychiatry, School of Medicine, University of California at San Diego, La Jolla, Ca.

EDITH G. McGEER, Department of Psychiatry, University of British Columbia, Vancouver, B. C., Canada

PAUL L. McGEER, Department of Psychiatry, University of British Columbia, Vancouver, B. C., Canada

CHARLENE A. McQUEEN, Department of Pharmacology, School of Medicine, New York University, New York, New York

JOSE M. MUSACCHIO, Department of Pharmacology, School of Medicine, New York University, New York, New York

FRANZ OESCH, Department of Pharmacology, Biocenter of the University, Basel, Switzerland

CANDACE B. PERT, Department of Pharmacology, School of Medicine, The Johns Hopkins University, Baltimore, Maryland

FREDERICK E. SCHON, Physiological Laboratory, The University of
          Cambridge, England

GEORGE R. SIGGINS, Laboratory of Neuropharmacology, National Insti-
          tute of Mental Health, St. Elizabeth's Hosp., Wash., D.C.

SOLOMON H. SNYDER, Departments of Pharmacology and Psychiatry,
          School of Medicine, The Johns Hopkins Univ., Baltimore, Md.

HANS THOENEN, Department of Pharmacology, Biocenter of the University,
          Basel, Switzerland

E. LEONG WAY, The Langley Porter Neuropsychiatric Institute,
          San Francisco, California

NORMAN WEINER, Department of Pharmacology, School of Medicine,
          University of Colorado, Denver, Colorado

HENRY I. YAMAMURA, Biomedical Laboratory, Edgewood Arsenal, Edgewood,
          Maryland

CONTENTS

NEUROTRANSMITTER REGULATION AND ENZYME SYNTHESIS

NEUROTRANSMITTER REGULATION AND ENZYME ACTIVITY

MULTIPLE MEASURES OF COMPENSATORY ADAPTATION IN

CATECHOLAMINE BIOSYNTHESIS

Wallace Dairman

Roche Institute of Molecular Biology

Nutley, New Jersey

INTRODUCTION

It has become apparent that the in vivo rate of catecholamine synthesis is subject to control by a variety of factors. The first such regulating influence to be described, and probably the most important, was the acute effect of sympathetic nerve activity on the catecholamine synthetic rate. Work from a number of different laboratories has demonstrated that changes in sympathetic tone result in an immediate and corresponding alteration of the rate of catecholamine synthesis (Alousi and Weiner, 1966; Gordon et al., 1966; Sedvall and Kopin, 1967; Dairman and Udenfriend, 1970 a). Evidence has been presented that the activity of tyrosine hydroxylase, the rate limiting enzyme in catecholamine synthesis (Levitt et al., 1965), is being reversibly modified through a mechanism thought to involve end-product inhibition by catecholamines (Alousi and Weiner, 1966; Neff and Costa, 1966; Spector et al., 1967). This occurs without an actual change in the level of tyrosine hydroxylase enzyme (Dairman et al., 1968).

Recently, Shiman et al. (1971) proposed that the concentration of the substrate, tyrosine, could potentially exert a regulatory influence on the activity of tyrosine hydroxylase. This suggestion was based on the in vitro finding that bovine tyrosine hydroxylase was subject to substrate inhibition by tyrosine. This was demonstrable when the enzyme activity was assayed with tetrahydrobiopterin, the putative natural cofactor (Lloyd and Weiner, 1970). The first section of this paper presents the results of experiments designed to test whether the in vitro findings of Shiman et al. function under in vivo conditions.

1

In 1969 experiments by Mueller et al. (1969 a) and Viveros et al. (1969) demonstrated that when animals were subjected to chronically maintained stressful conditions the activity of adrenal tyrosine hydroxylase could be elevated. Subsequent work showed that this effect was dependent on a chronic increased sympathetic nerve activity (Thoenen et al., 1969; Weiner and Mosimann, 1970; Patrick and Kirshner, 1971) and that it probably represented an induction of tyrosine hydroxylase enzyme protein (Mueller et al., 1969 b). Evidence has also been presented that an induction of tyrosine hydroxylase can be correlated with a corresponding increase in catecholamine synthesis in the intact animals (Dairman and Udenfriend, 1970 b). The second portion of this paper discusses a mechanism(s) whereby the tissue levels of tyrosine hydroxylase can be reduced in response to certain pharmacological agents.

RESULTS AND DISCUSSION

Tyrosine Levels as a Regulatory Factor in Catecholamine Synthesis

The aim of the following experiments was to increase the in vivo concentration of L-tyrosine and then to evaluate the effect on the catecholamine synthesis rate. Based on the in vitro data of Shiman et al. (1970) an in vivo increase in tyrosine concentration might be expected to result in substrate inhibition of tyrosine hydroxylase and thus a corresponding decrease in the catecholamine synthesis rate. If this occurred the tissue levels of catecholamines would be expected to fall, since the synthetic rate would not be able to keep pace with catecholamine release and degradation (Gordon et al., 1966).

Large amounts of L-tyrosine were administered intraperitoneally to a group of rats housed at 4°C. The imposition of a cold stress will result in an increased sympathetic nerve activity and an increased release of norepinephrine. Under these conditions an inhibition of tyrosine hydroxylase should result in decreased tissue catecholamine levels. Following the administration of tyrosine, the plasma and tissue levels of this amino acid were double that of the controls (Table 1). However, this did not result in a diminution of norepinephrine levels in either the heart or the brain in comparison to saline injected controls.

A somewhat more effective method of elevating endogenous tyrosine levels is by the administration of a protein synthesis inhibitor. Under these conditions amino acid incorporation into protein is halted while the reverse process, the degradation of protein and peptides to amino acids, remains functional. As

TABLE 1

Catecholamine Concentrations After Increases in Tissue and
Plasma Tyrosine Concentrations Produced by Cycloheximide or L-tyrosine

| | Tyrosine | | Noradrenaline | | Dopamine |
	Brain (µg/g)	Plasma (µg/ml)	Brain (µg/g)	Heart (µg/g)	Brain (µg/g)
Exp. I					
Control	14.2 + 0.5	14.6 + 1.7	0.52 + 0.01	1.40 + 0.08	
L-tyrosine	26.7 + 2.0‡	27.2 + 2.6‡	0.56 + 0.3	1.48 + 0.1	
Exp. II					
Control	--	13.4 + 1.64	0.39 + 0.01	1.03 + 0.05	--
Cycloheximide 2.5 mg/kg	--	23.4 + 2.78*	0.44 + 0.04	1.19 + 0.25	--
Exp. III					
Control	13.5 + 2.3	11.8 + 1.0	--	0.96 + 0.09	0.93 + 0.1
Cycloheximide	60.7 + 1.5†	88.1 + 4.5†	--	1.19 + 0.14	0.80 + 0.08

Exp. I – Rats were given either 0.9% NaCl or 1,000 mg/kg of L-tyrosine intraperitoneally and placed in the cold at 4°C. Two and one-half hours later the drug
treatment was repeated. The animals were killed 3 hours later.

Exp. II – Rats were injected intraperitoneally with either 0.9% NaCl or cycloheximide (2.5 mg/kg) and killed 6.5 hours later. Five animals were used per group.

Exp. III – Rats were injected intraperitoneally with either 0.9% NaCl or cycloheximide (5 mg/kg) and killed 4.5 hours later. Four animals were used in each group.

*P <0.02; †P <0.001; ‡P <0.005. Student's t test; from Dairman (1972).

shown in Table 1, the protein synthesis inhibitor, cycloheximide elevated the tissue and plasma concentration of tyrosine by as much as seven-fold. However, under these conditions, no decrease in the catecholamine content of either heart or brain could be demonstrated.

The effect of raising the tyrosine concentration on the rate of catecholamine synthesis was evaluated by a second method. The cardiac stores of norepinephrine were labelled by the intravenous administration of ^{3}H-norepinephrine and the decline in specific activity was followed with time. One and a half hours after the injection of 5 μc of ^{3}H-L-norepinephrine, 3 mg/kg of cycloheximide were administered to the rats. As shown in Figure 1, the cyclo-heximide elevation of tyrosine levels did not result in a slowing of cardiac norepinephrine turnover. In fact, roughly a two-fold increase in the turnover rate of the cycloheximide-treated group was noted. This result could indicate that the normal neuronal tyrosine concentration may not be saturating with respect to tyrosine hydroxylase. A more likely explanation might be that protein synthesis inhibition imposed a stress, which resulted in an increased sympathetic nerve activity and by this mechanism increased turnover.

The results of our experiments indicate that raising the in vivo concentration of tyrosine 2 to 7-fold does not appear to result in inhibition of tyrosine hydroxylase, as reflected by the animals' ability to synthesize catecholamines. The lack of agree-ment between the in vitro data of Shiman et al. (1970) and our in vivo data could have several possible explanations. Substrate inhibition of tyrosine hydroxylase was investigated only with enzyme prepared from bovine adrenal. Thus this phenomenon might be peculiar to this species or tissue. Secondly, substrate inhibition by tyrosine was not observed with all tetrahydropteridines although tetrahydrobiopterin is the natural cofactor for tyrosine hydroxylase in beef adrenal (Lloyd and Weiner, 1970). A similar role for this pteridine has as yet not been unequivocally estab-lished in other tissues and species. Finally, despite the elevation of tyrosine concentration in tissue and plasma, the level of the amino acid in the sympathetic nerve endings may be unaltered.

There is also evidence that in the guinea pig an elevated concentration of tyrosine does not result in an inhibition of tyrosine hydroxylase. In 1956, Levitt et al. (1965), using an isolated guinea pig heart preparation showed that the maximum incorporation of ^{14}C-L-tyrosine into norepinephrine occurred at a perfusion concentration of about 8×10^{-5} M. This is close to the levels found in our control rats (7.4×10^{-5} M). Increasing the concentration of tyrosine in the perfusion fluid up to 1×10^{-3} M did not result in a diminution of norepinephrine synthesis. Since

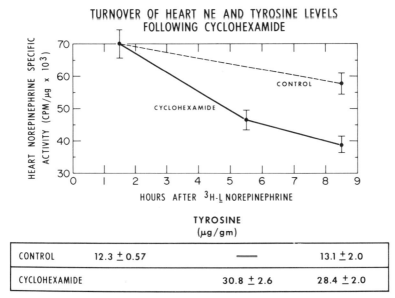

Figure 1. Female Sprague Dawley rats (200 g) were administered 5 μ Ci of ^{3}H-L-norepinephrine (6.41 Ci/mM) intravenously. One and one-half hours later some of these animals were killed. The remaining animals received either 3 mg/kg of cycloheximide or 0.9% sodium chloride intraperitoneally and the animals sacrificed at the indicated times thereafter. The cardiac norepinephrine was isolated by alumina absorption and the specific activity determined.

the studies of Levitt were carried out in an isolated organ, the possibility of an increase in sympathetic nerve activity releasing tyrosine hydroxylase from end product inhibition can be ruled out.

Decreases of Tyrosine Hydroxylase Levels Mediated by Pharmacological Agents

We have previously reported that the administration of L-dopa to rats, guinea pigs, and gerbils, for periods of from two to seven days resulted in a decreased activity of tyrosine hydroxylase as measured in vitro (Dairman and Udenfriend, 1971; Dairman and Udenfriend, 1972) (Table 2). A decrease in the mesenteric artery tyrosine hydroxylase activity of both rats and rabbits has also been demonstrated following L-dopa administration (Tarver, Berkowitz and Spector, 1971).

The decrease in tyrosine hydroxylase activity seen following the administration of L-dopa need not reflect an actual decrease in enzyme content. For example, L-dopa administration could result in an altered form of the enzyme or in the accumulation of

TABLE 2

Tyrosine Hydroxylase Activity of Tissues from Rat, Gerbil,
and Guinea Pig Following Administration of L-Dopa

Species	Tissue	Control	Tyrosine Hydroxylase Activity[a] L-Dopa
Rat	Adrenal	(10) 20.8 $\pm$ 1.05	(10) $10.24^{d}\pm$ 0.25
Gerbil	Adrenal	(8) 45.73 $\pm$ 1.05	(9) 33.9^{c} $\pm$ 2.6
		(10) 34.2	(9) 25.3^{d} $\pm$ 1.29
Guinea Pig	Adrenal	(7) 172.5 $\pm$ 19.07	(5) 99.7^{b} $\pm$ 5.0
	Heart	(7) 6910 $\pm$ 460	(6) 3835^{d} $\pm$ 298

Female Mongolian gerbils (50 g) and female Sprague Dawley rats
(200 g) were given 1000 mg/kg of L-Dopa (s.c.) daily for four consecutive days and killed on the fifth day. Male, Hartley strain
guinea pigs (500 g) were given L-Dopa 1000 mg/kg (s.c.) daily for
five consecutive days, and then no drug for two days followed by
two additional days of L-Dopa administration (1000 mg/kg/day s.c.).
The animals were then killed 1 day later. The number in parentheses
refers to the number of animals used. From Dairman and Udenfriend
(1972).

[a] Adrenal data expressed as n moles $\pm$ (S.E.M.) of tyrosine
hydroxylated to L-Dopa per adrenal pair per 15 minutes. Heart data
expressed as CPM of tritiated water released from 300,000 CPM of
tritiated tyrosine per 100 λ of heart puss juice per 15 minutes.

[b] Significantly different from control ($p < 0.01$)
[c]   ($p < 0.005$)
[d]   ($p < 0.001$)

----

inhibitory substances or the removal of activators. This however,
appears not to be the case. At times when adrenal tyrosine
hydroxylase activity was found to be depressed following L-dopa
administration, the mixing of enzyme extracts from these animals
and control animals yielded tyrosine hydroxylase activities which
were additive (Dairman et al., 1972; Table 3). These results
are consistent with the concept that L-dopa administration does
not result in accumulation of inhibitory substances or the
removal of activators. Km values were also determined for both

TABLE 3

Additivity of Tyrosine Hydroxylase Activity from Adrenal
Extracts of Control of L-Dopa Treated Rats

| Enzyme | Tyrosine Hydroxylated | | |
	Control	L-Dopa	Control & L-Dopa
ml			
0.05	0.32	0.20	0.53
0.10	0.74	0.39	1.10
0.20	1.44	0.84	
0.30	1.92	1.09	

Rats (female Sprague Dawley 200 g) were given L-Dopa s.c.,
1000 mg/kg/day for 4 consecutive days. The controls received
0.9% sodium chloride. One day following the last dose the
animals were killed. The adrenals from five L-Dopa treated
rats were pooled and homogenized in 10 ml of 0.13 m potassium
phosphate buffer, as were the adrenals from five control
animals. Various amounts of a 30,000 x g (10 min) supernatant
fraction for each group of rats and various combinations of the
two enzymatic fractions were assayed for tyrosine hydroxylase
activity.

tyrosine and 6,7-dimethyltetrahydropteridine following L-dopa
treatment and were found to be essentially identical to the
control values (Dairman et al., 1972):

Controls: Tyrosine, 3.7×10^{-5} M, pteridine, 3.3×10^{-4} M,
L-dopa treated: Tyrosine, 4.4×10^{-5} M, pteridine, 3.6×10^{-4} M.

Finally, since activity measurements were carried out on a
high speed supernatant fraction of adrenal homogenates, the distribution of tyrosine after L-dopa treatment was determined. The
enzyme distribution was found to be unaltered following L-dopa
administration in that all of the activity still remained in
the supernatant fraction. In addition the same decrease in
tyrosine hydroxylase activity could be observed with assay of
the crude homogenate.

The above results indicate that the decreased activity of
tyrosine hydroxylase observed following L-dopa administration
most likely represents an actual decrease in enzyme protein.
Whether this effect represents a repression of enzyme protein
synthesis or an increased degradation of the enzyme is not known.

Investigations were carried out to determine if either the endocrine system or sympathetic nerve activity were involved in the L-dopa mediated decrease of tyrosine hydroxylase. It had been reported that hypophysectomy resulted in a significant reduction in adrenal tyrosine hydroxylase (Mueller et al., 1970; Kvetnanský et al., 1970). It was therefore conceivable that L-dopa could exert its effect on tyrosine hydroxylase by interfering with pituitary function. An alternate possibility was that the administration of L-dopa resulted in a chronic decrease in sympathetic activity, for which some evidence exists (Whitsett et al., 1970). Since it is well known that a chronic increase in sympathetic nerve activity will result in an induction of tyrosine hydroxylase, perhaps a decrease in sympathetic tone would have the opposite effect. However, this seems unlikely in that reports have also appeared demonstrating that adrenal tyrosine hydroxylase activity does not fall following transection of the splanchnic nerve (Thoenen et al., 1969; Weiner and Mosimann, 1970; Patrick and Kirshner, 1971). Thus it was not surprising to find that L-dopa administration was capable of reducing tyrosine hydroxylase in a denervated adrenal (Dairman et al., 1972; Figure 2). In a similar fashion the involvement of

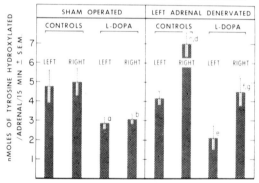

EFFECT OF L-DOPA ON TYROSINE HYDROXYLASE
ACTIVITY IN DENERVATED RAT ADRENALS

Figure 2.   Sham-denervated rats and animals with the left adrenal denervated received s.c. injections daily of either L-dopa 1000 mg/kg or saline for 4 consecutive days. The animals were killed on the fifth day and each adrenal assayed for tyrosine hydroxylase activity. Surgery was performed 5 days prior to initiation of dosing.   Seven to ten animals were used per group. Taken from Dairman and Udenfriend (1972). [a]Statistically different from sham saline, left adrenal (P <.05); [b]statistically different from sham saline, right adrenal (P <.02); [c]statistically different from denervated saline, left adrenal (P <.01); [d]statistically different from sham saline, right adrenal (P <.05); [e]statistically different from denervated saline, left adrenal (P <.01); [f]statistically different from innervated saline, right adrenal (P <.025); [g]statistically different from denervated dopa, left adrenal (P <.05).

the pituitary endocrine system in the mediation of L-dopa's effect
on tyrosine hydroxylase, was investigated by the use of hypophysectomized rats. The results of these experiments confirmed the
findings of other laboratories (Mueller et al., 1970; Kvetnansky
et al., 1970), in that they demonstrated that hypophysectomy
resulted in about a 50% reduction of adrenal tyrosine hydroxylase.
However, the administration of L-dopa to hypophysectomized rats
resulted in an additional 50% decrease in activity (Dairman et
al., 1972; Figure 3). These results clearly rule out the involvement of pituitary influences or decreases in sympathetic nerve
activity as required factors in the L-dopa mediated decrease of
tyrosine hydroxylase.

Another factor which merits attention would be the possible
formation of 6-hydroxydopa that might arise from the autoxidation
of L-dopa. 6-Hydroxydopa, if it were indeed formed, could be
decarboxylated to 6-hydroxydopamine by aromatic L-amino acid
decarboxylase (Ong et al., 1969). This latter compound is capable
of destroying sympathetic nerve endings (Thoenen and Tranzer, 1968)
and thus can decrease the tissue levels of tyrosine hydroxylase
(Mueller et al., 1969 a). If these compounds were formed in
functionally significant amounts, then their effects should be
demonstrable in the heart. This tissue is very susceptible to the
destruction of its sympathetic nerve endings following either the
administration of the precursor, 6-hydroxydopa, or 6-hydroxydopa-
mine. The depletion of cardiac norepinephrine and the destruction
of the heart's capability to take up circulating catecholamines
are the result of 6-hydroxydopamine's ability to destroy sympathetic
nerve endings (Stone et al., 1963; Theonen et al., 1968; Berkowitz
et al., 1970). However, when tyrosine hydroxylase levels are
depressed by L-dopa administration, the ability of the heart to
take up exogenously administered norepinephrine is unimpaired
(Table 4). This finding makes it very unlikely that L-dopa
administration causes its effect on tyrosine hydroxylase via
formation of 6-hydroxydopamine.

The question remained as to whether L-dopa itself, or a
metabolic product, was responsible for the effect on tyrosine
hydroxylase. The two principle routes for the metabolism of L-
dopa are O-methylation to 3-methoxydopa and decarboxylation to
catecholamines and their metabolites (Bartholini and Pletscher,
1968; Wurtman, Chou and Rose, 1970). A number of potent inhibitors
of aromatic L-amino acid decarboxylase, the enzyme responsible for
the conversion of L-dopa to dopamine, are currently available. By
the use of such an inhibitor, RO 4-4602 (N'-[DL-SERYL]-N^2-[2,3,4-
trihydroxybenzyl] hydrazine) (Burkhard et al., 1964), it was
possible to differentiate between the effects of L-dopa itself and
products beyond the decarboxylation step. As shown in Figure 4,
the administration of RO 4-4602 concomitantly with L-dopa prevented

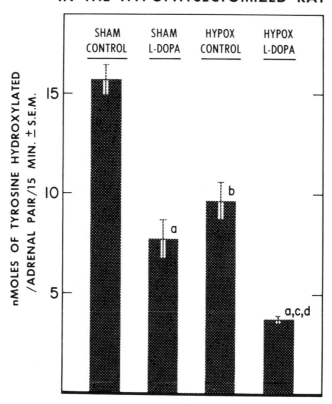

EFFECT OF L-DOPA ON
ADRENAL TYROSINE HYDROXYLASE
IN THE HYPOPHYSECTOMIZED RAT

Figure 3. Hypophysectomized and sham-operated rats were prepared
8 days prior to the initiation of dosing. These animals received
1000 mg/kg/day of L-dopa s.c. or 0.9% NaCl for two consecutive days
and then 500 mg/kg of L-dopa s.c. or 0.9% NaCl for an additional
day. The animals were killed one day following the last dose and
the adrenals assayed for tyrosine hydroxylase activity. Five
animals were used in each group except the hypophysectomized saline
group in which 10 were used. All the animals were kept from the
time of the surgical manipulation until the termination of the
experiment in a 30°C room and maintained on a low iodine test diet
and drinking water containing 5% sucrose. [a]Significantly different
from control (p< 0.001). [b]Significantly different from control
(p< 0.005). [c]Significantly different from sham-L-dopa (p< 0.005).
[d]Significantly different from hypox-saline (p< 0.001).

PREVENTION OF L-DOPA INDUCED DECREASE
OF ADRENAL TYROSINE HYDROXYLASE
BY DECARBOXYLASE INHIBITION

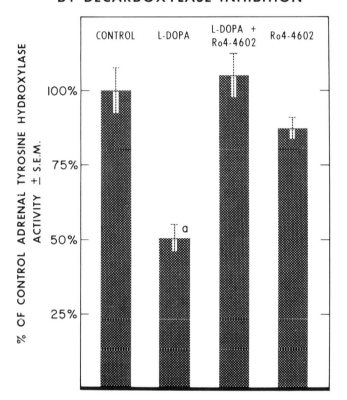

Figure 4.   Rats were administered the following compounds for four
consecutive days; L-dopa 1000 mg/kg s.c. (once daily) plus 0.9%
NaCl i.p. (twice daily) or L-dopa 1000 mg/kg s.c. (once daily) plus
RO 4-4602 50 mg/kg i.p. (twice daily or RO 4-4602 50 mg/kg i.p.
(twice daily) plus 0.9% NaCl s.c. (once daily). Controls received
0.9% NaCl s.c. (once daily) and i.p. (twice daily). The animals
were killed one day following the last dose and the adrenals assayed
for tyrosine hydroxylase activity. Eight animals were used in each
group. Taken from Dairman and Udenfriend (1972).
   [a]Significantly different from all other groups (p< 0.005)

TABLE 4

Uptake of ^{3}H-Norepinephrine by the Heart Following
Four Days of L-Dopa Administration

	Heart Norepinephrine	
	DPM/gm Heart + S.E.M.	DPM/µg N.E.
Control	365,515 ± 63,600	406,312 ± 59,000
L-Dopa	465,707 ± 56,300	505,910 ± 62,000

Female Sprague-Dawley rats (200 g) were dosed with L-Dopa
(1000 mg/kg/day, s.c.) or 0.9% NaCl for four consecutive days.
Twenty-four hours following the last dosing, the animals were
administered 10 µCi of ^{3}H-DL norepinephrine (5 Ci/mmole) intravenously and killed five minutes later. Five animals were used
per group. From Pharmacological Reviews (Dairman, Christenson,
and Udenfriend, 1972).

the L-dopa mediated decrease in adrenal tyrosine hydroxylase
(Dairman et al., 1972). RO 4-4602, when given alone, was without
effect on tyrosine hydroxylase but did result in greater than an
85% inhibition of liver decarboxylase activity.

Bartholini and Pletscher (1968) have reported that following
the administration of L-dopa, the inhibition of aromatic L-amino
acid decarboxylase by RO 4-4602, elevates the tissue levels of L-
dopa and its methylated metabolite, 3-methoxydopa. Inhibition of
aromatic L-amino acid decarboxylase spares the administered L-dopa
from one of its principle metabolic routes. Consistent with these
findings is the observation that the administration of high doses
of 3-methoxydopa to rats (1000 mg/kg/day s.c. for 4 days) failed
to reduce mesenteric artery or adrenal tyrosine hydroxylase. It
seems clear that L-dopa itself or 3-methoxydopa are not the causative agents in the reduction of tyrosine hydroxylase but since the
administered L-dopa must first be decarboxylated to dopamine, it
would seem that dopamine or a metabolite of dopamine must be the
compound(s) responsible for this effect.

The finding that dopamine appeared to be an obligatory intermediate in the formation of the compound(s) responsible for
reducing tyrosine hydroxylase prompted us to investigate whether
the conversion of dopamine to norepinephrine was also a necessary
requirement. It should be emphasized that while dopamine synthesis
and levels are markedly elevated following the administration of
L-dopa, norepinephrine turnover is also increased (Dairman et al.,

1971). Our initial aim was to administer a dopamine-β-hydroxylase
inhibitor in conjunction with L-dopa and determine if this would
attenuate the reduction in tyrosine hydroxylase seen following
L-dopa administration. The results of such an experiment proved
to be difficult to interpret. The administration of dopamine-β-
hydroxylase inhibitor, U14-624 (1-phenyl-3-[2-thiazolyl]-2-
thiourea), (Johnson et al., 1970) 75 mg/kg/day for 4 consecutive days
resulted in a decrease of adrenal tyrosine hydroxylase which was
of the same magnitude as that seen following L-dopa administration
(1000 mg/kg/day for 4 consecutive days) or the concomitant administration of U14-624 and L-dopa. As shown in Figure 5 the ability
of U14-624 to reduce adrenal tyrosine hydroxylase activity is
not unique to this compound but is a property of several other
dopamine-β-hydroxylase inhibitors. This reduction in adrenal
tyrosine hydroxylase activity is probably the consequence of a
decreased amount of enzyme protein. The compounds themselves do
not inhibit tyrosine hydroxylase directly at concentration as high
as 1×10^{-4} M. The administration of a large single dose of
U14-624, 200 mg/kg did not decrease adrenal tyrosine hydroxylase
activity either 1 or 7 hours following its administration, making
it unlikely that an inhibitory metabolite was being formed. As

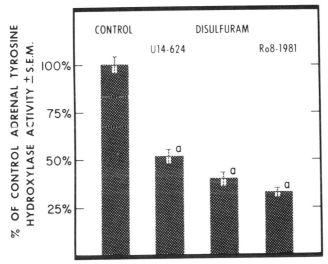

Figure 5. Rats were administered i.p. the following compounds for
4 consecutive days: Disulfiram, 100 mg/kg/day; RO 8-1981, 100
mg/kg for the first day and thereafter 50 mg/kg/day; U14-624,
35 mg/kg twice daily; or 0.9% NaCl. The animals were killed one day
following the last dose and the adrenals assayed for tyrosine
hydroxylase activity. From 7-10 animals were used in each group.
[a]Significantly different from control (p< 0.001)

TABLE 5

Additivity of Tyrosine Hydroxylase from Adrenal
Extracts of Control and U14-624 Treated Rats

Enzyme	Control	U14-624	Control & U14-624
ml		n moles/15 min	
0.1	.82	.36	1.25
0.1	.82		
0.2		.76	1.63
0.1		.36	
0.2	1.65		2.05

U14-624 35 mg/kg/twice daily was administered s.c. for 4 consecutive days to female Sprague Dawley rats (200 g). The controls received 0.9% sodium chloride. On the fifth day the animals were killed. Five adrenal pairs from each set of animals were pooled and the high speed supernatant fractions assayed for tyrosine hydroxylase individually and in various combinations with one another.

shown in Table 5 when adrenal extracts obtained from rats treated for 4 days with U14-624 were mixed with extracts obtained from control rats, the tyrosine hydroxylase activities were additive. This indicates that neither tyrosine hydroxylase inhibitors were formed nor activators removed as a consequence of U14-624 administration.

It was tempting to speculate that excess dopamine, arising from the administered L-dopa or by inhibition of dopamine-β-hydroxylase, triggered the reduction in tyrosine hydroxylase. If dopamine itself was the causative agent, then one might expect the administration of a small amount of L-dopa given together with a monoamine oxidase inhibitor to result in a decrease of tyrosine hydroxylase. As shown in Table 6 this proved not to be the case. The combination of 10 mg/kg L-dopa given together for 5 consecutive days with the monoamine oxidase inhibitor marsilid failed to result in a reduction of adrenal tyrosine hydroxylase. This amount of L-dopa was close to maximally tolerated amount when given together with a MAO inhibitor. These negative results necessitated the formulation of a somewhat modified hypothesis. Dopamine itself is

TABLE 6

Activity Following the Administration of L-Dopa
and a Monoamine Oxidase Inhibitor (Marsalid)

	Tyrosine Hydroxylase Activity + S.E.M.
	n moles of tyrosine hydroxylated/ 15 min/adrenal pair
Control	(7) 24.5 $\pm$ .79
L-Dopa	(7) 24.6 $\pm$ .90
Marsalid	(7) 23.7 $\pm$ 1.20
L-Dopa + Marsalid	(7) 26.2 $\pm$ .73

Female Sprague Dawley rats (200 g) were dosed with 10 mg/kg s.c.
of L-dopa daily for five days, or L-dopa plus 50 mg/kg i.p. of
marsalid on days one and three and 20 mg/kg i.p. of marsalid on
day four. Marsalid animals received the above doses of marsalid.
Controls received 0.9% sodium chloride. The animals were killed
on the fifth day six hours after the last administration of drugs
or saline. The numbers in parentheses refer to the number of
animals used.

not responsible for the reduction of tyrosine hydroxylase, but
the causative factor might be a deaminated metabolite of this
catecholamine, such as 3,4-dihydroxyphenylacetaldehyde. Generally,
the catecholamine metabolites have been considered inactive.
However, a recent report has appeared by Prasad (1971) indicating
that 3,4-dihydroxyphenylacetaldehyde is capable of reducing the
growth of neuroblastom in tissue culture. Thus, the aldehyde
formed from dopamine as a result of monoamine oxidase activity
has been demonstrated to affect neuronal tissue. In addition,
under in vitro conditions it has been shown that this aldehyde
is capable of condensing with dopamine to form tetrahydropaperoline
(Walsh et al., 1970) a compound having many beta sympathomimetic
actions (Holtz et al., 1964).

It is well established that reserpine induces tyrosine
hydroxylase through a mechanism involving the increased sympathetic nerve activity (Thoenen et al., 1969), invoked in response
to the catecholamine depleting effect of this drug. The administration of dopamine-β-hydroxylase inhibitor in addition to
reserpine would be expected to increase the norepinephrine depletion and thus enhance the reserpine mediated induction of

tyrosine hydroxylase. However, the opposite effect occurred. As
shown in Figure 6 disulfiram administration resulted in a decrease
in the reserpine mediated induction of adrenal tyrosine hydroxylase.
These experiments were carried out over 48 hours in which disulfiram
administration caused a small reduction in tyrosine hydroxylase in
comparison to the controls. However, the magnitude of this decrease
was far below that observed when comparing the reserpine plus
disulfiram group to the reserpine group. It is known that reserpine
by virtue of its ability to block dopamine vesicle uptake (Potter and
Axelrod, 1963; Stjarne et al., 1967) will result in a large increase
in the urinary excretion of the deaminated dopamine metabolite
homovanillic acid (Kopin and Weise, 1968). This compound is formed
via the oxidation of the corresponding aldehyde by aldehyde dehydrogenase (Erwin and Deitrich, 1966). Since disulfiram is an
inhibitor of both dopamine-β-hydroxylase (Goldstein et al., 1964)

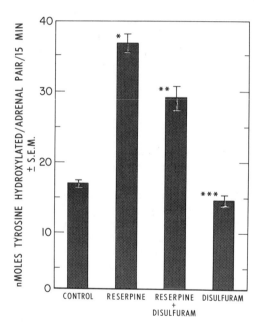

Figure 6. Decrease in the reserpine mediated induction of tyrosine
hydroxylase by disulfiram. Female Sprague Dawley rats (200 g) received either reserpine, 2.5 mg/kg s.c. daily for 2 consecutive days
or this dosage of reserpine plus 100 mg/kg i.p. of disulfiram daily
for two days, or disulfiram 100 mg/kg i.p. daily for two days. The
animals were killed on the third day and the adrenals assayed for
tyrosine hydroxylase activity. * Significantly different from
controls (p< 0.001). **Significantly different from reserpine
(p< 0.005). ***Significantly different from control (p< 0.02).

and aldehyde dehydrogenase (Deitrich and Hellerman, 1962). The combined administration of these two drugs should create conditions favorable for the formation of 3,4-dihydroxyphenylacetaldehyde. These data are compatible with the concept that both L-dopa and dopamine-β-hydroxylase inhibitors reduce tyrosine hydroxylase levels by virtue of 3,4-dihydroxyphenylacetaldehyde formation.

Further support for this hypothesis was obtained by the use of a monoamine oxidase inhibitor. The formation of 3,4-dihydroxy-phenylacetaldehyde is dependent upon monoamine oxidase activity. Therefore, inhibition of this enzyme should prevent the reduction in tyrosine hydroxylase brought about by dopamine-β-hydroxylase inhibitors. As shown in Figure 7, treatment of rats with the mono-amine oxidase inhibitor, marsilid, prevented U14-624's ability to reduce tyrosine hydroxylase.

Although these data support a role for 3,4-dihydroxyphenyl-acetaldehyde in the reduction of tyrosine hydroxylase levels, this hypothesis should be considered as only tentative. Additional studies will be required to either confirm or reject this hypothesis.

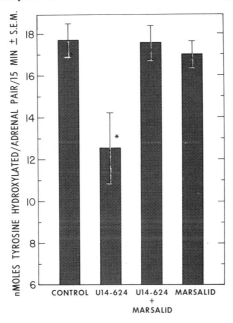

Figure 7. Effects of Marsalid treatment on the ability of U14-624 administration to decrease adrenal tyrosine hydroxylase. Female Sprague Dawley rats (200 g) were administered i.p. 35 mg/kg of U14-624 plus 120 mg/kg of marsalid i.p. on days one and three or marsalid alone. The animals were killed on the fifth day and the adrenals assayed for tyrosine hydroxylase activity.
*Statistically significant from all other groups ($p < 0.025$).

REFERENCES

Alousi, A. and Weiner, N. 1966. The regulation of norepinephrine synthesis in sympathetic nerves: Effects of nerve stimulation, cocaine, and catecholamine-releasing agents. Proc. Nat. Acad. Sci. USA 56: 1491-1496.

Bartholini, G. and Pletscher, A. 1968. Cerebral accumulation and metabolism of C^{14}-dopa after selective inhibition of peripheral decarboxylase. J. Pharmacol. Exp. Ther. 161: 14-20.

Berkowitz, B.A., Spector, S., Brossi, A., Focella, A. and Teitel, S. 1970. Preparation and biological properties of (-) and (+)-6-hydroxydopa. Experimentia 26: 982-983.

Burkard, W.P., Gey, K.F., and Pletscher, A. 1964. Inhibition of decarboxylase of aromatic amino acids by 2,3,4-trihydroxy-benzylhydrazine and its seryl derivative. Arch. Biochem. Biophys. 107: 187-196.

Dairman, W. 1972. Catecholamine concentration and the activity of tyrosine hydroxylase after an increase in the concentration of tyrosine in rat tissues. Brit. J. Pharmacol. 44: 307-310.

Dairman, W., Gordon, R., Spector, S., Sjoerdsma, A. and Udenfriend, S. 1968. Increased synthesis of catecholamines in the intact rat following administration of α-adrenergic blocking agents. Mol. Pharmacol. 4: 457-464.

Dairman, W. and Udenfriend, S. 1970 a. Effect of ganglionic blocking agents on the increased synthesis of catecholamines resulting from α-adrenergic blockade on exposure to cold. Biochem. Pharmacol. 19: 979-984.

Dairman, W. and Udenfriend, S. 1970 b. Increased conversion of tyrosine to catecholamines in the intact rat following elevation of tissue tyrosine hydroxylase levels by administered phenoxybenzamine. Mol. Pharmacol. 6: 350-356.

Dairman, W. and Udenfriend, S. 1971. Decrease in adrenal tyrosine hydroxylase and increase in norepineprhine synthesis in rats given L-dopa. Science 171: 1022-1024.

Dairman, W. and Udenfriend, S. 1972. Studies on the mechanism of the L-3,4-dihydroxyphenylalanine induced decrease in tyrosine hydroxylase activity. Mol. Pharmacol. 8: 293-299.

Deitrich, R.A. and Hellerman, L. 1963. Diphosphopyridine nucleo-tide-linked aldehyde dehydrogenase II inhibitors. J. Biol. Chem. 238: 1683-1689.

Erwin, G.V. and Deitrich, R.A. 1965. Brain aldehyde dehydrogenase localization, purification, and properties. J. Biol. Chem. 241: 3533-3539.

Gordon, R., Spector, S., Sjoerdsma, A. and Udenfriend, S. 1966. Increased synthesis of norepinephrine and epinephrine in the intact rat during exercise and exposure to cold. J. Pharmacol. Exp. Ther. 153: 440-447.

Holtz, P., Stock, K. and Westermann, E. 1964. Pharmakologies des tetrahydropapaerolins und weine entstehung aus dopamin naunyn-Schmeideberg. Arch. Pharmakol. Exp. Pathol. 248: 387-405.

Johnson, G.A., Boukma, S.J. and Kim, E.G. 1970. In vivo inhibition of dopamine-β-hydroxylase by 1-phenyl-3-(2-thiazolyl)-2-thiourea (U-14-624). J. Pharmacol. Exp. Ther. 171: 80-87.

Kvetnansky, R., Gewirtz, G.P., Weise, V.K. and Kopin, I.J. 1970. Effect of hypophysectomy on immobilization-induced elevation of tyrosine hydroxylase and phenylethanolamine-N-methyl transferase in the rat adrenal. Endocrinology 87: 1323-1329.

Levitt, M., Spector, S., Sjoerdsma, A. and Udenfriend, S. 1965. Elucidation of the rate limiting step in norepinephrine biosynthesis using the perfused guinea pig heart. J. Pharmacol. Exp. Ther. 148: 1-8.

Lloyd, T. and Weiner, N. 1970. Isolation and characterization of the tyrosine hydroxylase cofactor from bovine adrenal medulla. Pharmacologist 12: 287.

Mueller, R.A., Thoenen, K. and Axelrod, J. 1969 a. Adrenal tyrosine hydroxylase: Compensatory increase in activity after chemical sympathectomy. Science 163: 468-469.

Mueller, R.A., Thoenen, H. and Axelrod, J. 1969 b. Inhibition of transsynaptically increased tyrosine hydroxylase activity by cycloheximide and actinomycin D. Mol. Pharmacol. 5: 463-469.

Mueller, R.A., Thoenen, H. and Axelrod, J. 1970. Effect of pituitary and ACTH on the maintenance of basal tyrosine hydroxylase activity in the rat adrenal gland. Endocrinology 86: 751-755.

Neff, N.H. and Costa, E. 1966. A study of the control of catecholamine synthesis. Fed. Proc. 25: 259.

Ong, H.H., Creveling, C.R. and Daly, J.W. 1969. The synthesis of 2,4,5-trihydroxyphenylalanine (6-hydroxydopa) a centrally active norepinephrine-depleting agent. J. Med. Chem. 12: 458-461.

Patrick, R.L. and Kirshner, N. 1971. Effect of stimulation on the levels of tyrosine hydroxylase and catecholamines in intact and denervated rat adrenal glands. Mol. Pharmacol. 7: 87-96.

Potter, L.T. and Axelrod, J. 1963. Properties of norepinephrine storage particles of the rat heart. J. Pharmacol. Exp. Ther. 142: 299-305.

Sedvall, G.C. and Kopin, I. 1967. Acceleration of norepinephrine synthesis in the rat submaxillary gland in vivo during sympathetic nerve stimulation. Life. Sci. 6: 45-51.

Shiman, R., Akino, M. and Kaufman, S. 1971. Solubilization and partial purification of tyrosine hydroxylase from bovine adrenal medulla. J. Biol. Chem. 246: 1330-1340.

Spector, S., Gordon, R., Sjoerdsma, A. and Udenfriend, S. End product inhibition of tyrosine hydroxylase as a possible mechanism for regulation of norepinephrine synthesis. Mol. Pharmacol. 3: 549-555.

Stjarne, L., Roth, H.L. and Lishajko, F. 1967. Noradrenaline formation from dopamine in isolated subcellular particles from bovine splenic nerve. Biochem. Pharmacol. 16: 1729-1739.

Stone, C.A., Stavorski, J.M., Ludden, C.T., Wenger, H.C., Ross, C.A., Totaro, J.A. and Porter, C.C. 1963. Comparison of some pharmacologic effects of certain 6-substituted dopamine derivatives with reserpine, guanethidine and metaramenol. J. Pharmacol. Exp. Ther. 142: 147-156.

Tarver, J., Berkowitz, B. and Specotr, S. 1971. Alteration in tyrosine hydroxylase and monoamine oxidase activity in blood vessels. Nature (New Biology) 231: 252-253.

Thoenen, H., Mueller, R.A. and Axelrod, J. 1969. Trans-synaptic induction of adrenal tyrosine hydroxylase. J. Pharmacol. Exp. Ther. 169: 249-254.

Thoenen, H. and Tranzer, J.P. 1968. Chemical sympathectomy by selective destruction of adrenergic nerve endings with 6-hydroxydopamine. Arch. Pharmacol. Exp. Path. 261: 271-288.

Viveros, O.H., Argqueros, L., Connett, R.J. and Kirshner, N. 1969. Mechanism of secretion from the adrenal medulla IV. The fate of the storage vesicles following insulin and reserpine administration. Mol. Pharmacol. 5: 69-82.

Walsh, M.J., Davis, V.E. and Yasumitsu, Y. 1970. Tetrahydro-papaveroline: An alkaloid metabolite of dopamine in vitro. J. Pharmacol. Exp. Ther. 174: 388-400.

Weiner, N. and Mosimann, W.F. 1970. The effect of insulin on the catecholamine content and tyrosine hydroxylase activity of cat adrenal glands. Biochem. Pharmacol. 19: 1189-1199.

Whitsett, T.L., Halushka, P.V. and Goldberg, L.I. 1970. Attenuation of post-ganglionic sympathetic nerve activity by L-dopa. Circ. Res. 27: 561-570.

Wurtman, R.J., Chou, C. and Rose, C. 1970. The fate of C^{14}-dihydroxyphenylalanine (L-dopa) in the whole mouse. J. Pharmacol. Exp. Ther. 174: 351-356.

CONTROL OF SYNTHESIS, TRANSPORT AND RELEASE OF DOPAMINE-BETA-HYDROXYLASE AND TYROSINE HYDROXYLASE

Irwin J. Kopin

Laboratory of Clinical Science, National Institute of

Mental Health, Bethesda, Maryland 20014

Adrenergic neuronal function is dependent on stimulation-induced release of norepinephrine (NE) from the synaptic vesicles of terminal varicosities of the axons. When neuronal activity is increased, there is an immediate acceleration of NE formation (Weiner, 1970). The enhanced rate of catecholamine synthesis appears to be regulated by a feedback control of tyrosine hydroxylase (TH) activity. In addition to this short-term, rapidly responsive method for regulation of levels of enzyme activity, the amount of enzymes present in the adrenergic tissue can also be altered. A variety of pharmacological agents or physiologic stresses which produce increased adrenal medullary or adrenergic neuronal activity have been shown to elevate tissue levels of TH and dopamine-beta-hydroxylase (DBH). It is the purpose of the present paper to review current concepts regarding the regulation of TH and DBH, which are essential to the synthesis of catecholamines in the adrenal medulla, sympathetic nerves and brain.

Neuronal control of adrenal medullary TH and DBH. When drugs such as reserpine, phenoxybenzamine or 6-hydroxydopamine interfere with the function of the sympathetic nervous system, there is an increase in the levels of TH (Mueller, Thoenen and Axelrod, 1969 a,b) and DBH (Molinoff, et al., 1970) in the adrenal medulla. Because the elevation of activity of the enzymes is blocked by inhibitors of protein synthesis (Mueller, Thoenen and Axelrod, 1969 c), formation of new enzyme molecules is presumed to occur. A direct measure of incorporation of radioactive ^{3}H-leucine into adrenal DBH, which was isolated by immunological techniques (Hartman, Molinoff and Udenfriend, 1970), confirmed the acceleration by reserpine of enzyme synthesis. Interference with the arrival of splanchnic nerve impulses at the adrenal, however,

21

prevents the elevation of DBH and TH. Exposure to cold (Kvetnansky et al., 1971 a) or repeated immobilization (Kvetnansky, Weise and Kopin, 1970; Kvetnansky et al., 1971 b) of rats results in a neuronally mediated elevation of adrenal TH and DBH. Because the increase in TH levels of adrenal medullae cultured in a medium containing high levels of potassium could be prevented by blocking release of the catecholamines (Silberstein et al., 1972 a), the induction of TH appears to be related to release of NE. Furthermore, administration of acetylcholine in combination with eserine also elevates TH and DBH levels in the adrenal medulla (Patrick and Kirshner, 1971). Thus, in the adrenal medulla, release of catecholamines appears to be related to induction of the enzymes required for the catecholamines' synthesis rather than any factor derived from the presynaptic neuron.

Hormonal control of adrenal medullary TH and DBH. Hypophysectomy results in atrophy of both the adrenal cortex and adrenal medulla. Levels of TH (Mueller, Thoenen and Axelrod, 1970) and DBH (Gewirtz et al., 1971 a; Weinshilboum and Axelrod, 1970) are markedly diminished in the adrenals of hypophysectomized animals. Treatment with ACTH or dexamethasone (in large doses) restores the levels of adrenal DBH, but only ACTH is effective in restoring levels of TH to normal. Immobilization of hypophysectomized rats results in elevation of levels of adrenal TH and DBH; however, the levels attained, although two- to threefold greater than non-immobilized hypophysectomized animals, are much lower than in the immobilized intact control animals (Kvetnansky et al., 1970). Thus, both hormonal and neuronal factors influence the levels of TH and DBH in the adrenals of hypophysectomized animals without altering levels of phenylethanolamine-N-methyltransferase (PNMT), the effect of ACTH on the adrenal medullary ACTH may be mediated by cyclic-AMP and not by steroids derived from the cortex. PNMT, however, is very sensitive to adrenal cortical control of levels of hormones (Gewirtz et al., 1971 b). If dibutyryl cyclic-AMP acted solely by enhancing production of hormones from the adrenal cortex, elevation of PNMT, as well as TH and DBH, would result.

TH and DBH in sympathetic neurons. Alteration of sympathetic neuronal activity also produces changes in levels of catecholamine-synthesizing enzymes in sympathetic neurons. Administration of reserpine results in elevation of TH (Mueller, Thoenen and Axelrod, 1969 b) and DBH (Kvetnansky et al., 1971 a). The fact that elevation of TH in the ganglia precedes the changes in the peripheral organs (Thoenen, Mueller and Axelrod, 1970) suggests that the increase in enzyme activity at the nerve terminals is a consequence of increased formation of the enzyme in the perikaryon. The cell body contains the genetic information and protein synthetic mechanisms; the nerve ending is specialized to carry out the functional aspects of neurotransmitter release.

The axon is the route for flow of substances from the cell body to
the nerve terminals. The mechanism for transfer of information
from the nerve ending to the cell body, however, is poorly
understood although there is some evidence for retrograde axonal
flow. When sympathetic ganglia are grown in vitro in media
containing elevated levels of potassium, there is an elevation
of DBH levels in the ganglia (Silberstein et al., 1972 b).
Because the elevation of DBH is prevented by cycloheximide, it
appears that depolarization, possibly by inducing NE release,
may lead to enzyme induction.

Axonal transport of TH and DBH. In addition to conducting
nerve impulses from the perikaryon to the nerve ending, the axon
is a route for continual flow of substances produced in the cell
body which are necessary for maintenance of the nerve endings
(Weiss, 1970). Isotopic techniques (Droz and Leblond, 1963) have
revealed the existence of at least two rates of axonal transport.
The slower rate (1-3 mm/day) appears to be the result of bulk
flow; a faster rate (1-10 mm/day) is dependent on the integrity of
the neurotubules (Schmitt, 1968). Proximal to the site of ligation of sympathetic axons, NE (Kapeller and Mayor, 1967; Banks,
Kapeller and Mayor, 1969; Laduron and Belpaire, 1968), granular
vesicles (Kapeller and Mayor, 1967; Banks, Kapeller and Mayor,
1969; Geffen and Ostberg, 1969), DBH (Laduron and Belpaire,
1968; Livett, Geffen and Rush, 1969; Laduron, 1968), TH (Coyle and
Wooten, 1972)   and chromagranin (Livett, Geffen and Rush, 1969)
are found to accumulate. Dahlström (1968, 1970) and Keen and
Livingstone (1969) found that colchicine and vinblastine, drugs
known to disrupt neurotubules (Schmitt, 1968), inhibit the
proximo-distal migration of NE storage vesicles. In the lamprey
nervous system, Smith et al. (1970) demonstrated a close association of vesicular structures with microtubules, but the mechanism
for vesicular transport remains unknown.

Colchicine or vinblastine applied to the superior cervical
ganglion of a rat results in a rapid increase in levels of DBH
and a slower increase in levels of TH. The increases in enzyme
levels are prevented by inhibition of protein synthesis. The
rate of DBH accumulation in a ganglion treated with colchicine
or vinblastine, drugs which inhibit axonal transport, can be used
to estimate the rate of synthesis of the enzyme (Lamprecht,
Weise and Kopin, 1972; Kopin and Silberstein, 1972). The initial
rate of increase of DBH in a colchicine-treated ganglion corresponds to approximately 50% of the enzyme content of the ganglion
each hour; this agrees well with estimates of the turnover of DBH
based on the rate of decline of DBH in the ganglion after inhibition of protein synthesis (Axelrod, 1972).

The levels of DBH in the salivary gland innervated by a

colchicine- or vinblastine-treated ganglion decline slowly during
the first day and decline more rapidly thereafter (Kopin and
Silberstein, 1972). The apparent rate of transport of DBH from
the ganglion to the salivary gland is equivalent to a turnover
rate (T-1/2 = 4.1 days) which is in close agreement with the rate
of catecholamine repletion after treatment with reserpine (Iversen,
Glowinski and Axelrod, 1965; Dahlström and Häggendal, 1966). The
latter has been used as an index of the rate of reappearance of
intact vesicles at the nerve ending.

After the initial increase in enzyme activity in colchicine-
or vinblastine-treated ganglia, there is a fall in levels of DBH.
A similar decline in ganglionic DBH is found after postganglionic
section (Kopin and Silberstein, 1972) or treatment with 6-hydroxy-
dopamine (Kopin and Silberstein, 1972; Brimijoin and Molinoff,
1971). The decline in levels of DBH does not appear to be a
result of death of the cell bodies. After vinblastine treatment,
the protein content of the ganglion continues to rise even after
the DBH levels are strikingly decreased and uptake of ^{3}H-NE
increases (Figure 1). The uptake of ^{3}H-NE, assessed by incubation

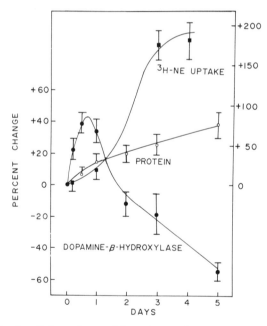

Figure 1. Effect of local application of vinblastine on dopamine-
beta-hydroxylase and protein content of the superior cervical
ganglia, and uptake of ^{3}H-norepinephrine (^{3}H-NE) in vitro by the
superior cervical ganglia.

in vitro of the ganglia in a physiologic media containing the
labelled catecholamine, is unchanged for several days. At about
the time DBH levels begin to fall, however, an increase in uptake
of the labelled amine becomes apparent. Histological examination
of the ganglia indicates that, when DBH levels begin to decrease,
the perikaryon of the neurons is swollen, but no new axonal sprouts
have formed (Hanbauer, Bloom and Kopin, unpublished observations).
Similar correlations of the decline of DBH levels and enhancement of amine uptake have been found after axonal section or
administration of 6-hydroxydopamine (Kopin and Silberstein, 1972).
The enhanced uptake of amines appears to be a consequence of an
increase in membrane surface. Apparently, the metabolic changes
which occur in the perikaryon after axonal damage result in a
switch from production of the enzymes concerned with maintenance
of function (neurotransmitter replenishment and storage) to
formation of structural components necessary for regrowth of the
axon and restoration of the nerve ending. The signal for the
change in protein-synthetic mechanisms is unknown, but the rapidity
of transmission of the information regarding nerve-ending damage
to the ganglion from the nerve ending is consistent with rapid
axonal transport.

Release of DBH from the adrenal medulla and sympathetic
nerve ending. There is now considerable evidence that release
of catecholamines from the adrenal medulla occurs by a process of
exocytosis and is accompanied by release of the entire soluble
contents of the vesicles, which include adenine nucleotides,
chromogranin and DBH (Kirshner and Viveros, 1972). More recently,
it has been found that DBH (Gewirtz and Kopin, 1970; Geffen,
Livett and Rush, 1969; Smith et al., 1970) and chromogranin
(Geffen, Livett and Rush, 1969; Smith et al., 1970; Smith, 1970)
are released from perfused organs by sympathetic nerve stimulation
and that the ratio of NE to DBH released is similar to that found
in the soluble contents of the vesicles (Weinshilboum et al.,
1971 a). Release of DBH is prevented in the absence of calcium
and by prostaglandin E_2. Phenoxybenzamine increases the release
of DBH during nerve stimulation, presumably by a presynaptic
action (Johnson et al., 1971). Phenoxybenzamine also enhances
stimulation-induced release of NE from cultured ganglia where
there are only presynaptic structures (Johnson et al., 1971;
DePotter et al., 1971).

The mechanism for exocytosis requires fusion of the vesicular
and neuronal membranes by an unknown process. It is probable that
there are several discrete steps involved in the sequence of
events which lead from membrane depolarization to calcium entry
to approximation of the vesicle and nerve terminal membrane and
finally to membrane fusion, opening of a channel to the synaptic
cleft, extrusion of the vesicular contents and termination of the

release process with reconstitution or disposal of the remainder
of the vesicle. The process of exocytosis appears to be similar
in a variety of secreting cells. Colchicine and vinblastine interfere with release of insulin from the pancreas (Lacy et al., 1968),
histamine from mast cells (Gillespie et al., 1968), catecholamines
from the adrenal medulla (Poisner and Bernstein, 1971) and NE and
DBH from the sympathetic nerves in the isolated guinea-pig vas
deferens (Thoa et al., 1972). The above results suggest that
microtubules are involved in the release of a variety of substances
from vesicular storage sites. Cytochalasin B, a fungal metabolite
which disrupts microfilaments, also prevents release of DBH from
stimulated sympathetic neurons, possibly by interfering with a
calcium-activated contractile mechanism involved in extrusion of
the vesicular contents.

Demonstration of release by stimulation of DBH from sympathetic
nerves and adrenal medulla led to examination of blood plasma for
DBH. DBH activity was found in the plasma of humans as well as
experimental animals (Weinshilboum and Axelrod, 1971 a; Friedman
et al., 1972). The DBH derived from the plasma has the same
electrophoretic mobility, requirements for ascorbic acid, fumarate
and oxygen as DBH derived from the tissues (Weinshilboum and
Axelrod, 1971 a).

Serum DBH appears to derive mainly from the sympathetic nerves
since adrenalmedullectomy failed to decrease levels of the enzyme;
however 6-hydroxydopamine, which destroys many sympathetic
nerve endings, produces a 25% decrease in serum DBH (Friedman
et al., 1972). There is an increase in serum DBH levels of rats
subjected to immobilization which is still apparent after adrenalmedullectomy (Weinshilboum and Axelrod, 1971 b).

In man, Wooten and Cardon (1972) have found that a variety of
procedures associated with increased sympathetic nerve activity
elevate circulating levels of DBH. Thus, DBH levels are increased
during the elevation in blood pressure provoked by either immer-
sion of a hand in ice-water or during postural adjustment to assuming a vertical position after reclining. The levels of DBH are
significantly diminished in patients with familial dysautonomia
(Weinshilboum and Axelrod, 1971 c; Weinshilboum et al., 1971 b),
but no significant alterations have been found in hypertensive
subjects or depressed patients.

In a variety of types of experimental hypertension, serum
levels of DBH are diminished (Lamprecht, Williams and Kopin, 1972).
Rats made hypertensive by administration of DOCA and salt, spontaneously hypertensive rats and Dahl's strain of rats (which

develop hypertension when placed on a high-salt diet) all have low
levels of serum DBH. The diminished levels of DBH may reflect
compensatory diminution in sympathetic neuronal activity in the
presence of other causes of elevated blood pressure.

Serum DBH levels appear to reflect the level of adrenergic
neuronal activity, but the degree of change in enzyme levels is
less marked than the changes observed in catecholamine content of
the plasma. It is likely that the large protein molecules enter
the circulation more slowly than the relatively small molecules
of catecholamines and that the enzyme is removed much more slowly
than the amines which are selectively taken up by adrenergic
tissues and readily metabolized in the liver and kidney. The
difference in half-life of the enzyme and the catecholamine would
result in relatively transient, but more striking, changes in
amine concentration when compared to changes in DBH levels. The
assessment of the wide range of DBH levels in the plasma of normal
individuals, the variation in enzyme levels with age, and the
alterations found in clinical states will involve determination of
factors which control removal of the circulating enzyme, as well
as its release, from adrenergic tissue.

SUMMARY

The levels of TH and DBH in the adrenal medulla and in
adrenergic neurons are altered in response to requirements for
synthesis of the catecholamines, but are also subject to hormonal
influences. The signals for control of both TH and DBH levels
are complex and involve cell depolarization, catecholamine
release, cyclic-AMP formation and requirements for synthesis of
structural components. In adrenergic neurons, enzyme synthesis
occurs mainly in the perikaryon; and levels of the enzymes are a
net result of formation and transport down the axon. When the
axon is damaged or when interference with axonal transport occurs,
there is a switch of priorities in protein synthesis to renew the
structural components at the expense of formation of enzymes
involved in formation of catecholamines.

The process of neurotransmitter release appears to involve
extrusion of the contents of the synaptic vesicles, including
DBH. The release of DBH from the adrenal medulla and from
sympathetic neurons into the systemic circulation may provide a
means for assessing peripheral adrenergic function, which is less
sensitive to rapid fluctuations than is measurement of the
circulating catecholamines.

REFERENCES

Axelrod, J. 1972. Dopamine-beta-hydroxylase: regulation of its
    synthesis and release from nerve terminals. Pharmacol. Rev.
    24: 233-243.
Banks, P., Kapeller, K. and Mayor, D. 1969. The effects of
    iproniazid and reserpine on the accumulation of granular
    vesicles and noradrenaline in constricted adrenergic nerves.
    Brit. J. Pharmacol. 27: 10-18.
Brimijoin, S. and Molinoff, P.B. 1971. Effects of 6-hydroxy-
    dopamine on the activity of tyrosine hydroxylase and dopamine-
    beta-hydroxylase in the sympathetic ganglia of the rat. J.
    Pharmacol. Exp. Ther. 178: 417-425.
Coyle, J.T. and Wooten, G.F. 1972. Rapid axonal transport of
    tyrosine hydroxylase and dopamine-beta-hydroxylase. Brain
    Res. 44: 701-704.
Dahlström, A. 1968. Effect of colchicine on transport of amine
    storage granules in sympathetic nerves of rat. Eur. J.
    Pharmacol. 5: 111-113.
Dahlström, A. 1970. Effects of drugs on axonal transport of
    amine storage granules. In: New Aspects of Storage and
    Release Mechanisms of Catecholamines, (Eds. Schumann, H.G.
    and Kroneberg, G.) Berlin: Springer-Verlag, pp. 20-36.
Dahlström, A. and Häggendal, J. 1966. Studies on the transport
    and life-span of amine storage granules in a peripheral
    adrenergic neuron system. Acta Physiol. Scand. 67: 278-288.
DePotter, W.P., Chubb, I.W., Post, A. and DeSchaepdryver, A.F.
    1971. Facilitation of release of noradrenaline and dopamine-
    beta-oxidase at low stimulation frequencies by alpha-
    blocking agents. Arch. Int. Pharmacodyn. Ther. 194: 191-197.
Droz, B. and Leblond, C.P. 1963. Axonal migration of proteins in
    the central nervous system and peripheral nerves as shown
    by radioautography. J. Comp. Neurol. 121: 325-346.
Friedman, L.S., Ouchi, T. and Goldstein, M. 1972. Changes in serum
    dopamine-beta-hydroxylase activity with age. Nature (New
    Biology), in press.
Geffen, L.B., Livett, B.G. and Rush, R.A. 1969. Immunological
    chemical localization of chromogranins in sheep sympathetic
    nerves. J. Physiol. (London) 204: 58-59.
Geffen, L.B. and Ostberg, A. 1969. Distribution of granular
    vesicles in normal and constricted sympathetic neurones.
    J. Physiol. (London) 204: 583-592.
Gewirtz, G.P. and Kopin, I.J. 1970. Release of dopamine-beta-
    hydroxylase with norepinephrine by splenic nerve stimulation.
    Nature 227: 406-407.
Gewirtz, G.P., Kvetnansky, R., Weise, V.K. and Kopin, I.J. 1971 a.
    Effect of hypophysectomy on adrenal dopamine-beta-hydroxylase
    activity in the rat. Molec. Pharmacol. 7: 163-171.

Gewirtz, G.P., Kvetnansky, R., Weise, V.K. and Kopin, I.J. 1971 b.
    Effect of ACTH and dibutyryl cyclic-AMP on catecholamine-
    synthesizing enzymes in the adrenals of hypophysectomized
    rats. Nature 230: 462-464.
Gillespie, E., Levine, R.J. and Malawista, S.E. 1968. Histamine
    release from rat peritoneal mast cells: inhibition by colchi-
    cine and potentiation by deuterium oxide. J. Pharmacol. Exp.
    Ther. 164: 158-165.
Hartman, B.K., Molinoff, P.B. and Udenfriend, S. 1970. Increased
    rate of synthesis of dopamine-beta-hydroxylase in adrenals
    of reserpinized rats. Pharmacologist 12: 470.
Iversen, L.L., Glowinski, J. and Axelrod, J. 1965. The uptake and
    storage of ^{3}H-norepinephrine in the reserpine-pretreated rat
    heart. J. Pharmacol. Exp. Ther. 150: 173-183.
Johnson, D.G., Thoa, N.B., Weinshilboum, R., Axelrod, J. and Kopin,
    I.J. 1971. Enhanced release of dopamine-beta-hydroxylase
    from sympathetic nerves by calcium and phenoxybenzamine and
    its reversal by prostaglandins. Proc. Nat. Acad. Sci. USA
    68: 2227-2230.
Kapeller, K. and Mayor, D. 1967. The accumulation of noradrenaline
    in constricted sympathetic nerves as studied by fluorescence
    and electron microscopy. Proc. Roy. Soc. (Biol.) 167: 282-292.
Keen, P. and Livingstone, A. 1969. Intraneuronal transport of
    noradrenaline in the rat. Mem. Soc. Endocrinol. 19: 671-682.
Kirshner, N. and Viveros, O.H. 1972. The secretory cycle in the
    adrenal medulla. Pharmacol. Rev. 24: 385-398.
Kopin, I.J. and Silberstein, D.S. 1972. Axons of sympathetic
    neurons: transport of enzymes in vivo and properties of axonal
    sprouts in vivo. Pharmacol. Rev. 24: 245-254.
Kvetnansky, R., Gewirtz, G.P., Weise, V.K. and Kopin, I.J. 1970.
    Effect of hypophysectomy on immobilization-induced elevation
    of tyrosine hydroxylase and phenylethanolamine-N-methyl
    transferase in the rat adrenal. Endocrinology 87: 1323-1339.
Kvetnansky, R., Gewirtz, G.P., Weise, V.K. and Kopin, I.J. 1971 a.
    Catecholamine-synthesizing enzymes in the rat adrenal gland
    during exposure to cold. Amer. J. Physiol. 220: 928-931.
Kvetnansky, R., Gewirtz, G.P., Weise, V.K. and Kopin, I.J. 1971 b.
    Enhanced synthesis of adrenal dopamine-beta-hydroxylase
    induced by repeated immobilization in rats. Molec. Pharmac.
    7: 81-86.
Kvetnansky, R., Weise, V.K. and Kopin, I.J. 1970. Elevation of
    adrenal tyrosine hydroxylase and phenylethanolamine-N-methyl
    transferase by repeated immobilization of rats. Endocrinology
    87: 744-749.
Lacy, P.E., Howell, S.L., Young, D.A. and Fink, C.J. 1968. New
    hypothesis of insulin secretion. Nature 219: 1177-1179.
Laduron, P. 1968. Axonal flow of dopamine-beta-hydroxylase con-
    taining granules in splenic nerves. Arch. Int. Pharmacodyn.
    Ther. 171: 233-234.

Laduron, P. and Belpaire, F. 1968. Transport of noradrenaline and dopamine-beta-hydroxylase in sympathetic nerves. Life Sci. 7: 1-7.

Lamprecht, F., Weise, V.K. and Kopin, I.J. 1972. Effect of colchicine and vinblastine on the tyrosine hydroxylase and dopamine-beta-hydroxylase content of the rat superior cervical ganglion and salivary gland. Fed. Proc. 31: 544.

Lamprecht, F., Williams, R.B. and Kopin, I.J. 1972. Serum dopamine-beta-hydroxylase (DBH) during development of immobilization-induced and genetic hypertension in rats. Naunyn Schmiedebergs Arch. Exp. Path., Suppl. 274.

Livett, B.G., Geffen, L.B. and Rush, R.A. 1969. Immunohisto-chemical evidence for the transport of dopamine-beta-hydroxylase and a catecholamine-binding protein in sympa-thetic nerves. Biochem. Pharmacol. 18: 923-924.

Molinoff, P.B., Brimijoin, W.S., Weinshilboum, R.M. and Axelrod, J. 1970. Neurally mediated increase in dopamine-beta-hydroxylase activity. Proc. Nat. Acad. Sci. USA 66: 453-458.

Mueller, R.A., Thoenen, H. and Axelrod, J. 1969 a. Adrenal tyrosine hydroxylase: compensatory increase in activity after chemical sympathectomy. Science 163: 468-469.

Mueller, R.A., Thoenen, H. and Axelrod, J. 1969 b. Increase in tyrosine hydroxylase activity after reserpine administration J. Pharmacol. Exp. Ther. 169: 74-79.

Mueller, R.A., Thoenen, H. and Axelrod, J. 1969 c. Inhibition of trans-synaptically increased tyrosine hydroxylase activity by cycloheximide and actinomycin D. Mol. Pharmac. 5: 463-469.

Mueller, R.A., Thoenen, H. and Axelrod, J. 1970. Effect of pituitary and ACTH on the maintenance of basal tyrosine hydroxylase activity in the rat adrenal gland. Endocrinology 86: 751-755.

Patrick, R.L. and Kirshner, N. 1971. Effect of stimulation on the levels of tyrosine hydroxylase, dopamine-beta-hydroxylase and catecholamine in intact and denervated rat adrenal glands. Mol. Pharmac. 7: 87-96.

Poisner, A.M. and Bernstein, J. 1971. A possible role of micro-tubules in catecholamine release from the adrenal medulla: effect of colchicine, vinca alkaloids and deuterium oxide. J. Pharmacol. Exp. Ther. 177: 102-108.

Schmitt, F.O. 1968. The molecular biology of neural fibrous proteins. Neurosci. Res. Program Bull. 6: 119-144.

Silberstein, S.D., Brimijoin, S., Molinoff, P.B. and Lemberger, L. 1972 a. Induction of dopamine-beta-hydroxylase (DBH) in rat superior cervical ganglia in organ culture. J. Neurochem. 19: 919-921.

Silberstein, S.D., Lemberger, L., Klein, D.C., Axelrod, J. and Kopin, I.J. 1972 b. Induction of adrenal tyrosine hydroxylase in organ culture. Neuropharmacol. (in press).

Smith, A.D. 1970. Proteins of vesicles from sympathetic axons: chemistry, immunoreactivity and release upon stimulation. Neurosci. Res. Prog. Bull. 8: 337-382.

Smith, A.D., DePotter, W.P., Moerman, E.J. and DeSchaepdryver, A.F. 1970. Release of dopamine-beta-hydroxylase and chromogranin upon stimulation of the splenic nerves. Tissue and Cell 2: 2547-2568.

Smith, O.S., Jarlfors, U. and Beranek, R. 1970. The organization of synaptic axoplasm in the lamprey (Petromyzon marinus) central nervous system. J. Cell. Biol. 46: 199-210.

Thoa, N.B., Wooten, G.F., Axelrod, J. and Kopin, I.J. 1972. Inhibition of release of dopamine-beta-hydroxylase and noradrenaline from sympathetic nerves by colchicine, vinblastin and cytochalasin B. Proc. Nat. Acad. Sci. USA 69: 520-522.

Thoenen, H., Mueller, R.A. and Axelrod, J. 1970. Phase difference in the induction of tyrosine hydroxylase in cell body and nerve terminals of sympathetic neurones. Proc. Nat. Acad. Sci. USA 65: 58-62.

Weiner, N. 1970. Regulation of norepinephrine biosynthesis. Ann. Rev. Pharmacol. 10: 273-290.

Weinshilboum, R.M. and Axelrod, J. 1970. Dopamine-beta-hydroxylase activity in the rat after hypophysectomy. Endocrinology 87: 894-899.

Weinshilboum, R.M. and Axelrod, J. 1971 a. Serum dopamine-beta-hydroxylase activity. Circ. Res. 28: 307-315.

Weinshilboum, R.M. and Axelrod, J. 1971 b. Serum dopamine-beta-hydroxylase: decrease after chemical sympathectomy. Science 173: 931-934.

Weinshilboum, R.M. and Axelrod, J. 1971 c. Reduced plasma dopamine-beta-hydroxylase in familial dysautonomia. New Eng. J. Med. 285: 938-942.

Weinshilboum, R.M., Thoa, N.B., Johnson, D.G., Kopin, I.J. and Axelrod, J. 1971 a. Proportional release of norepinephrine and dopamine-beta-hydroxylase from sympathetic nerves. Science 174: 1349-1351.

Weinshilboum, R.M., Kvetnansky, R., Axelrod, J. and Kopin, I.J. 1971 b. Elevation of serum dopamine-beta-hydroxylase activity with forced immobilization. Nature (New Biology) 230: 287-288.

Weiss, P. 1970. Neuronal dynamics and neuroplasmic flow. In: The Neurosciences: Second Study Program. (Ed. Schmitt, F.O.) New York:Rockefeller University Press, pp. 840-850.

Wooten, G.F. and Cardon, P.V. 1972. Elevation of plasma dopamine-beta-hydroxylase activity in man during cold pressor test and exercise. Arch. Neurol. (in press).

NEW ENZYME SYNTHESIS AS A LONG-TERM ADAPTATION TO INCREASED TRANSMITTER UTILIZATION

Hans Thoenen and Franz Oesch

Department of Pharmacology, Biocenter of the

University, Basel, Switzerland

INTRODUCTION

Adequate regulatory function of the peripheral autonomous nervous system depends on both prompt liberation and prompt inactivation of the neurohumoral transmitter substances.

In the cholinergic nervous system the transmitter action is terminated mainly by enzymatic degradation of acetylcholine to choline and acetate (for references see Koelle, 1970). In the adrenergic system the corresponding major mechanism of transmitter inactivation is the reuptake of liberated norepinephrine into the nerve terminals (for references see Iversen, 1967; Thoenen, 1969; Molinoff and Axelrod, 1971). This mechanism is not only of crucial importance for the termination of transmitter action on the effector organ but it also represents a major mechanism of transmitter preservation, since the rate of norepinephrine synthesis cannot keep pace with the rate of loss by liberation and subsequent enzymatic degradation (Haefely, Hürlimann and Thoenen, 1965). In spite of this efficient mechanism of transmitter preservation, an increased activity of the adrenergic neurons is instantaneously followed by an increase in the rate of catecholamine synthesis (for references see Costa, 1970; Weiner, 1972). This immediate adaptation to increased transmitter utilization is not accompanied by an increase in the in vitro activity of the enzymes involved in the synthesis of norepinephrine. The possible factors determining this immediate regulation have recently been reviewed (Udenfriend and Dairman, 1971; Weiner, 1972).

However, a prolonged increase in the activity of peripheral and central adrenergic neurons and adrenal chromaffin cells brings

33

into play a second mechanism of adaptation, i.e. a neuronally
mediated induction of enzymes involved in the synthesis of
norepinephrine (for references see Molinoff and Axelrod, 1971;
Thoenen, 1972). This trans-synaptic induction is of particular
interest, since the increased activity of the preganglionic
cholinergic neurons provokes characteristic changes in the enzyme
pattern of the adrenergic neuron rather than merely a general
increase in RNA and/or protein synthesis (Thoenen et al., 1971;
Thoenen, 1972). This system thus offers the opportunity of
studying the relationship between the functional state of the
neuronal membrane, effected by the cholinergic transmitter
acetylcholine, and the regulation of the expression of the available genetic information of the adrenergic neuron. It is the aim
of this paper to evaluate the importance of this trans-synaptic
enzyme induction as a mechanism of long-term adaptation to increased
transmitter utilization.

TRANS-SYNAPTIC INDUCTION OF TYROSINE HYDROXYLASE

The neuronally mediated induction of tyrosine hydroxylase
was detected in the course of experiments designed to quantify
biochemically the extent of destruction of adrenergic nerve
terminals in the rat heart after administration of 6-hydroxy-
dopamine (Mueller, Thoenen and Axelrod, 1969 a). As was to be
expected from surgical denervation experiments (Sedvall and
Kopin, 1967), the activity of tyrosine hydroxylase, an enzyme
which is selectively located in adrenergic neurons and adrenal
chromaffin cells, was drastically reduced in the rat heart
(Figure 1). However, in the adrenal medulla, which is not
destroyed by 6-hydroxydopamine (Thoenen and Tranzer, 1968),
the activity of tyrosine hydroxylase was not only not reduced
but markedly increased (Mueller, Thoenen and Axelrod, 1969 a).
The functional significance of this increase in the in vitro
activity is demonstrated by the fact that both synthesis and
turnover of catecholamines in the adrenal medulla are increased
(Mueller, 1971), whereas the level of the adrenal catecholamines
remains unaltered, as shown in Figure 2. From a teleological
point of view, this increase in the in vitro activity of tyrosine
hydroxylase, with consequent increase in transmitter production,
could be considered as an attempt by the adrenal medulla to
compensate for the extensively destroyed peripheral adrenergic
nervous system. In further experiments it was demonstrated that
this increase in the in vitro activity of tyrosine hydroxylase
does not only occur after administration of 6-hydroxydopamine
but under a great variety of other experimental conditions
(for references see Molinoff and Axelrod, 1971; Thoenen, 1972),
and that it involves not only the adrenal medulla but also
peripheral (Mueller, Thoenen and Axelrod, 1969 b; Thoenen,
Mueller and Axelrod, 1969 a,b; Thoenen, 1970) and central
(Musacchio et al., 1969; Thoenen, 1970) adrenergic neurons.

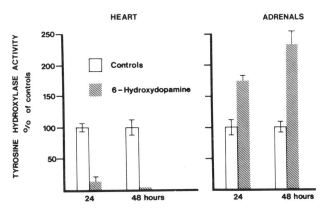

Figure 1. Effect of 6-hydroxydopamine on the in vitro activity of
tyrosine hydroxylase in the rat heart and adrenal medulla.
Male Sprague-Dawley rats were injected with 6-hydroxydopamine (2 x
200 mg/kg given intravenously) at 8 hour intervals and killed
24 and 48 hours after the first dose. The values given represent
the mean + S.E.M. (n = 4-5). (According to Mueller, Thoenen
and Axelrod, 1969 a.)

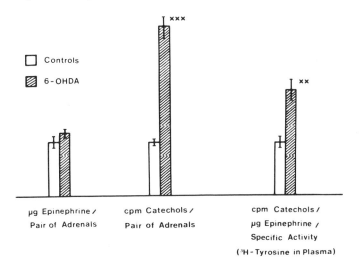

Figure 2. Effect of chemical sympathectomy on the synthesis of
adrenal ^{3}H-catechols from ^{3}H-tyrosine. Male Sprague-Dawley rats
weighing 90-100 g were injected intravenously with 2 x 200 mg/kg
of 6-hydroxydopamine at an interval of 8 hours. Sixteen hours
after the last injection the animals were infused with 25.2 μc of
^{3}H-tyrosine (duration of infusion 1 hour). At the end of the
infusion the animals were killed and the adrenals were assayed for
^{14}H-catechols and endogenous catecholamines (determined as epinephrine), and plasma was assayed for endogenous tyrosine. The
values given represent the mean + S.E.M. (n = 5-7). (According
to Mueller, 1971).

The common denominator in all these experimental conditions is a prolonged increase in the activity, and thus transmitter utilization, of the adrenergic neurons or chromaffin cells. The fact that inhibitors of protein synthesis abolish the increase in enzyme activity (Mueller, Thoenen and Axelrod, 1969 c) suggests, together with enzyme kinetic data (Mueller, Thoenen and Axelrod, 1969 b) that the increase in tyrosine hydroxylase activity results from an augmented synthesis of new enzyme protein. Furthermore, it has been shown that this enzyme induction is neuronally mediated since it can be prevented by trans-secting the preganglionic cholinergic trunk of the superior cervical ganglion (Thoenen, Mueller and Axelrod, 1969 a) or the splanchnic fibers supplying the adrenal medulla (Thoenen, Mueller and Axelrod, 1969 b; Kvetňanský et al., 1970; Patrick and Kirshner, 1971). All these findings suggest that in addition to the immediate adaptation to increased transmitter utilization, which is not accompanied by a change in the in vitro activity of enzymes involved in the synthesis of the adrenergic transmitter (Weiner, 1972), there is a second much slower mechanism which comes into play only after a prolonged increase in neuronal activity and which involves a trans-synaptic induction of tyrosine hydroxylase, the rate-limiting enzyme of norepinephrine synthesis (Levitt et al., 1965; Udenfriend and Dairman, 1971).

SELECTIVITY OF TRANS-SYNAPTIC ENZYME INDUCTION

From the point of view of long-term adaptation to increased transmitter utilization the availability of augmented amounts of tyrosine hydroxylase for transmitter synthesis seems to be of primary importance (Molinoff and Axelrod, 1971; Udenfriend and Dairman, 1971). However, the question arises as to whether the enhanced synthesis of the rate-limiting enzyme is a manifestation of a generally increased neuronal protein synthesis or whether it represents a more specific process. It is a well known fact, established in many species and under various experimental conditions, that an increased activity of all kinds of neurons is followed by an increased synthesis of RNA and protein (for references see Gisiger and Gaide-Huguenin, 1969; Larrabee, 1969; Richter, 1970). However, these investigations do not distinguish whether the observed changes reflect the selective increase in synthesis of one or a group of specific proteins or whether they reflect a nonspecific overall increase. In the case of the trans-synaptic enzyme induction in adrenergic neurons the several-fold increase in tyrosine hydroxylase in sympathetic ganglia (Mueller, Thoenen and Axelrod, 1969 b), together with the absence of detectable changes in their total protein content is barely compatible with the assumption that the rise in tyrosine hydroxylase is a manifestation of a general increase in ganglionic protein synthesis. However, there still remains the question as to whether

the induction is selectively confined to tyrosine hydroxylase or
whether, analogous to bacterial systems (Ames and Martin, 1964),
the enzymes engaged in the synthesis of the adrenergic transmitter
are located in adjacent chromosomal areas and are regulated as an
operational unit. Both after cold exposure of rats and after
administration of reserpine, experimental conditions which lead to
an increase in the in vitro activity of tyrosine hydroxylase and
dopamine β-hydroxylase (Mueller, Thoenen and Axelrod, 1969 b;
Molinoff et al., 1970; Thoenen et al., 1971), no increase has
been observed in the activity of DOPA decarboxylase, the third
enzyme engaged in the synthesis of norepinephrine (Black, Hendry
and Iversen, 1971; Thoenen et al., 1971). These findings do not
support the assumption that all the enzymes involved in the
synthesis of the adrenergic transmitter are regulated by a
common mechanism as an operational unit. However, it has to be
taken into account that the level of a given enzyme is the summation of its synthesis and degradation and that differences in the
increase of enzyme protein could result from differences in
degradation rather than synthesis. For instance, in the superior
cervical ganglion of the rat the increase in dopamine β-hydroxylase
after cold stress and reserpine administration is considerably
smaller than that of tyrosine hydroxylase (Mueller, Thoenen and
Axelrod, 1969 b; Molinoff et al., 1970; Thoenen et al., 1971).
This discrepancy in the increase of the two enzymes could be
explained, at least partially, by differences in degradation
rather than synthesis since the turnover of tyrosine hydroxylase
is much smaller than that of dopamine β-hydroxylase as far as can
be judged from the rate of decay of the in vitro activity of
these enzymes during inhibition of protein synthesis. For tyrosine
hydroxylase no consistent decrease in the in vitro activity was
observed within 6 to 8 hours after administration of an initial
dose of 10 mg/kg of cycloheximide followed by 5 mg/kg every 3 hours,
which is sufficient to reduce the incorporation of ^{3}H-leucine into
protein by more than 90% (Thoenen et al., 1971). However, the
activity of dopamine β-hydroxylase showed a gradual decay, from
which a t 1/2 of 13 hours was calculated (Thoenen et al., 1971).
Cold stress or administration of reserpine did not change the
rate of decay.

The absence of an increase in the activity of DOPA decarboxylase
in adrenals and sympathetic ganglia cannot be explained by differences
in turnover since the decay rate of DOPA decarboxylase during inhibition of protein synthesis with cycloheximide was very similar to
that of dopamine β-hydroxylase. The t 1/2 of DOPA decarboxylase
amounted to 12 hours versus 13 hours for that of dopamine β-
hydroxylase (Thoenen et al., 1971).

The turnover of an enzyme, determined by inhibition of protein
synthesis or immunological methods after pulse labelling with inert
radioactive aminoacids, may not only depend on the proteolytic

degradation of the enzyme but on additional factors such as loss
of enzyme protein from the cell body by neurosecretion, or transport into remote, peripheral parts of the neuron, which for
technical reasons cannot be included into the determination. Such
differences in the rate of transport from the cell body to the
peripheral parts of the neuron may represent a relevant factor for
the differences between the turnover rate of dopamine β-hydroxylase
and tyrosine hydroxylase in the superior cervical ganglion of the
rat. Although there is convincing evidence for axonal transport of
both tyrosine hydroxylase and dopamine β-hydroxylase in adrenergic
neurons (Laduron and Belpaire, 1968; Livett, Geffen and Rush, 1969;
Thoenen, Mueller and Axelrod, 1970) the rate of transport for
dopamine β-hydroxylase is faster than that of tyrosine hydroxylase,
as will be shown below.

RELATIONSHIP BETWEEN THE SITE OF SYNTHESIS OF THE ADRENERGIC TRANSMITTER AND THAT OF THE CORRESPONDING ENZYMES

In the peripheral adrenergic neuron the nerve terminals
contain not only the majority of the transmitter present in the
whole neuron (Dahlström and Häggendal, 1966) but they are also the
principal site of its synthesis (for references see Geffen and
Livett, 1971). In the cat spleen Geffen and Rush (1968) have
shown that the amount of norepinephrine transported from the cell
body to the periphery amounts to less than 2% of the quantity of
norepinephrine synthesized in the nerve terminals.

Thus, if trans-synaptic induction of enzymes involved in the
synthesis of the adrenergic transmitter should represent a relevant
factor for the long-term adaptation to increased transmitter
utilization, the rise in enzyme activity in the nerve terminals
rather than the cell body is of primary importance. Moreover,
the relationship between the increase in enzyme activity in the
cell body and the nerve terminals is not only of importance for
the long-term adaptation as such, but also for the time point of
its functional occurrence. The appearance of increased amounts
of enzyme protein in the nerve terminals depends not only on the
time-lag between the beginning of increased neuronal activity and
the manifestations of an enhanced enzyme synthesis, as judged by a
measurable rise in the in vitro activity in the cell body, but also
on the rate of transport from the perikaryon to the periphery
where increased enzyme levels are of functional importance.

Although exposure of animals to extensive stress, such as
swimming to exhaustion, produces a small rise in tyrosine
hydroxylase and dopamine β-hydroxylase activity within 4 to 6 hours
both in adrenals and sympathetic ganglia, this increase is so small
(10 to 20%) and variable that it reaches statistically significant
levels only by use of a large number of animals (unpublished

observation). However, a consistent rise in enzyme activity,
particularly tyrosine hydroxylase can be observed after 18 to
24 hours of cold exposure (Thoenen, 1970; Thoenen et al., 1971)
or administration of reserpine (Mueller, Thoenen and Axelrod,
1969 b). However, in the nerve terminals the time-lag between
the beginning of increased neuronal activity and the increase in
the in vitro activity of enzymes is much longer (Figure 3). After
subcutaneous administration of a single dose of 5 mg/kg of reserpine, the increase in tyrosine hydroxylase activity in the rat
heart does not reach statistically significant ($P < 0.05$) levels
before 72 hours, whereas in the stellate ganglion, containing
the corresponding cell bodies, there is already a marked increase
in enzyme activity after 24 hours (Thoenen, Mueller and Axelrod,
1970). However, the enzyme levels remain elevated much longer in
the heart than in the stellate ganglion, indicating that the
assembled active enzyme, and possibly also enzyme precursors,
are synthesized in the cell body and are transported to the
periphery. In this context the situation in the adrenal medulla

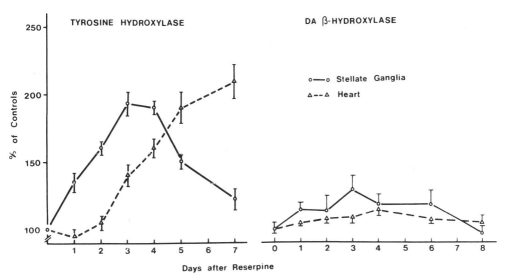

Figure 3. Comparison between the time course of induction of tyrosine hydroxylase and dopamine β-hydroxylase in stellate ganglia and
heart. Male Sprague-Dawley rats (120-130 g) were injected subcutaneously with 5 mg/kg reserpine 1-8 days before they were killed.
Dopamine β-hydroxylase activity was determined according to Molinoff,
Weinshilboum and Axelrod (1971) with 1 mM phenylethylamine as substrate.
Zero time activity amounted to 166 ± 17 nmoles phenylethanolamine/mg
protein/hr in the stellate ganglion and to 0.68 ± 0.03 nmoles/mg
protein/hr in the heart. The values given represent means ± S.E.M.
(n = 6). Data for tyrosine hydroxylase from Thoenen, Mueller and
Axelrod (1970).

is of particular interest. The adrenal medullary cells have the
same ontogenetic origin as the adrenergic neurons, i.e. the neural
crest. They can be considered as neurons without neuronal processes,
and thus, the sites of enzyme and transmitter synthesis are not as
remote as in the adrenergic neuron. This is also reflected by the
time-course of the changes in adrenal tyrosine hydroxylase activity
after administration of a single dose of 5 mg/kg of reserpine. The
rate of increase is about the same as in stellate and superior
cervical ganglia (Mueller, Thoenen and Axelrod, 1969 b; Thoenen,
Mueller and Axelrod, 1970) but the return to control levels is
much slower and resembles that in the rat heart, i.e. two weeks
after administration of reserpine the enzyme levels are still
significantly (P < 0.05) higher than those of untreated controls
(Mueller, Axelrod and Thoenen, unpublished results). Dopamine
β-hydroxylase, the second enzyme selectively located in adrenergic
neurons (for references see Geffen and Livett, 1971), does not show
a clear cut phase-difference between the activity changes in cell
body and nerve terminals as does tyrosine hydroxylase (Figure 3).
This may indicate that the transport of dopamine β-hydroxylase is
considerably faster than that of tyrosine hydroxylase. However, the
factors determining the level of dopamine β-hydroxylase are particularly complex, since in addition to the rate of synthesis, transport
and proteolytic degradation, there is loss of enzyme protein by
exocytosis (Viveros, Arqueros and Kirshner, 1968; Viveros et al.,
1969; Gewirtz and Kopin, 1970; Smith et al., 1970).

    In view of the great importance of the transport of enzyme from
the cell body to the periphery for the long-term adaptation to
increased transmitter utilization by increased neuronal activity,
this aspect will be discussed in more detail. In the rat, the
species predominantly used for studies on trans-synaptic enzyme
induction, the distance between the neuronal cell bodies and their
effector organs is generally too short to allow the determination
of possible changes in enzyme activity within the postganglionic
adrenergic axon. However, the sciatic nerve offers favorable
conditions for such studies since the main part of the postganglionic
adrenergic nerve originating in the 4th to the 6th lumbar ganglia,
run to the periphery in the sciatic nerve.

    In previous experiments it has been shown that after administra-
tion of a single dose of reserpine the rise in tyrosine hydroxylase
activity in the lumbar ganglia is followed by a gradual proximo-
distal rise in enzyme activity in the sciatic nerve (Thoenen,
Mueller and Axelrod, 1970). From the progress of this "wave of
induced enzyme" a proximo-distal transport rate of 2-3 cm/day has
been calculated. However, for an accurate determination of the
transport velocity this procedure did not seem to be optimal,
since the proximo-distal rise in tyrosine hydroxylase activity
in the sciatic nerve was preceded by an initial general decrease,

the cause of which has not been elucidated so far. Furthermore, preliminary experiments have shown that there is no corresponding "dopamine β-hydroxylase wave" in the sciatic nerve which would allow a similar determination of the rate of transport of this enzyme.

In view of these facts we have determined the rate of transport of all enzymes involved in the synthesis of norepinephrine by measuring the time-course of enzyme accumulation above a ligature of the right sciatic nerve at the hip joint where it crosses the sacrotubular ligament. This procedure has already been used for the determination of the rate of transport of norepinephrine from the cell body to the periphery (for references see Geffen and Livett, 1971). These studies were based on the assumption that the ligature of postganglionic nerves neither influences the synthetic function of the cell body nor the axoplasmic transport proximal to the ligature. These aspects deserve serious consideration, since it is known that trans-section or ligature of axons have severe functional consequences on the cell body and even produce marked morphological alterations (for references see Cragg, 1970). To judge possible functional consequences, particularly those concerning enzyme synthesis, the level of tyrosine hydroxylase and dopamine β-hydroxylase, as well as their inducibility, were determined in the lumbar ganglia of both ligated and non-ligated sides and compared with unoperated animals. Within a time-period twice as long as was necessary to determine the rate of enzyme accumulation above the sciatic ligature, no differences in either enzyme level or inducibility could be detected between the three experimental groups in the lumbar ganglia (Table 1, Figure 4). This indicates that at least during the first 24 hours after ligation of the sciatic nerve there does not seem to be an impaired ability of the lumbar ganglia to maintain the normal rate of enzyme synthesis, and to respond with an increased synthesis to the enhanced activity of the preganglionic cholinergic nerves. However, one week after ligation of the sciatic nerve both tyrosine hydroxylase and dopamine β-hydroxylase are markedly reduced and also the trans-synaptic induction of these enzymes seems to be impaired (Table 1, Figure 4).

For the determination of the rate of transport the enzyme activity was measured at different time-points after ligation in the 1 cm-segments just proximal to the ligation. The determination of enzyme activity was confined to this single segment since preliminary experiments had shown that ligations had no effect on the enzyme level in the more proximal parts of the sciatic nerve. As shown in Figure 5, the increase in enzyme activity is linear up to 12 hours for tyrosine hydroxylase, dopa decarboxylase and dopamine β-hydroxylase. The transport velocity calculated from the rate of rise in this linear part of the curve amounted to

TABLE 1

Effect of ligation of rat sciatic nerve on tyrosine hydroxylase
and dopamine β-hydroxylase levels in lumbar ganglia *

	Tyrosine hydroxylase activity after ligation**				Dopamine β-hydroxylase activity after ligation**			
	12 hr	24 hr	96 hr	192 hr	12 hr	24 hr	96 hr	192 hr
Ligated Side	101 ± 6	105 ± 7	32 ± 3	28 ± 2	101 ± 6	98 ± 7	44 ± 5	38 ± 5
Non-Ligated Side	105 ± 8	96 ± 5	48 ± 1	45 ± 2	96 ± 8	99 ± 6	67 ± 6	55 ± 5

*   Right sciatic nerves were ligated in 100-120 g male Sprague-Dawley rats and enzyme activity
     determined in lumbar ganglia IV-VI. Tyrosine hydroxylase was assayed according to Levitt
     et al. (1967) as modified by Mueller, Thoenen and Axelrod (1969 b) with 15 μM L-tyrosine and
     720 μM 6,7-dimethyl-5,6,7,8-tetrahydropteridine·HC1 and dopamine β-hydroxylase according to
     Molinoff, Weinshilboum and Axelrod (1971) with 1 mM phenylethylamine.

** Enzyme activities are expressed in percent of zero time controls. The latter amounted to
     0.73 ± 0.06 nmoles DOPA/mg protein/hr for tyrosine hydroxylase and 129 ± 11 nmoles phenyl-
     ethanolamine/mg protein/hr for dopamine β-hydroxylase. Contralateral controls did not
     differ significantly from each other at 0 time. The values given represent means ± S.E.M.
     (n = 6-12).

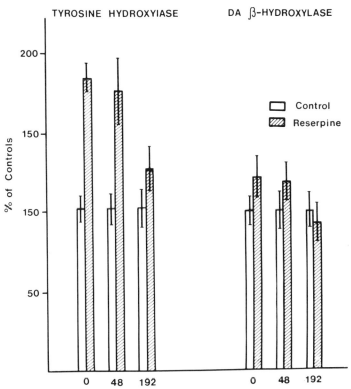

Figure 4. Inducibility of tyrosine hydroxylase and dopamine β-hydroxylase in rat lumbar ganglia after ligation of the sciatic nerve. The right sciatic nerve of 100-120 g male Sprague-Dawley rats was ligated at zero time. The animals were injected subcutaneously with 5 mg/kg reserpine 48 hours before they were killed. Enzyme activities were determined in lumbar ganglia IV-VI. Tyrosine hydroxylase activity in untreated controls was 0.82 ± 0.09 nmoles DOPA/mg protein/hr at 0 hour, 0.68 ± 0.09 at 48 hours and 0.23 ± 0.03 at 192 hours, and dopamine β-hydroxylase activity 145 ± 13 nmoles phenylethanolamine/mg protein/hour at 0 hour, 134 ± 14 at 48 hours and 55 ± 4.6 at 192 hours after ligation. No statistically significant (P < 0.05) differences were noticed between the lumbar ganglia of ligated and nonligated sides. The values given represent means ± S.E.M. (n = 6).

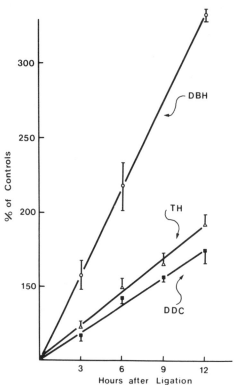

Figure 5. Rate of accumulation of dopamine β-hydroxylase, tyrosine
hydroxylase and DOPA decarboxylase. Sciatic nerves of 110-115 g
male Sprague-Dawley rats were ligated at the hip joint. Enzyme
activities were determined in 1 cm segments proximal to the ligature.
Tyrosine hydroxylase was assayed according to Levitt et al. (1967)
as modified by Mueller, Thoenen and Axelrod (1969 b) with 15 μM
L-tyrosine and 720 μM 6,7-dimethyl-5,6,7,8-tetrahydropteridine·HCl,
          DOPA decarboxylase according to Håkanson and Owman (1966) as
modified by Thoenen et al. (1971) with 1 mM L-DOPA, and dopamine
β-hydroxylase according to Molinoff, Weinshilboum and Axelrod (1971)
with 1 mM phenylethylamine. The values given represent means $\pm$ S.E.M.
(n = 8-16). Accumulation of enzyme activities with time is expressed
as percent of controls. Enzyme activities in sciatic segments taken
from unoperated controls did not differ from those in segments taken
from the unligated contralateral sciatic nerve of unilaterally
ligated animals. The activities in controls amounted to 17.4 $\pm$ 1.1
pmoles DOPA/hr/cm of sciatic for tyrosine hydroxylase, 6.2 $\pm$ 0.25
nmoles dopamine/hr/cm of sciatic for DOPA decarboxylase and 1.39 $\pm$
0.10 nmoles phenylethanolamine/hr/cm of sciatic for dopamine β-
hydroxylase. The correlation coefficients of the regression lines
were 0.98 for tyrosine hydroxylase, 0.97 for DOPA decarboxylase and
0.99 for dopamine β-hydroxylase. Each slope is significantly
(P < 0.005) different from the other two.

4.65 ± 0.08 cm/day for dopamine β-hydroxylase, 1.80 ± 0.04 cm/day
for tyrosine hydroxylase and 1.51 ± 0.04 cm/day for DOPA decarboxylase.

Although it cannot be decided with certainty whether ligation
of the sciatic has any effect on enzyme transport, the linearity
of enzyme accumulation within the first 12 hours speaks against
a severe impairment. Moreover, the rate of transport determined
by this method is very similar to that calculated from the proximo-
distal progress of increased tyrosine hydroxylase levels after
administration of reserpine (Thoenen, Mueller and Axelrod, 1970).

The rate of dopamine β-hydroxylase accumulation above the
sciatic ligature observed in our experiments is considerably slower
than that of norepinephrine, which was taken as a measure of transport for the storage vesicles (Dahlström and Häggendal, 1966).
The rate of dopamine β-hydroxylase accumulation corresponds to a
transport rate of 1.94 ± 0.03 mm/hr and that of norepinephrine
accumulation to a rate of 5-6 mm/hr (Dahlström and Häggendal, 1966).
It is possible that part of this discrepancy results from differences
in animal size, since the male Sprague-Dawley rats used by Dahlström
and Häggendal (1966) weighed 200-300 g whereas ours weighed only
100-120 g. However, since all the enzymes necessary for the
synthesis of norepinephrine are present in the adrenergic axon, it
cannot be excluded that norepinephrine synthesis also continues in
the ligated part of the axon in which the storage vesicles are
piling up, and that this in loco synthesis mimics a more rapid
transport of storage vesicles. Furthermore, it has to be taken
into account that dopamine β-hydroxylase could be transported
in both particulate and cytoplasmic form and that the determined
rate of transport represents a summation of both forms of transport. Thus, neither the rate of accumulation of dopamine β-
hydroxylase nor that of norepinephrine would be fully representative
for the rate of transport of storage vesicles.

This assumption is not completely irrational, since preliminary
experiments on subcellular distribution of dopamine β-hydroxylase
have shown considerable differences between the cell body, axon
and nerve terminals. In organs such as the heart and vas deferens
("stripped" preparation) containing mainly terminal parts of the
adrenergic neuron, most of the dopamine β-hydroxylase activity is
localized in the particulate fraction. In contrast, in lumbar,
stellate and superior cervical ganglia up to 50% of the activity
is found in the high speed (100,000 x g) supernatant. The distribution in the sciatic is intermediate, i.e. about 25-30% of the
activity is in the high speed supernatant. Although it cannot
definitely be decided whether the dopamine β-hydroxylase present
in the high speed supernatant represents really non-particulate
enzyme or whether it represents a moiety which is easily released

from the particulate fraction during the experimental procedure,
definite differences between cell body and nerve terminals seem to
exist, since repeated rehomogenization of the microsomal fraction
of the rat heart brought only a relatively small part of dopamine
β-hydroxylase into solution. Differences between the subcellular
distribution in cell body and nerve terminals are not confined to
dopamine β-hydroxylase but have also been reported for norepinephrine,
which in nerve terminals is predominantly located in the microsomal
fraction, whereas in the cell body the main part is found in the
supernatant (Fischer and Snyder, 1965; Geffen and Livett, 1971).
Thus, the norepinephrine storage vesicles could perhaps change their
properties on the way down from the cell body to the periphery both
with respect to their binding capacity for norepinephrine and to
the strength of binding of dopamine β-hydroxylase. It could be
assumed that in the cell body part of the dopamine β-hydroxylase is
still in its native form i.e. not yet incorporated into the
"transport-packages" of the storage vesicles. Furthermore, in
the nerve terminals norepinephrine is liberated together with
dopamine β-hydroxylase, and thus a continuous loss of less tightly
bound dopamine β-hydroxylase by nervous activity would lead to a
shift in the subcellular distribution.

It has also been suggested that only the large dense core
vesicles contain soluble dopamine β-hydroxylase, which can be
liberated from adrenergic nerve terminals by exocytosis, whereas
in the small vesicles dopamine β-hydroxylase is either absent or
membrane-bound (for references see Geffen and Livett, 1971). The
latter assumption suggests that the large dense core vesicles are
transformed into small ones by losing their soluble proteins,
although they retain the ability to store catecholamines.

The rate of transport of tyrosine hydroxylase calculated from
the rate of rise of the enzyme activity in the first 1-cm segment
proximal to the sciatic ligature, amounts to 1.80 ± 0.04 cm/day.
This rate of transport is intermediate, being at the upper limit
of the slow component of axoplasmic flow, which is generally thought
to be representative for the transport of cell constituents not
associated with particles. The latter are transported by a specific,
more rapid mechanism (for references see Geffen and Livett, 1971).
This slower rate of transport of tyrosine hydroxylase is in agreement with the subcellular distribution of this enzyme. Both in the
sympathetic ganglia (stellate, superior cervical and lumbar) of the
rat and organs such as heart and "stripped" vas deferens containing
mainly adrenergic nerve terminals, the greatest part of enzyme
activity is located in the high-speed supernatant. In view of the
great difficulties of accurately assaying tyrosine hydroxylase in
peripheral organs of the rat (Mueller, Thoenen and Axelrod, 1969 a),
it cannot be decided whether the 10% of total activity detected in
the microsomal fraction is an artifact or represents a true small

moiety of enzyme associated with particulate constituents of the cell.

These findings are in distinct contrast to the observations of Kuczenski and Mandell (1972) in the rat brain. In the mid-brain where tyrosine hydroxylase is located mainly in cell bodies of catecholaminergic neurons the majority of enzyme activity ($\sim$ 75%) is found in the high speed supernatant. However, in the corpus striatum, where tyrosine hydroxylase is located mainly in dopaminergic nerve endings, the activity is not only located in the particulate fraction ($\sim$ 85%) but seems to be tightly associated with membranes.

The fact that the rate of accumulation of DOPA decarboxylase, an enzyme generally accepted to be cytoplasmic (for references see Geffen and Livett, 1971) is little but significantly (P < 0.005) slower than that of tyrosine hydroxylase could support the assumption that the small, but consistently found moiety of tyrosine hydroxylase in the microsomal fraction of the sciatic nerve is not an artifact, but reflects the true physiological subcellular distribution. This would imply that a small part of the enzyme is transported in association with subcellular particles and thus at a faster rate. This could also explain the slight discrepancy between the rate of transport calculated in the present experiments (1.8 cm/day) from that obtained in previous ones ($\sim$ 2.5 cm/day) by measuring the proximo-distal progress of enzyme activity in the sciatic nerve after trans-synaptic induction of tyrosine hydroxylase in lumbar ganglia (Thoenen, Mueller and Axelrod, 1970). The progress of the front of the induced enzyme would then be determined by the faster component, whereas the rate of accumulation would represent the summation of fast and slow moieties.

However, in view of the great complexity of the factors determining the rate of axoplasmic transport (Davison, 1970; Karlsson and Sjöstrand, 1971) it seems to be hazardous to draw definite conclusions on differences in the subcellular distribution of enzymes from such small differences in the rate of axoplasmic transport as is found between tyrosine hydroxylase and DOPA decarboxylase.

From the present results it can be concluded that the long-term adaptation of the sympathetic nervous system to increased transmitter utilization involves an increased synthesis of tyrosine hydroxylase and dopamine β-hydroxylase in the cell body of the adrenergic neuron, and that both enzymes are transported to the nerve terminals, the main sites of transmitter synthesis.

It is worth noticing that the increased rate of enzyme synthesis takes place in the perikaryon, a part of the neuron in which increased neuronal activity is not accompanied by increased turnover and synthesis of norepinephrine. At least in the superior cervical ganglia of the cat, the stimulation of preganglionic cholinergic nerves produces an immediate increase in synthesis and turnover of norepinephrine in the nerve terminals of the adrenergic neuron but not in the cell body (Bhatnagar and Moore, 1971). Although most experiments on neuronally mediated enzyme induction in the sympathetic nervous system have been performed in rats, it has also been shown in cats that electrical stimulation of the posterior hypothalamus leads to an increase in the in vitro activity of tyrosine hydroxylase in the adrenal medulla, implying that trans-synaptic enzyme induction is also present in this species (Reis et al., 1971).

Therefore, it appears that the trans-synaptic induction in the cell bodies of the adrenergic neurons does not depend on an increased turnover of the transmitter in this part of the neuron.

ADDITIVE EFFECT OF IMMEDIATE AND LONG-TERM ADAPTATION TO INCREASED TRANSMITTER UTILIZATION

In experiments with 6-hydroxydopamine Mueller (1971) has shown that in the adrenal medulla an increased level of tyrosine hydroxylase is accompanied by an increased synthesis and turnover of catecholamines (Figure 2). These experiments have been performed under experimental conditions in which the reflex increase in the activity of splanchnic fibers supplying the adrenal medulla was still in play, and it cannot be decided to what extent the increased synthesis is due to the immediate or the long-term adaptation, i.e. the induction of tyrosine hydroxylase. However, in recent experiments Dairman and Udenfriend (1970) have shown that the increased synthesis of norepinephrine in the rat heart and adrenal chromaffin cells occurring after repeated administration of phenoxybenzamine is only partially blocked by chlorisandamine, a ganglionic blocking agent. This indicates that both the mechanism of immediate adaptation, based on the increased activity of the neuron, and the increased level of the rate-limiting enzyme contribute to the increased synthesis.

SUMMARY

An increased activity of peripheral and central adrenergic neurons leads to an instantaneous augmentation of transmitter synthesis which is not accompanied by changes in the in vitro activity of enzymes engaged in norepinephrine synthesis. However, in addition to this immediate adaptation to the increased transmitter utilization, there is a long-term adaptation which involves a trans-synaptic induction of tyrosine hydroxylase and dopamine β-hydroxylase, enzymes which are selectively located in adrenergic

neurons and adrenal chromaffin cells. Since the nerve terminals in
adrenergic neurons are not only the main sites of transmitter storage
but also the main sites of transmitter synthesis, the enzyme levels
in the nerve terminals, rather than cell bodies, are of primary
functional importance for the long-term adaptation to increased
transmitter utilization. The enzyme levels in various parts of the
adrenergic neuron are not only determined by the rate of synthesis
and proteolytic degradation of enzymes but also by the rate of
their transport from the cell body to the periphery and possible
loss by neurosecretion. In view of the great importance of enzyme
transport from the cell body to the peripheral parts of the neuron
for the long-term adaptation to increased transmitter utilization
this aspect has been treated in more detail. The rates of transport
of the enzymes involved in the biosynthesis of norepinephrine have
been determined in the rat sciatic nerve by determining their rate
of accumulation in a 1 cm segment proximal to a ligature at the
level of the sacrotuberal ligament. For the first 12 hours after
ligation the rate of accumulation was linear, and both the enzyme
levels and trans-synaptic induction was not altered in the corresponding lumbar ganglia, suggesting that both transport in the axon
and the synthetic properties of the cell body were not impaired by
ligation of the post-ganglionic adrenergic axon, at least within
the time necessary to determine the rate of accumulation. The rate
of transport for tyrosine hydroxylase amounted to 1.80 ± 0.04 cm/day,
for dopamine β-hydroxylase to 4.65 ± 0.08 cm/day and to 1.51 ± 0.04
cm/day for DOPA decarboxylase. The differences in the rate of
transport are discussed in connection with the subcellular distribution of these enzymes in cell body, axon and nerve terminals.

ACKNOWLEDGEMENTS

    This work was supported by the Swiss National Foundation for
Scientific Research (Grant Nr. 3.653.71). We wish to express
our thanks to Miss Vreni Forster, Mrs. Hilary Wood and Mr. Ueli
Jäggi for their excellent technical assistance.

REFERENCES

Ames, B.N. and Martin, R.G. 1964. Biochemical aspects of genetics:
    the operon. Ann. Rev. Biochem. 33: 235.
Bhatnagar, R.K. and Moore, K.E. 1971. Effects of electrical stimu-
    lation, α-methyltyrosine and desmethylimipramine on the
    norepinephrine contents of neuronal cell bodies and terminals.
    J. Pharmacol. Exp. Ther. 178: 450.
Black, I.B., Hendry, I., and Iversen, L.L. 1971. Differences in
    the regulation of tyrosine hydroxylase and DOPA decarboxylase
    in sympathetic ganglia and adrenals. Nature New Biol. 231: 27.

Costa, E. 1970. Simple neuronal models to estimate turnover rate
    of noradrenergic transmitter in vivo. Adv. Biochem.
    Psychopharmacol. 2: 169.
Cragg, B.G. 1970. What is the signal for chromatolysis? Brain
    Res. 23: 1.
Dahlström, A. 1967. The interneuronal distribution of nor-
    adrenaline and the transport and life-span of amine storage
    granules in the sympathetic adrenergic neuron. Naunyn-
    Schmiedebergs Arch. Exp. Path. Pharmakol. 257: 93.
Dahlström, A. and Häggendal, J. 1966. Studies on the transport
    and life-span of amine storage granules in a peripheral
    adrenergic neuron system. Acta physiol. Scand. 67: 278.
Dairman, W. and Udenfriend, S. 1970. Increased conversion of
    tyrosine to catecholamines in the intact rat following
    elevation of tissue tyrosine hydroxylase levels by administered
    phenoxybenzamine. Mol. Pharmacol. 6: 350.
Davison, P.F. 1970. Axoplasmic transport: Physical and chemical
    aspects. In: The Neurosciences. New York: The Rockefller
    Univ. Press, pp. 851.
Fischer, J.E. and Snyder, S. 1965. Disposition of norepinephrine-
    H^3 in sympathetic ganglia. J. Pharmacol. Exp. Ther. 150: 190.
Geffen, L.B. and Livett, B.G. 1971. Synaptic vesicles in
    sympathetic neurons. Physiol. Rev. 51: 98.
Geffen, L.B. and Rush, R.A. 1968. Transport of noradrenaline in
    sympathetic nerves and the effect of nerve impulses on its
    contribution to transmitter stores. J. Neurochem. 15: 925.
Gewirtz, G.P. and Kopin, I.J. 1970. Release of dopamine β-
    hydroxylase with norepinephrine during cat splenic nerve
    stimulation. Nature 227: 406.
Gisiger, V. and Gaide-Huguenin, A.-C. 1969. Effect of preganglionic
    stimulation upon RNA synthesis in the isolated sympathetic
    ganglion of the rat. Progr. Brain Res. 31: 125.
Haefely, W., Hürlimann, A. and Thoenen, H. 1965. Relation between
    the rate of stimulation and the quantity of noradrenaline
    liberated from sympathetic nerve endings in the isolated
    perfused spleen of the cat. J. Physiol. 181: 48.
Håkanson, R. and Owman, C. 1966. Pineal DOPA decarboxylase and
    monoamine oxydase activities as related to the monoamine stores.
    J. Neurochem. 13: 597.
Iversen, L.L. 1967. The Uptake and Storage of Noradrenaline in
    Sympathetic Nerves. London: Cambridge Univ. Press.
Karlsson, J.O. and Sjöstrand, J. 1971. Characterization of the
    fast and slow components of axonal transport in retinal
    ganglion cells. J. Neurobiol. 2: 135.
Koelle, G.B. 1970. Neurohumoral transmission and the autonomic
    nervous system. In: The Pharmacological Basis of Therapeutics.
    (Eds., Goodman, L.S. and Gilman, A.) 4th Ed. London: The
    MacMillan Company, p. 402.
Kuczenski, R.T. and Mandell, A.J. 1972. Regulatory properties of
    soluble and particulate rat brain tyrosine hydroxylase.
    J. Biol. Chem. 247: 3114.

Kvetnanský, R., Gewirtz, G.P., Weise, V.K. and Kopin, I.J. 1970. Effect of hypophysectomy on immobilization-induced elevation of tyrosine hydroxylase and phenylethanolamine-N-methyl transferase in the rat adrenal. Endocrinology 87: 1323.

Laduron, P. and Belpaire, F. 1968. Transport of noradrenaline and dopamine β-hydroxylase in sympathetic nerves. Life Sci. 7:1.

Larrabee, M.G. 1969. Metabolic effects of nerve impulses and nerve-growth factor in sympathetic ganglia. Progr. Brain Res. 31: 95.

Levitt, M., Gibb, J.W., Daly, J.W., Lipton, M. and Udenfriend, S. 1967. A new class of tyrosine hydroxylase inhibitors and a simple assay of inhibition in vivo. Biochem. Pharm. 16: 1313.

Levitt, M., Spector, S., Sjoerdsma, A. and Udenfriend, S. 1965. Elucidation of the rate-limiting step in norepinephrine biosynthesis in the perfused guinea-pig heart. J. Pharmacol. Exp. Ther. 148: 1.

Livett, B.G., Geffen, L.B. and Rush, R.A. 1969. Immunohistochemical evidence for the transport of dopamine β-hydroxylase and a catecholamine binding protein in sympathetic nerves. Biochem. Pharmacol. 18: 923.

Molinoff, P.B. and Axelrod, J. 1971. Biochemistry of catechol-amines. Ann. Rev. Biochem. 40: 465.

Molinoff, P.B., Brimijoin, S., Weinshilboum, R. and Axelrod, J. 1970. Neurally mediated increase in dopamine β-hydroxylase activity. Proc. Nat. Acad. Sci. USA 66:453.

Molinoff, P.B., Weinshilboum, R. and Axelrod, J. 1971. A sensitive enzymatic assay for dopamine β-hydroxylase. J. Pharmacol. Exp. Ther. 178: 425.

Mueller, R.A. 1971. Effect of 6-hydroxydopamine on the synthesis and turnover of catecholamines and protein in the adrenal. In: 6-Hydroxydopamine and Catecholamine Neurons (Eds., Malmfors, T. and Thoenen, H.) Amsterdam-London: North-Holland Publishing Company, pp. 291.

Mueller, R.A., Thoenen, H. and Axelrod, J. 1969 a. Adrenal tyrosine hydroxylase; compensatory increase in activity after chemical sympathectomy. Science 158: 468.

Mueller, R.A., Thoenen, H. and Axelrod, J. 1969 b. Increase in tyrosine hydroxylase activity after reserpine administration. J. Pharmacol. Exp. Ther. 169: 74.

Mueller, R.A., Thoenen, H. and Axelrod, J. 1969 c. Inhibition of trans-synaptically increased tyrosine hydroxylase activity by cycloheximide and actinomycin D. Mol. Pharmacol. 5: 463.

Musacchio, J.M., Julou, L., Kety, S.S. and Glowinski, J. 1969. Increase in rat brain tyrosine hydroxylase activity produced by electroconvulsive shock. Proc.Nat.Acad.Sci.USA 63: 1117.

Patrick, R.L. and Kirshner, N. 1971. Effect of stimulation on the levels of tyrosine hydroxylase, dopamine β-hydroxylase, and catecholamines in intact and denervated rat adrenal glands. Mol. Pharmacol. 7: 87.

Reis, D.J., Moorhead, D.T., Rifkin, M., Joh, T.H. and Goldstein, M. 1971. Changes in adrenal enzymes synthesizing catecholamines in attack behavior evoked by hypothalamic stimulation in the cat. Nature 229:562.

Richter, D. 1970. Protein metabolism and functional activity. In: Protein Metabolism of the Nervous System (Ed. Lajtha, A.) London: Plenum Press, pp. 241.

Sedvall, G.C. and Kopin, I.J. 1967. Influence of sympathetic denervation and nerve impulse activity on tyrosine hydroxylase in the rat submaxillary gland. Biochem. Pharmacol. 16: 39.

Smith, A.D., De Potter, W.P., Moerman, E.J. and De Schaepdryver, A.F. 1970. Release of dopamine β-hydroxylase and chromogranin A upon stimulation of the splenic nerve. Tissue and Cell 2: 547.

Thoenen, H. 1969. Bildung und funktionelle Bedeutung adrenerger Ersatztransmitter. Berlin-Heidelberg-New York: Springer-Verlag.

Thoenen, H. 1970. Induction of tyrosine hydroxylase in peripheral and central adrenergic neurons by cold-exposure of rats. Nature 228: 861.

Thoenen, H. 1972. Comparison between the effect of neuronal activity and nerve growth factor on enzymes involved in the synthesis of norepinephrine. Pharmacol. Rev. 24:255.

Thoenen, H., Kettler, R., Burkard, W. and Saner, A. 1971. Neurally mediated control of enzymes involved in the synthesis of norepinephrine: Are they regulated as an operational unit? Naunyn-Schmiedebergs Arch. Pharmak. 270: 146.

Thoenen, H., Mueller, R.A. and Axelrod, J. 1969 a. Increased tyrosine hydroxylase activity after drug-induced alteration of sympathetic transmission. Nature 221: 1264.

Thoenen, H., Mueller, R.A. and Axelrod, J. 1969 b. Trans-synaptic induction of adrenal tyrosine hydroxylase. J. Pharmacol. Exp. Ther. 169: 249.

Thoenen, H., Mueller, R.A. and Axelrod, J. 1970. Phase difference in the induction of tyrosine hydroxylase in cell body and nerve terminals of sympathetic neurones. Proc.Nat.Acad.Sci.USA 65: 58.

Thoenen, H. and Tranzer, J.P. 1968. Chemical sympathectomy by selective destruction of adrenergic nerve endings with 6-hydroxydopamine. Naunyn-Schmiedebergs Arch. Pharmak. 261: 271.

Udenfriend, S. and Dairman, W. 1971. Regulation of norepinephrine synthesis. Adv. Enzyme Regul. 9: 145.

Viveros, O.H., Arqueros, L. and Kirshner, N. 1968. Release of catecholamines and dopamine β-oxidase from the adrenal medulla. Life Sci. 7: 609.

Viveros, O.H., Arqueros, L., Connett, R.J. and Kirshner, N. 1969. Mechanism of secretion from the adrenal medulla IV. The fate of storage vesicles following insulin and reserpine administration. Mol. Pharmacol. 5: 69.

Weiner, N. 1972. Modification of norepinephrine synthesis in intact tissue during short-term adrenergic nerve stimulation. Pharmacol. Rev. (in press).

SOME CHARACTERISTICS OF BRAIN TYROSINE HYDROXYLASE

Edith G. McGeer and Paul L. McGeer

Division of Neurological Sciences, Department of
Psychiatry, University of British Columbia
Vancouver, Canada

There is general agreement as to the properties of tyrosine
hydroxylase from the adrenal medulla, but the properties of brain
tyrosine hydroxylase are more controversial. This is perhaps not
so surprising when one considers that the adrenal medullary cells
are secretory cells which do not possess the long axons and multi-
plicity of nerve endings characteristic of central catecholaminergic neurons. The relatively complex structure of the neuron has
complicated the problem of defining the properties of brain
tyrosine hydroxylase and will probably prove important to an
understanding of the factors which control or modify enzyme
activity in vivo.

Adrenal tyrosine hydroxylase is, as you have heard, an
easily solubilized, supernatant enzyme which, whether homogenized
in isotonic or hypertonic medium, requires oxygen and an exogenous
pteridine cofactor for in vitro activity; it is markedly stimulated
by ferrous ion. Nagatsu, Levitt and Udenfriend (1964 a,b) and Cote
and Fahn (1969; Fahn, Rodman and Cote, 1969) indicated that brain
tyrosine hydroxylase was like adrenal tyrosine hydroxylase and
required exogenous pteridine cofactor for maximal activity. Based
on comparative experiments such as shown in Table 1, we suggested
that tyrosine hydroxylase activity in fresh rat brain sucrose
homogenates differed from adrenal tyrosine hydroxylase activity
in that it is particle-bound, not activated by exogenous $DMPH_4$
(2-amino-4-hydroxy-6,7-dimethyltetrahydropteridine) and rapidly
loses activity post-mortem (McGeer, Gibson and McGeer, 1967).
The hydroxylating activity in this form was in fact slightly
inhibited in the fortified system used for the adrenal enzyme, due
to the 2-mercaptoethanol used to protect the $DMPH_4$. A number of
other thiol compounds have also been found to be slightly

53

TABLE 1

Comparative Activities of Rat Brain and Beef Adrenal
Homogenates in 0.25 M Sucrose Under Various Assay Conditions

	Rat Brain		Beef Adrenal	
	0.2 M NaAc pH 6	0.09 M PO_4 pH 6.2	0.2 M NaAc pH 6	0.09 M PO_4 pH 6.2
None	55	100[*][†]	100[*]	76
1 mM $DMPH_4$ + 20 mM 2-mercaptoethanol (SH)	74-90[†]	92	1520[†]	1160
1 mM $DMPH_4$ + 20 mM SH, pre-incubated 10 min	–	75	1190	–
0.1 mM $DMPH_4$ + 20 mM SH	–	86	1495	–
1 mM $DMPH_4$	–	98	280	–
20 mM SH	–	79	89	–
0.1 mM Fe^{++}	–	100	–	–
0.1 mM Fe^{++}, 0.1 mM $DMPH_4$ + 20 mM SH	92	94	1900	1450

[*] Chosen as reference condition

[†] When portions of these homogenates were centrifuged at 20,000 g for 20 min most of the brain tyrosine hydroxylating activity was found in the sediment (96% without $DMPH_4$ and 75% with) while 88% of the adrenal activity (analyzed with $DMPH_4$) was in the supernatant fraction.

inhibitory towards rat brain tyrosine hydroxylase activity in such in vitro assay systems (McGeer and McGeer, 1967).

Using sucrose homogenates in an unfortified medium (Condition A; Table 3), we found the highest activity per unit weight of brain tissue to be in the striatum (Table 2) (McGeer et al., 1967 The particle-bound enzyme in the striatum was highly localized to the nerve ending or synaptosomal fraction (McGeer, Bagchi and McGeer, 1965). This localization was subsequently confirmed by others using somewhat different assay conditions (Fahn, Rodman and Cote, 1969; Nagatsu and Nagatsu, 1970; Fahn and Cote, 1968).

The concentration of tyrosine hydroxylase in the nerve ending fraction of the striatum is perfectly consistent with histo-chemical studies. Such studies have established that this struc-ture contains no catecholaminergic cell bodies (Anden et al., 1964), but only nerve endings which come primarily from cell bodies in the substantia nigra.

In order to learn more about the details of hydroxylating activity in the nigral-striatal dopaminergic tract, we examined normal human material obtained within 2 hours of accidental death. The results, while initially surprising, seem readily explainable on the basis of our current knowledge of cellular structure. Small sections of tissue were taken along the length of the tract (Figure 1), homogenized in sucrose and assayed both with and without added cofactor. It was found (Figure 1 and Table 3) that tyrosine hydroxylation in tissue from the substantia nigra was markedly stimulated by added cofactor, from the globus pallidus it was mildly stimulated, while from the caudate and putamen it was slightly inhibited. On centrifugation of these sucrose homogenates of both human and baboon tissue, the hy-droxylating activity of the cell bodies of the substantia nigra was found primarily in the supernate while that of the nerve endings in the caudate and putamen sedimented with the particulate fraction. The activity in the globus pallidus was divided between particulate and supernatant form. The supernatant enzyme required exogenous $DMPH_4$ while the particle-bound enzyme was not stimulated by this added cofactor (McGeer, McGeer and Wada, 1971). The supernatant enzyme seemed to have considerably more stability than the particle-bound enzyme (Table 4).

Axons and nerve terminals are believed not to synthesize protein. Thus enzymes must be synthesized in the cell bodies and transported along the axons to the nerve endings. The large cell bodies of the substantia nigra are probably easily ruptured during the homogenation process, releasing both enzyme and co-enzyme into the medium. Dilution of the endogenous cofactor by the medium could thus be responsible for the $DMPH_4$-mercaptoethanol

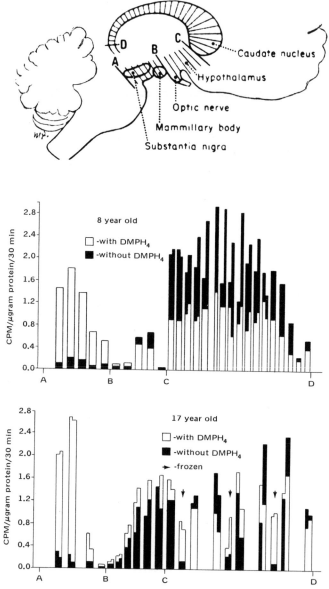

Figure 1. Activities of tyrosine hydroxylase in sections taken from human substantia nigra and caudate nucleus. The left half of double columns denotes the medial aspect of these areas and the right half denotes the lateral aspect. Where no differentiation existed a medial/lateral division was not made. The homogenate of the medial part of the 17th section in the 8 year old subject was lost.

TABLE 2

Activity of the Tyrosine Hydroxylase Systems in Various Areas of the
Human Brain and Brains of Other Species in nmol g^{-1} of wet tissue, h^{-1}

	Human	Baboon (P. papio)	Monkey (M. mulatta)	Cat	Rat
Putamen	15–198 (14)	141 ± 18	112	–	100–120
Caudate nucleus	16–121 (14)	136 ± 15	109	98.5	100–120
Substantia nigra	8–52 (12)	50 ± 32	141	–	50–110
Globus pallidus	4.6–23 (12)	25 ± 6	36	–	50– 55
Accumbens	8–56 (6)	95 ± 29	–	19	105
Septal area	2– 9 (3)	–	–	19	10– 17
Red nucleus	8–33 (6)	–	–	–	–
Amygdala	2– 7 (3)	–	–	4.2	–
Hypothalamus	2–12 (9)	–	8	3.9	11
Thalamus	1– 6 (3)	–	4	2.7	–
Cerebral cortex	n.d.	n.d.	0.5	2.5	<1
Hippocampus	3– 8 (3)	–	–	1.6	4
Cerebellum	0– 1 (3)	–	–	1.4	–

The human values are the ranges found for a given area in the brains of accident victims with the number of cases indicated in parentheses. The baboon values are averages (± S.D.) of analyses on brain samples from 3 baboons. The values for cat (McGeer et al., 1967) and for monkey (Cote and Fahn, 1969) have been previously reported. The rat values are indicative only since there is some variation between strains and, in certain cases, with the fineness of the dissection.

n.d. = no detectable activity (< 0.5).   – = not analyzed.

TABLE 3

Relative Activity of Sucrose Homogenates of Various Brain Areas
Assayed with and without DMPH4 and Distribution of Activity
Between Supernatant and Particulate Fraction[†]

	Activity of total homogenate assayed with DMPH4 as per cent of activity in unfortified assay	Ratio of particulate activity to supernatant activity[*]
Human		
Caudate nucleus	84%	4.5 : 1[*]
Putamen	94%	6.1 : 1[*]
Globus pallidus	185%	0.4[*] : 1[*]
Substantia nigra	1500%	0.3[*] : 1[*]
Baboon		
Caudate nucleus	42%	5.7 : 1[*]
Putamen	36%	10.1 : 1[*]
Globus Pallidus	123%	1.8[*] : 1[*]
Substantia nigra	890%	0.4[*] : 1[*]

[*] The homogenates were centrifuged in the cold at 10,000 g for 15 min.
To calculate this ratio the higher value obtained for each fraction
was used. An asterisk is placed by each number based on an assay
with DMPH4. Thus the higher value with supernatant enzyme was
always obtained with DMPH4 while the higher value with the sedimented enzyme was obtained in the caudate and putamen without
DMPH4 and in the substantia nigra with DMPH4 in 2 out of 4 instances.

[†] Tyrosine hydroxylase assays without DMPH4 were done using 9.1 mg of
tissue or fractionated equivalent and 57,000–76,000 cpm of L-[U-^{14}C]
tyrosine (specific activity 440–513 mCi/mmol) in a total volume of
0.3 ml of incubation medium which was 0.09 M in phosphate buffer,
pH 6.2; 0.08 M in sucrose and 1 mM in NSD-1034 (conditions A). The
assays "with DMPH4" used the same volume and identical amounts of
tissues, radioactive tyrosine, sucrose and NSD-1034 but the solution
was 0.2 M in acetate buffer, pH 6.0, 0.1 mM in DMPH4; 0.3 mM in
FeSO4 and 0.1 M in 2-mercaptoethanol, as described by Cote and
Fahn (1969; Fahn, Rodman and Cote, 1969) (conditions B). The data
for humans was based on 2–4 brains and for baboons on 2 brains; the
details have been reported previously (McGeer, McGeer and Wada, 1971)

cofactor requirement. The situation with regard to synaptosomes
seems to be more complicated. Synaptosomes are not usually
ruptured by homogenization in isotonic media, and tyrosine hydroxylase assays of sucrose homogenates of the caudate nucleus and
putamen are presumably values for intact nerve endings. These
nerve endings may already possess near optimal concentrations of
cofactor and thus be insensitive to the fortification system. It
is also possible that added $DMPH_4$ is not taken up by the synaptosomes.

It seems probable from the results with solubilized enzyme
from both the adrenal medulla and brain (Poillon, 1971) that the
enzyme has an absolute requirement for pteridine cofactor in
vivo. Tetrahydrobiopterin is a strong candidate for such an
endogenous cofactor. This compound has been isolated from liver
and is believed to be the endogenous cofactor for phenylalanine
hydroxylase (Kaufman, 1963). It has also been reported to be the
natural in vivo cofactor for hydroxylations in the adrenal
medulla (Brenneman and Kaufman, 1964; Kaufman, 1964). Its origin
in the body is still obscure. Cofactor activity showing the
chemical characteristics of tetrahydrobiopterin has been measured
in brain and kidney as well as in liver (Guroff, Rhoads and
Abramowitz, 1967), which suggests its ubiquitous nature. Dihydropteridine reductase, an enzyme that reduces the oxidized pteridine
cofactor, has been reported to be present in the brain (Musacchio,
Craviso and Wurzburger, 1972).

So far only the barest outlines of the in vivo cofactor
system have emerged. However, there is every indication that this
system may be considerably more complex than the hydroxylation
system itself. If the cofactor itself, as well as its reductase,
need to be synthesized by the same cells which produce tyrosine
hydroxylase, then each of these factors would need to be considered
in assessing the action of any drug or the etiology of any disease
influencing catecholamine synthesis.

Treating the corpus striatum by methods which disrupt
synaptosomes or disrupt the membrane integrity as, for example,
freezing and thawing, osmotic shock or shaking with ether, led to
apparent substantial losses of activity which could not be
completely restored by the addition of $DMPH_4$, even when the buffered conditions were adjusted to those favorable for the
hydroxylation in the presence of $DMPH_4$ (Table 4). The work of
others, and subsequent comparative studies of sucrose and aqueous
homogenates of rat brain tissue, indicated that this apparent loss
of activity with osmotic shock is probably only due to a change
in the apparent Km of the system towards substrate (Figure 2) and
to the very low concentrations of tyrosine used for the experiments
in Table 4. The Km measured in sucrose homogenates undoubtedly

TABLE 4

Stability of the Tyrosine Hydroxylating
System in Caudate Nucleus and Midbrain

	Assayed under	
	Condition A[*]	Condition B[*]
Human (55 yr. old) caudate dissected 4 hrs. post-mortem and portions homogenized:		
- immediately	100%[†]	71%
- 2 hrs. later	59%	83%
- 4 hrs. later	33%	83%
Rat striatum		
sucrose homogenate:		
- fresh	100%[†]	85%
- on ice 3 hrs.	96%	89%
- 18 hrs. at 5°C	15%	67%
- 18 hrs. at -15°C	47%	89%
- ether treated	<1%	29%
tissue 18 hrs. at -15°C	27%	74%
water homogenate	<1%	87%
Rat midbrain		
sucrose homogenate:		
- fresh	100%[†]	142%
- 18 hrs. at 5°C	63%	143%
- 18 hrs. at -15°C	90%	170%
- ether treated	<1%	95%

[*] For description of conditions see Table 3.

[†] Chosen as reference condition.

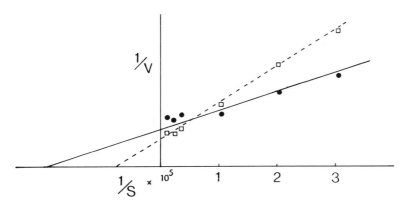

Figure 2. Measured activities of tyrosine hydroxylating system in rat brain homogenates at various concentrations of substrate tyrosine. □ — — Water homogenate, Conditions B, Table 3
              ●——— Sucrose homogenate, Conditions A, Table 3

reflects uptake of tyrosine into the particles and possibly other factors as well as the true Km of the enzyme. These various factors may play a role in regulating the _in vivo_ hydroxylating capacity and reported changes in such capacity due to drugs or environmental influences may reflect changes in enzyme form rather than in the quantity of enzyme _per se_.

Fahn et al. (1969) suggested that caudate tyrosine hydroxylase was associated with synaptic vesicles contained in synaptosomes and reported substantial losses of enzyme activity on synaptosomal disruption. Kuczenski and Mandell (1972) recently suggested that the physical form of the enzyme in its binding to the synaptosomal membrane is indeed essential to its activity. They based this suggestion on the particulate characteristics of caudate tyrosine hydroxylase, its tendency to become membrane bound when activated by drugs (Mandell et al., 1972) and the activating effect of specific sulfated mucopolysaccharides on canine hypothalamic tyrosine hydroxylase. Heparin, for example, did not change the Km of tyrosine hydroxylase towards substrate but decreased the Km towards $DMPH_4$ approximately 7-fold and slightly increased the measurable Vmax.

The objective of _in vitro_ assays has been to design a system which measures the total tyrosine hydroxylating capacity of the tissue. It is probable, however, that this total capacity is not normally used _in vivo_. This presumption is based on two considerations: first that the hydroxylating capacity is probably at least 5-6 fold greater than the estimated catecholamine turnover in most areas of brain (McGeer et al., 1967); and, second, that the probable concentrations of catecholamines in nerve endings are

sufficient to inhibit the enzyme partially and thus provide a
mechanism for the rapid regulation of catecholamine synthesis
(Spector et al., 1967; Gordon, Spector, and Sjoerdsma, 1967;
Reis, 1971). Hormonal control of tyrosine hydroxylase has also
been suggested, particularly by thyroid hormones (Harrison, 1964;
Prange, Meek, and Lipton, 1970; Emlen, Segal and Mandell, 1972), and
by ACTH (Kvetnansky et al., 1970), but the situation is still
unclear (McGeer and McGeer, 1972). Previous papers at this
Meeting have been concerned with the probability that a slower
(interneuronal feedback) mechanism of control also exists
involving adaptive changes in enzyme synthesis.

The fact that changes in rat caudate tyrosine hydroxylating
capacity are manifest after only two days of treatment with
certain drugs such as thioproperazine and methamphetamine (Fibiger
and McGeer, 1971; cf. Emlen et al., 1972) suggests that, if adaptive changes in synthesis are really involved, this enzyme system
probably has a relatively short half-life. This possibility
receives some support from the very rapid fall in caudate hydroxylating activity following axonal transection (Figure 3)(McGeer
et al., 1972), and from the demonstration of rapid and

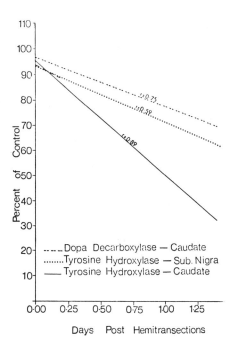

Figure 3. Lines of regression calculated from data on some enzyme
activities in rats 0, 3, 6, 12, 18, 24, 36, and 48 hours after a
hemitransection at the mid-hypothalamic level.

relatively massive axonal transport of protein along the dopaminergic nigral striatal tract. Only three hours after stereotaxic
injection of labelled leucine into the rat substantia nigra substantial amounts of labelled protein appear in the ipsilateral
striatum. The amount of such protein at 3 h - 30 days is more
than 3 times as much as found in the ipsilateral thalamus, which
is well known to receive projections from the nigra. Experiments
with 6-hydroxydopamine-treated rats indicate that most of the
nigral striatal flow is along catecholaminergic neurons (Fibiger
et al., 1972 a,b). These indications are by no means conclusive
and the enzymic half life, as well as the rate and mechanism of
synthesis and transport of newly formed tyrosine hydroxylase,
remain challenging problems for future research.

An interesting question relevant to control mechanisms is
raised by the reports of diurnal or ultradian variations in
catecholamine concentrations in various parts of brain (Scheving
et al., 1968; Graziani and Montanaro, 1967; Reis, Weinbren and
Corvell, 1968; Matussek and Patschke, 1963; Reis and Wurtman,
1968; Kanshardt and Wurtman, 1967), in the rate of norepinephrine
depletion following reserpine treatment (Black, Parker and Axelrod,
1969) and in the rate of in $vivo$ synthesis of ^{3}H-catecholamines
from circulating ^{3}H-tyrosine in some areas of brain (Zigmond and
Wurtman, 1970). These changes might be due to a diurnal rhythm
in release or catabolism rather than to a rhythm in synthesis
per se. Some years ago, however, we did in $vitro$ measurements
of the tyrosine hydroxylating system in sucrose homogenates of
the brains of rats sacrificed at different times of day. In 6 out
of 7 such series there was a significant difference between the
peak hydroxylating activity measured at 3 p.m. and the low measured
at 3 a.m. (Figure 4), but the magnitude of the effect varied
greatly from series to series and presumably involved unidentified
factors other than the duration of the light-dark cycle. The
rhythm for the in $vitro$ hydroxylating capacity indicated in
Figure 4 is in general accord with the data of Zigmond and Wurtman
(1970) who found that the accumulation of ^{3}H-catecholamines in
brain after administration of ^{3}H-tyrosine was twice as great in
the middle of the daily light period as in the middle of the dark
period. Since the in $vitro$ assays were all done with sucrose
homogenates and the non-fortified incubation medium (Condition A,
Table 3), these changes may reflect rhythmic variations in the
amount of particle-bound cofactor or in membrane characteristics
which affect either the measurable activity of the enzyme or the
uptake of tyrosine into the particles.

The tyrosine hydroxylating system also shows long-term variations. There is an appreciable fall of the activity of this system
with age in the striatum. This has been seen both with humans and
rats (McGeer et al., 1971). In humans, the measurements were all

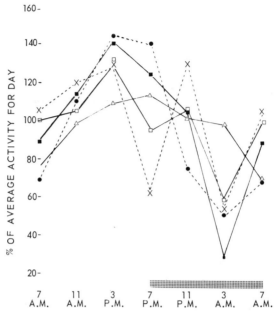

Figure 4. Apparent diurnal variation in tyrosine hydroxylase
activity of rat brain stem (dotted lines) or whole brains minus
cerebella (solid lines); the species of rat, season of year, and
p value for the difference between data for 3 a.m. and 3 p.m.
groups are listed below.

    x - - - -   Female, Brown; 12/66; p<0.01
    ● - - - -   Female, Wistar, 12/66 and 5/67 (2 series) p<0.05
    ■ ————   Female, Wistar, 5/67 and 6/67 (2 series) p<0.001
    □ ————   Female, Wistar, 2/67, p<0.001
    Δ ————   Female, Sprague-Dawley, 12/68-1/69, p<0.05

done both with and without added cofactor and the nigral as well as
the striatal tyrosine hydroxylating activities were measured.
Interestingly, no significant age effect was evident in the nigra.
The differences noted in the caudate could, therefore, reflect a
slow down of axonal transport and/or a drop-out of nerve endings
rather than a primary defect in enzyme synthesis. This "normal"
aging process for the striatal tyrosine hydroxylating system is
apparently quite different from the situation in Parkinsonian
cases where the data (Figure 5) would suggest a primary defect in
nigral enzyme synthesis. This is consistent with the known drop-
out of cells in this body in Parkinson's disease and the frequently
noted pallor of the substantia nigra.

We have tried to emphasize in this presentation some of the
practial and theoretical considerations involved in brain tyrosine
hydroxylase measurements. The finding that tyrosine hydroxylase is
produced in a soluble form in the cell body but is held in particles

in the nerve endings has now been paralleled by work on tryptophan
hydroxylase (Mandell and Knapp, 1972). It may be true of a number
of key enzymes for neurotransmitter synthesis. Assay systems need
to be designed to take into account these differing forms of the
enzymes. The fascinating evidence adduced by Kuczenski and Mandell
(1972) that the activity of synaptosomal tyrosine hydroxylase may
be altered by allosteric shifts suggests another possible mechanism
for both rapid control of catecholamine synthesis and drug action.
Cofactor and substrate availability must also be taken into consideration. Finally, it must be remembered that there is both
rapid synthesis of new protein and transport of that protein along
axons to nerve endings. Moreover, the sulfated mucopolysaccharides,
which cause allosteric shifts in synaptosomal tyrosine hydroxylase
(Kuczenski and Mandell, 1972), are also rapidly transported along
axons (Elam et al., 1970). The site of synthesis of various
materials important to enzymic activity may, therefore, be remote,
in neurons, from the site where activity is being measured. It is
important in designing experiments that the total aspects of the
catecholaminergic cell be considered.

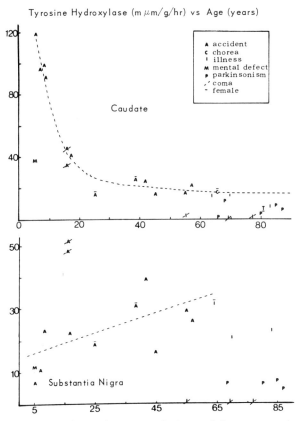

Figure 5. Tyrosine hydroxylase activity of human striatum and
substantia nigra as a function of age.

REFERENCES

Anden, N.E., Carlsson, A., Dahlstrom, A., Fuxe, K., Hillarp, N.A., Larsson, K. 1964. Demonstration and mapping out of nigrostriatal dopamine neurons. Life Sci. 3: 523.

Black, I.B., Parker, L., and Axelrod, J. 1969. A daily rhythm in the rate of depletion of brain NA by reserpine. Biochem. Pharmacol. 18: 2688.

Brenneman, A.R. and Kaufman, S. 1964. The role of tetrahydro-pteridines in the enzymatic conversion of tyrosine to 3,4-di-hydroxyphenylalanine. Biochem. Biophys. Res. Commun. 17: 177.

Cote, L.J. and Fahn, S. 1969. Some aspects of the biochemistry of the substantia nigra of the rhesus monkey. In: Progress in Neuro-Genetics (Ed. A. Barbeau and J.R. Brunette) Amsterdam: Excerpta Medica Foundation, p. 311.

Elam, J.S., Goldberg, J.M., Radin, N.S., and Agranoff, B.W. 1970. Rapid axonal transport of sulfated mucopolysaccharide proteins. Science 170:458.

Emlen, W., Segal, D.W., and Mandell, A.J. 1972. Thyroid state: effects on pre and postsynaptic central noradrenergic mechanisms. Science 175:79-82.

Fahn, S. and Cote, L. J. 1968. Regional and subcellular distribution of tyrosine hydroxylase. Neurology 18: 293.

Fahn, S., Rodman, J.S., and Cote, L.J. 1969. Association of tyro-sine hydroxylase with synaptic vesicles in bovine caudate. J. Neurochem. 16: 1293.

Fibiger, H.C. and McGeer, E.G. 1971. Effect of acute and chronic methamphetamine treatment on tyrosine hydroxylase activity in brain and adrenal medulla. Eur. J. Pharmacol. 16: 176.

Fibiger, H.C., Pudritz, R.E., McGeer, P.L., and McGeer, E.G. (1972a) Axonal transport in nigrostriatal neurons. Nature New Biology 237: 177.

Fibiger, H.C., Pudritz, R.E., McGeer, P.L., and McGeer, E.G. (1972b) Axonal transport in nigrostriatal and nigrothalamic neurons: Effects of medial forebrain bundle lesions and 6-hydroxydopa-mine. J. Neurochem. 19: 1697.

Gordon, R., Spector, S. and Sjoerdsma, A. 1967. Regulation of norepinephrine (NE) synthesis at the rate-limiting step by endogenous NE. Fed. Proc. 26: 463.

Graziani, G. and Montanaro, N. 1967. Variations of the cerebral concentration of noradrenaline in the albino rat during the day. Boll Soc. Ital. Sper. 43: 46.

Guroff, G., Rhoads, C.A., and Abramowitz, A. 1967. A simple radio-isotope assay for phenylalanine hydroxylase cofactor. Anal. Biochem. 21: 273.

Harrison, J.S. 1964. Adrenal medullary and thyroid relationships. Physiol. Rev. 44: 161.

Kaufman, S. 1963. The structure of the phenylalanine-hydroxylation cofactor. Proc. Natl. Acad. Sci. U.S.A. 50: 1085.

Kaufman, S. 1964. The role of pteridines in the enzymatic conversion
    of phenylalanine to tyrosine. Trans. N.Y. Acad. Sci. 26: 977.
Knapp, S. and Mandell, A.J. 1972. Some drug effects on the functions
    of the two physical forms of tryptophan-5-hydroxylase; influence
    on hydroxylation and uptake of substrate. In: Serotonin and
    Behavior (Ed: J. Barchus) U.S. Govt. Printing Office (in press).
Kuczenski, R.T. and Mandell, A.J. 1972. Allosteric activation of
    hypothalamic tyrosine hydroxylase by ions and sulphated muco-
    polysaccharides. J. Neurochem. 10: 131.
Kvetnansky, R., Gewirtz, G.P., Weiss, V.K., and Kopin, I.J. 1970.
    Effect of hypophysectomy on immobilization-induced elevation
    of tyrosine hydroxylase and phenylethanolamine-N-methyl trans-
    ferase in the rat adrenal. Endocrinology 87: 1323.
Mandell, A.J., Knapp, S., and Kuczenski, R.T. 1972. An amphetamine-
    induced shift in the subcellular distribution of caudate tyro-
    sine hydroxylase. In: Proc. 33rd Mtg. Drug Abuse Committee,
    Natl. Res. Council, Natl. Acad. Sci. U.S.A., pp. 742-766.
Manshardt, J., and Wurtman, R.J. 1967. Daily rhythm in the noradren-
    aline content of rat hypothalamus. Nature 217: 574.
Matussek, N. and Patschke, U. 1963. Beziehungen des Schlaf--und
    Wachrhythmus zum Noradrenalin--und Serotoningehalt im Zentral-
    nervensystem von Hamstern. Med. Exp. 11: 81.
McGeer, E.G., Gibson, S., and McGeer, P.L. (1967a) Some character-
    istics of brain tyrosine hydroxylase. Canad. J. Biochem. 45: 1557.
McGeer, E.G., Gibson, S., Wada, J., and McGeer, P.L. (1967b) Dis-
    tribution of tyrosine hydroxylase in adult and developing brain.
    Canad. J. Biochem. 45: 1943.
McGeer, E.G. and McGeer, P.L. 1967. In vitro screen of inhibitors
    of rat brain tyrosine hydroxylase. Canad. J. Biochem. 45: 115.
McGeer, E.G., Fibiger, H.C., McGeer, P.L., and Wickson, V. (1971a)
    Aging and brain amines. Exp. Gerontol. 6: 391.
McGeer, E.G., McGeer, P.L., and Wada, J.A. (1971b) Distribution of
    tyrosine hydroxylase in human and animal brain. J. Neurochem.
    18: 1647.
McGeer, E.G., Fibiger, H.C., McGeer, P.L., and Brooke, S. 1972
    Temporal changes in amine synthesizing enzymes of rat extra-
    pyramidal structures after hemitransections or 6-hydroxydopamine
    administration. Brain Research (in press).
McGeer, P.L., Bagchi, S.P., and McGeer, E.G. 1965. Subcellular local-
    ization of tyrosine hydroxylase in beef caudate nucleus.
    Life Sci. 4: 1859.
McGeer, P.L. and McGeer, E.G. 1972 Amino acid hydroxylase inhibi-
    tors. In: Metabolic Inhibitors New York: Academic Press
    Vol. IV (in press).
Musacchio, J.M., Craviso, G.L., and Wurzburger, R.J. 1972. Dihydro-
    pteridine reductase in the rat brain. Life Sci. 11-2: 267.
Nagatsu, T., Levitt, M., and Udenfriend, S. (1964a) Tyrosine hydroxy-
    lase. The initial step in norepinephrine biosynthesis. J. Biol.
    Chem. 239: 2910.

Nagatsu, T., Levitt, M., and Udenfriend, S. (1964b) A rapid and simple radioassay for tyrosine hydroxylase activity. Anal. Biochem. 9: 122.

Nagatsu, T. and Nagatsu, I. 1970. Subcellular distribution of tyrosine hydroxylase and monamine oxidase in the bovine caudate nucleus. Experientia 26: 722.

Poillon, W.N. 1971. Kinetic properties of brain tyrosine hydroxylase and its partial purification by affinity chromatography. Biochem. Biophys. Res. Commun. 44: 64.

Prange, A.J.,Jr., Meek, J.L., and Lipton, M.A. 1970. Catecholamines: Diminished rate of synthesis in rat brain and heart after thyroxine pretreatment. Life Sci. 9-2: 901.

Reis, D.J. and Wurtman, R.J. (1968) A circadian rhythm of norepinephrine regionally in cat brain: its relationship to environmental lighting and to regional diurnal variation in brain serotonin. Life Sci. 7: 91.

Reis, D. 1971. Fourth Annual Winter Conference on Brain Research, January 16-22.

Scheving, L.E., Harrison, W.H., Gordon, P., and Pauly, J.E. 1968. Daily fluctuation (circadian and ultradian) in biogenic amines in the rat brain. Am. J. Physiol. 214: 166.

Spector, S., Gordon, R., Sjoerdsma, A., and Udenfriend, S. 1967. End product inhibition of tyrosine hydroxylase as a possible mechanism for regulation of norepinephrine synthesis. Mol. Pharmacol. 3: 549.

Zigmond, M.J. and Wurtman, R. J. 1970. Daily rhythm in the accumulation of brain catecholamines synthesized from circulating ^{3}H-tyrosine. J. Pharmacol. Exptl. Therap. 172: 416.

TYROSINE HYDROXYLASE: SUBCELLULAR DISTRIBUTION AND MOLECULAR AND KINETIC CHARACTERISTICS OF THE DIFFERENT ENZYME FORMS

José M. Musacchio, Charlene A. McQueen and
Gale L. Craviso

Department of Pharmacology, New York University
School of Medicine, 550 First Ave., New York, N.Y.

Tyrosine hydroxylase (E.C. 1.10.3.1) catalyzes the first step in catecholamine biosynthesis, the conversion of tyrosine to dopa. Since this is considered the rate-limiting step in catecholamine biosynthesis (Levitt et al., 1965) this reaction is the most likely one to be regulated. The hydroxylation of tyrosine to dopa is quite complex and it is not known which of its components is actually the limiting factor in the overall reaction. There is, however, general agreement that one of the most important factors which regulate tyrosine hydroxylase activity is feedback inhibition by catecholamines. Therefore, in order to fully understand the regulation of catecholamine synthesis, it is necessary to know the subcellular distribution of tyrosine hydroxylase and the kinetic characteristics of this enzyme. Obviously, the catecholamine pool that modulates tyrosine hydroxylase activity has to be in contact with the enzyme, and the localization of the enzyme will indicate which catecholamine pool regulates catecholamine synthesis. The localization of tyrosine hydroxylase has more than academic importance because it will allow us to understand the mechanism of action of certain drugs which indirectly modify catecholamine biosynthesis.

In this article, we will review some of the aspects of the subcellular distribution of tyrosine hydroxylase and the effect of the different purification procedures on the molecular weight of the enzyme. We will also examine the kinetic characteristics of the different forms of the enzyme.

Subcellular distribution of tyrosine hydroxylase. Tyrosine hydroxylase was isolated from the brain and adrenal medulla by Nagatsu et al. (1964 a,b); the enzyme was described as particle bound and the fraction found in the supernatant was considered to have been solubilized by prolonged homogenization. We investigated the subcellular distribution of the enzyme in the rat adrenal gland and found that practically all of the enzyme was soluble (Musacchio, 1967). Since it is quite unlikely that there would be species differences in the distribution of a regulatory enzyme in a highly organized organ such as the adrenal gland, we decided to reinvestigate the problem using techniques specifically designed for subcellular fractionation. Adrenal medullae were homogenized in different buffers with a glass homogenizer or they were disrupted with a tissue press. The distribution of the enzyme was then studied in different sucrose density gradients. The results clearly indicated that the enzyme is not associated with the catecholamine storage granules and that the majority of tyrosine hydroxylase is found in the supernatant fraction (Figure 1). Particular attention was devoted to the probable existence of structure-linked enzyme latency in the chromaffin granules.

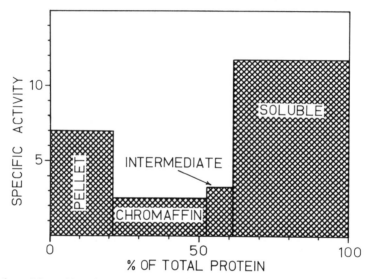

Figure 1. Distribution pattern of tyrosine hydroxylase in fractions obtained from a sucrose density gradient. Fresh adrenal medullae were homogenized in 5 vol isotonic KCl, 0.005 M Tris-Cl, pH 6.7 and the total homogenate, without any previous centrifugation, was layered on a 0.4-2.0 M discontinuous sucrose density gradient. The pellet formed at the bottom of the tube was resuspended and processed as the other fractions. Tyrosine hydroxylase activity was determined by a modification of the method of Nagatsu et al. (1964c) as described by Wurzburger and Musacchio (1971). Ordinate represents the specific activity of tyrosine hydroxylase measured as nmoles of tritiated water produced in 10 min per mg of protein. Abscissa represents the percentage of total recovered proteins. (From Wurzburger and Musacchio, 1971).

Several methods were used to disrupt subcellular particles, such as osmotic shock, dialysis against hypotonic buffers, treatment with a detergent and tryptic digestion. All these procedures failed to disclose any hidden stores of tyrosine hydroxylase (Musacchio, 1968; Wurzburger and Musacchio, 1971).

The composition of the buffer used in the homogenization of the adrenal medulla has a marked effect on the distribution of tyrosine hydroxylase between the coarse fraction of nuclei and cell debris and the low speed supernatant fraction. When the adrenal glands were homogenized in isotonic KCl, 13% of the tyrosine hydroxylase activity was found in the 700 x g sediment as compared with 36% when the glands were homogenized in isotonic sucrose (Wurzburger and Musacchio, 1971). The adsorption of tyrosine hydroxylase to coarse particles may explain why the enzyme was originally described as particle-bound. In addition to the adsorption to several subcellular particles, tyrosine hydroxylase aggregates to other macromolecules; soluble enzyme contained in the 100,000 x g supernatant fraction can be sedimented by centrifugation after fractionation with ammonium sulfate, gel filtration or just upon standing (Wurzburger and Musacchio, 1971).

Our results strongly suggest that adrenal tyrosine hydroxylase is a soluble enzyme which is not contained in the chromaffin granules (Musacchio, 1967 and 1968; Wurzburger and Musacchio, 1971). Independently, Laduron and Belpaire (1968) and more recently, Weiner et al. (1971) also concluded that the enzyme is localized in the high-speed supernatant fraction. Several reports also indicated that in sympathetic nerves tyrosine hydroxylase is almost exclusively localized in the high speed supernatant fraction (Stjarne and Lishajko, 1967).

The subcellular distribution of brain tyrosine hydroxylase is not as clearly defined as in other organs. A considerable fraction of rat brain tyrosine hydroxylase (60%) is contained in the synaptosomal fraction. When the synaptosomes are lysed with hypotonic shock, only 18% of the enzyme sediments at 100,000 x g (Coyle, 1972). Kuczenski and Mandell (1972 a) have studied the subcellular distribution of tyrosine hydroxylase in different regions of the brain and found that the enzyme isolated from the midbrain is localized mainly in the soluble fraction of the homogenate; in contrast, striatum tyrosine hydroxylase is found mainly in the synaptosomal fraction. Between 60 to 70% of the enzyme contained in the synaptosomes can be solubilized by hypotonic shock, while the rest remains bound to synaptosomal membranes (Kuczenski and Mandell, 1972 a). The fraction of tyrosine hydroxylase which remains adsorbed to synaptosomal membranes can not be resuspended by repeated washing; in this respect, the striatal enzyme is similar to the aggregated enzyme obtained from

the high-speed adrenal gland supernatant and to the adrenal enzyme
which is adsorbed onto subcellular particles. All these studies
strongly suggest that tyrosine hydroxylase has a similar intracellular distribution in all the tissues; the apparent differences
in the distribution of the enzyme are most likely related to the
existence of other macromolecules, membrane-bound or not, to
which tyrosine hydroxylase aggregates. We have previously stated
that: "The characteristic of tyrosine hydroxylase to aggregate
to other molecules under certain conditions and to adsorb to some
cellular organelles, may be a reflection of a basic characteristic
of the enzyme. The biologic significance of this property is,
for the moment, elusive, but it is conceivable that the enzyme
binds in vivo to membranes of cell organelles or forms macromolecular aggregates with other enzymes involved in catecholamine
biosynthesis, such as dihydropteridine reductase or dopa decarboxylase" (Wurzburger and Musacchio, 1971).

The location of tyrosine hydroxylase in the cytoplasm is
consistent with the pharmacological evidence which indicates that
there is a small cytoplasmic pool of catecholamines which, by
feedback inhibition, is an important regulatory factor for catecholamine biosynthesis (Alousi and Weiner, 1966); this view has been
supported by a considerable number of investigators (Weiner and
Selvaratnam, 1968; Kopin et al., 1969; Goldstein et al., 1970).
In a series of experiments performed in Dr. Glowinski's laboratory
(Besson et al., 1972; Musacchio, 1971), we found that thioproperazine and reserpine administered in vivo change the rate of catecholamine synthesis in rat caudate slices in vitro. As expected,
reserpine inhibits the hydroxylation of tyrosine to dopa, presumably by increasing the concentration of cytoplasmic catecholamines,
while thioproperazine increases catecholamine synthesis, presumably
by a physiological feedback which increases the rate of neuronal
firing. These changes occur without changes in the tissue content
of tyrosine hydroxylase assayed after cell disruption and partial
purification.

Different molecular forms of bovine adrenal tyrosine hydroxylase. In an effort to purify tyrosine hydroxylase, Petrack
et al. (1968) have solubilized, by trypsin digestion, the crude
adrenal enzyme fraction which sediments upon centrifugation. Since
the hydrolysis of peptide bonds could produce modifications in the
tyrosine hydroxylase molecule, we decided to study some of the
molecular parameters of the native and trypsin-treated enzyme.
The sedimentation coefficients of the different forms of tyrosine
hydroxylase were determined by sucrose density gradient centrifugation. The native form of tyrosine hydroxylase was found to have a
sedimentation coefficient of 9.20 S; that of trypsin-treated
tyrosine hydroxylase was only 3.45 S. The possibility that the
enzyme fragments obtained after trypsin digestion may be able to

reassociate was tested by incubating the enzyme with all and with different combinations of the substrates and stimulators used to detect enzyme activity; the sedimentation characteristics of the trypsin-treated enzyme, however, were not changed (Musacchio et al., 1971). Similar results have recently been obtained by Petrack et al. (1972 a). The failure to reconstitute the native enzyme was expected since the effects of trypsin on the enzyme are most likely due to the hydrolysis of peptide bonds.

An estimation of the molecular weight of the different forms of tyrosine hydroxylase can be obtained from their sedimentation coefficients. This procedure, however, requires several assumptions which introduce some errors into the calculations (Martin and Ames, 1961). A more accurate determination of the molecular weight can be obtained if, in addition to the sedimentation co-efficient, the Stokes radius of the protein is used in the calculations (Ackers, 1964). The Stokes radius of the trypsin-treated tyrosine hydroxylase was measured according to the method of Ackers (1964). The molecular weight of the trypsin-treated enzyme calculated from the sedimentation coefficient and the Stokes radius is 34,000 (Musacchio et al., 1971). The radius of the native form of the enzyme could not be measured due to aggregation during gel filtration, but all other measurements indicate that the native enzyme is about 4.4 fold larger than the trypsin-treated form; therefore, the molecular weight of the native enzyme can be estimated to be approximately 150,000. All these results indicate that the trypsin-treated enzyme is only a fragment of the native form; with the information available, however, it is not possible to establish whether the trypsin-produced fragments are equivalent to enzyme subunits. The questions about the number and nature (catalytic vs. regulatory) of the subunits of the native enzyme will remain unanswered until the enzyme is purified and appropriate experiments performed.

Kinetic studies on different forms of tyrosine hydroxylase. In view of the large difference in the molecular weight of both forms of tyrosine hydroxylase, it is reasonable to expect that they will have different kinetic characteristics. In attempting to determine the kinetic mechanism of an enzyme, three types of studies can be performed: initial velocity studies, determination of inhibition patterns and isotope exchange (Cleland, 1967). We are presenting in this paper results obtained by the first method; the study of the inhibition patterns has been delayed by technical difficulties.

Experiments were planned according to Cleland's method for three substrate systems: one substrate is varied at several fixed levels of the second, while the third substrate is held constant (Cleland, 1970). It was found that high tyrosine concentrations

were inhibitory and caused the double reciprocal plots to become
less convergent. Substrate concentrations were adjusted to avoid
inhibition.

Initial velocity studies were performed with both the native
and the trypsin-treated forms of tyrosine hydroxylase. The
following results were obtained with the native form: when
tyrosine was plotted as the variable substrate of the double
reciprocal plot, intersecting patterns resulted. The same
patterns were obtained whether $DMPH_4$ or oxygen was held at several
fixed levels (Figure 2A). Intersecting patterns also resulted
when $DMPH_4$ was plotted as the varied substrate with either oxygen
(Figure 2B) or tyrosine (Figure 2C) held at several fixed levels.

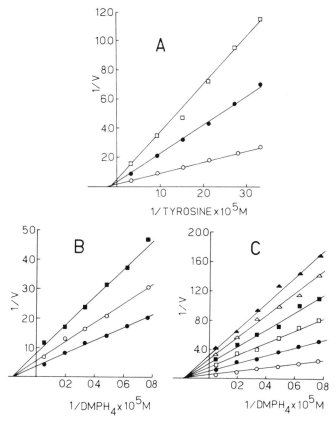

Figure 2A. Double reciprocal plot of tyrosine concentration against
the activity of native tyrosine hydroxylase in the presence of
several oxygen concentrations. The incubation mixture contained
0.2 M sodium acetate buffer, pH 6.0; 500 μM ferrous ammonium sulfate;
0.1 M 2-mercaptoethanol; native tyrosine hydroxylase; 3,5-H^3-L-

tyrosine, 3.0 to 30.0 μM; 200 μM $DMPH_4$ and water to 1 ml. Oxygen concentrations were 2.5% (□), 5.0% (●) and 20.0% (0).

All components, except $DMPH_4$ (dissolved in mercaptoethanol) and tyrosine, were added to incubation tubes kept in ice. These tubes, as well as those containing $DMPH_4$ and tyrosine, were gassed for 15 min with the desired oxygen concentration. After gassing, the reaction tubes were preincubated with $DMPH_4$ for 3 min at 25°C. The reaction was started with the addition of tyrosine and was carried out for 6 min at 25°C; 0.1 ml of 30% trichloroacetic acid was used to stop the reaction. Velocity was determined by measuring the amount of tritiated water released during the reaction and expressed as nmoles of product in 6 min.

Figure 2B. Double reciprocal plot of $DMPH_4$ concentration against the activity of native tyrosine hydroxylase in the presence of several oxygen concentrations. Assay as described for Figure 2A. $DMPH_4$ concentrations were 13–200 μM while tyrosine was held constant at 30 μM. Oxygen concentrations were 5.0% (▪), 10.0% (0) and 20.0% (●).

Figure 2C. Double reciprocal plot of $DMPH_4$ concentration against the activity of native tyrosine hydroxylase in the presence of several tyrosine concentrations. Assay as described for Figure 2A; incubation tubes were not gassed since atmospheric oxygen (20%) was used for all samples. $DMPH_4$ concentrations were 13–200 μM; tyrosine concentrations were 3.00 (▲), 3.66 (△), 4.69 (▪), 6.52 (□), 10.70 (●), and 30.00 (0) M. (From McQueen, 1972).

If, however, oxygen was taken as the variable substrate, the lines obtained were curved, concave downward. These curved patterns were obtained both at several different fixed concentrations of $DMPH_4$ and tyrosine.

When identical experiments were run using the trypsin-treated tyrosine hydroxylase, linear intersecting double reciprocal plots were obtained for all substrates, including oxygen. In order to rule out the possibility that the different patterns between the native and the trypsin-treated tyrosine hydroxylase may have resulted from artifacts due to the gassing of the samples, several experiments were conducted in which both forms of the enzyme were gassed at the same time and with the same gas mixture; one such experiment is shown in Figure 3.

The Michaelis constants (Km) of both enzyme forms were determined for each substrate (Table 1). The constant for $DMPH_4$ was about the same for both the native and the trypsin-treated enzyme; however, there were differences in the values obtained for tyrosine

TABLE 1

MICHAELIS CONSTANTS FOR THE SUBSTRATES OF NATIVE AND TRYPSIN-TREATED TYROSINE HYDROXYLASE

Substrate	Native Enzyme	Exp.[a]	Trypsin-Treated Enzyme	Exp.	S.S.[b]
DMPH$_4$	5.65×10^{-5}M (± 0.15)[c]	4	6.24×10^{-5}M (± 0.42)	4	NS[d]
Tyrosine	4.76×10^{-5}M (± 0.24)	3	2.38×10^{-5}M (± 0.08)	3	P< 0.01
Oxygen	12.33%[e] (± 1.53) 1.50×10^{-4}M (± 0.19)	3	4.20% (± 0.29) 5.12×10^{-5}M (± 0.35)	5	P< 0.01

The values given are the average of 3 to 5 experiments, as those described for Figure 2, and were calculated by determining the reciprocal of the Km directly from the double reciprocal plot (from McQueen, 1972).

[a] number of experiments
[b] statistical significance
[c] standard error of the mean

[d] not significant
[e] value obtained by extrapolation from curved plots as explained

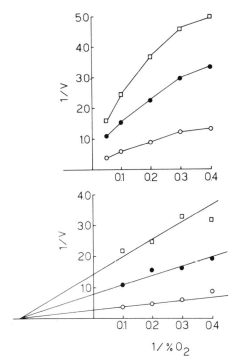

Figure 3. Double reciprocal plots of oxygen concentration against the initial velocity of native tyrosine hydroxylase (top) and trypsin-treated tyrosine hydroxylase (bottom). Assay as described for Figure 2A. Oxygen concentrations were 2.5%, 3.3%, 5.0%, 10.0% and 20.0% while tyrosine was held constant at 30 µM. DMPH$_4$ concentrations were 16.0 (□), 29.7 (●), and 200.0 (0) µM.

and for oxygen. The Km of tyrosine with the native form was almost twice that with the trypsin-treated form. In attempting to determine the constant for oxygen of the native enzyme form, it was necessary to extrapolate from the curved plots. The extrapolations were made and all the lines converged at a common point on the X-axis, giving a common value for the Michaelis constant, when either tyrosine or DMPH4 was held at several fixed levels. When the values for the two enzyme forms were compared, that of the native form was about three times that for the trypsin-treated form.

All of the initial velocity double reciprocal plots of both forms of tyrosine hydroxylase were intersecting; intersecting patterns can only be obtained in a sequential mechanism or in a ping-pong mechanism in the presence of fixed levels of product

(Cleland, 1970). Since product was not added to the initial
velocity experiments, the intersecting patterns are indicative of
a sequential mechanism. Ikeda et al. (1966), using the native
form of the enzyme, proposed a ping-pong mechanism for tyrosine
hydroxylase. On the other hand, Joh et al. (1969), using the
trypsin-treated tyrosine hydroxylase, indicated that the mechanism
is sequential. Our studies on both enzyme forms indicate that the
mechanism most likely is sequential for both enzyme forms
(McQueen, 1972).

Inhibition studies can be used to determine the order of
addition of substrates to an enzyme and they are obviously essential
to understand its regulatory properties. Native tyrosine hydroxylase
is inhibited by catecholamines and by dopa; this inhibition is
competitive with the artificial cofactor $DMPH_4$ (Udenfriend et al.
1965; Ikeda et al., 1966) and also with tetrahydrobiopterin
(Musacchio et al., 1971; Nagatsu et al., 1972). The inhibition
produced by α-methyl-L-tyrosine is competitive with tyrosine
(Nagatsu et al., 1964 b) and non-competitive with $DMPH_4$. Similar
patterns of inhibition are observed with the trypsin-treated form
of the enzyme (McQueen, 1972).

The relative effectiveness of dopamine, norepinephrine and
epinephrine to inhibit native tyrosine hydroxylase was measured.
The Ki for dopamine was found to be 2.1×10^{-5} M and the Ki for
norepinephrine and epinephrine was 4.6×10^{-5} M; this implies that
dopamine is twice as effective as a feedback inhibitor of tyrosine
hydroxylase than either norepinephrine or epinephrine. Since
dopamine is formed in the cytosol, it is tempting to speculate that
dopamine may be the amine that actually regulates catecholamine
synthesis.

In attempting to interpret the curved plots obtained with
oxygen, several possibilities can be considered. A possible
explanation for this type of curvature in a double reciprocal
plot is negative cooperativity (Cleland, 1970; Levitzki and
Koshland, 1969). Since such curved plots can be caused by several
other factors, a concave downward deviation is an indication rather
than a proof of negative cooperativity (Levitzki and Koshland,
1969). However, the fact that the concave downward deviation is
obtained only with the native enzyme and not with the trypsin-
treated form is consistent with the idea that native tyrosine
hydroxylase might be an allosteric enzyme (McQueen, 1972). The
four fold difference in the molecular weight between the two
enzyme forms would be consistent with a native enzyme made of
four subunits whose binding sites are destroyed by the trypsin
treatment. Obviously, further studies are necessary to fully
characterize the structure and kinetics of tyrosine hydroxylase.
The limiting factor in all these studies is the unavailability

of pure native enzyme.

Additional differences between native and trypsin-treated tyrosine hydroxylase can be demonstrated by studying the effects of Fe^{2+} on the enzyme activity. Adrenal tyrosine hydroxylase (Nagatsu et al., 1964 b) and the trypsin-digested enzyme (Petrack et al., 1968) are known to be stimulated by Fe^{2+}. The effect of different concentrations of iron on both enzymes is illustrated in Figure 4. It can be seen that only small concentrations of iron are necessary to stimulate the native enzyme and that inhibition results when the concentrations are increased. On the other

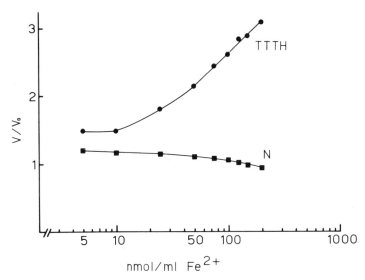

Figure 4. Effect of Fe^{2+} concentrations on the activity of native tyrosine hydroxylase (N) and trypsin-treated tyrosine hydroxylase (TTTH). The incubation mixture contained 0.11 M Tris acetate buffer to give a final pH of 6.1; 30 µM tyrosine-3,5-^{3}H; 200 µM DMPH4; 0.1 M 2-mercaptoethanol, 5-200 µM ferrous ammonium sulphate, water and enzyme in a final volume of 0.1 ml.
    All components, except DMPH4 (dissolved in mercaptoethanol) and tyrosine, were added to incubation tubes kept in ice. The samples were preincubated with DMPH$_4$ for 5 min at 37°C. The reaction was started with the addition of tyrosine and carried out for 6 min at 37°C. 0.4 ml of 3% trichloracetic acid was used to stop the reaction. Product was determined by measuring the amount of tritiated water released during the reaction and expressed as nmoles of product in 6 min. Ordinate represents the ratio between samples containing Fe^{2+} (V) and the corresponding control sample without Fe^{2+} (Vo).

hand, the trypsin-treated enzyme is stimulated several fold by
high concentrations of iron. This effect is unrelated to the
capacity of iron to destroy H_2O_2 since essentially the same results
are obtained in the presence of 2,000 units of catalase per ml.
In addition, there is only negligible catalase activity in the
ammonium sulfate fraction of native tyrosine hydroxylase. These
results are in contradiction with the results of Shiman et al. (1971)
who described that catalase can replace the need for iron in the
α-chymotrypsin digested enzyme. Petrack et al. (1972 a,b) have
described that, in addition to the catalase-like effect of iron,
this metal produces a marked stimulation of tyrosine hydroxylase
upon preincubation of the enzyme. It is possible, therefore, that
trypsin digestion either partially removes or oxidizes the Fe^{2+}
of tyrosine hydroxylase while α-chymotrypsin digestion does not.
This will be consistent with the inhibitory effect of iron chelating
agents on tyrosine hydroxylase (Nagatsu et al., 1964 b; Ellenbogen
et al., 1965).

It has recently been described by Kuczenski and Mandell (1972 a,
b) that ions and sulfated mucopolysaccharides stimulate the fraction of brain tyrosine hydroxylase found in the high speed supernatant. As illustrated in Figure 5, we have been able to confirm
these results. These authors reported that heparin activates

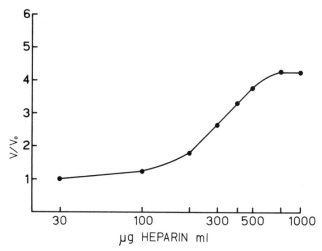

Figure 5. Effect of heparin on soluble rat brain tyrosine hydroxylase. Soluble rat brain tyrosine hydroxylase was prepared
by the method of Kuczenski and Mandell (1972 a). Assay as described
for Figure 4. The concentration of ferrous ammonium sulfate was
87.5 μM; heparin concentrations were 30-1000 μg/ml. Ordinate
represents the ratio between samples containing heparin (V) and
the control sample without heparin (Vo).

tyrosine hydroxylase by increasing the Vmax and the affinity of the enzyme for the synthetic cofactor, DMPH4, by nearly one order of magnitude. According to the same authors, the activation is allosteric in nature and the Hill plot yields a value of n_H near two. In contrast to the soluble enzyme, the membrane bound tyrosine hydroxylase is not activated by heparin and its Km for DMPH4 is similar to the Km of the soluble enzyme after heparin activation. Kuczenski and Mandell (1972 a,b) suggest that the effect of heparin on tyrosine hydroxylase in vitro may reflect an in vivo membrane-binding phenomenon which is involved in the regulation of this enzyme.

In view of these reports, we decided to test the effects of heparin on native and trypsin-treated tyrosine hydroxylase in an effort to further differentiate both enzyme forms. The results are shown in Figure 6 and they clearly indicate that native adrenal and brain tyrosine hydroxylase are stimulated by heparin and sulfate ions, while the trypsin-treated adrenal tyrosine hydroxylase is not. Similar results have been obtained by Kuczenski and Mandell (1972 c) using the native and the trypsin-treated rat brain enzyme.

In the course of the experiments with heparin and the native brain enzyme, we found that when low concentrations of DMPH4 are used, tyrosine hydroxylase is activated, but there are no changes in the Km for the cofactor; on the other hand, when high concentrations of DMPH4 are used, there is a change in the cofactor Km as described by Kuczenski and Mandell (1972 a,b). It is interesting to note that the Km for DMPH4 obtained in the presence of heparin and high pteridine concentrations is similar to the Km obtained when low pteridine concentrations are used (Figure 7). As shown in Figure 7 and Table 2, the apparent Km for DMPH4 of rat brain tyrosine hydroxylase does change when the concentration of the pteridine cofactor is increased. These changes are characteristic of a tyrosine hydroxylase preparation obtained from the whole brain excluding the brain cortex and the cerebellum. When tyrosine hydroxylase is prepared from carefully dissected caudate nuclei, this phenomenon is not observed. The caudate nucleus enzyme is actually inhibited by concentrations of DMPH4 higher than 200 µM, as indicated by a sharp upward deflection of the double reciprocal plots. The inhibition produced by high concentrations of DMPH4 cannot be overcome by heparin, but heparin produces a marked stimulation in the samples which contain non-inhibitory concentrations of the pteridine cofactor. In some experiments heparin decreases the Km for DMPH4 of caudate tyrosine hydroxylase by a factor of about three.

The concentration of heparin required for maximal stimulation of the different enzyme preparations is variable. Our preparation of brain (minus cortex and cerebellum) enzyme requires at least

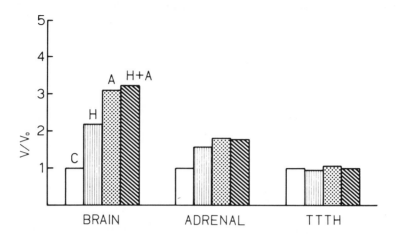

Figure 6. Effect of heparin and sulfate ions on native adrenal and brain tyrosine hydroxylase and on trypsin-treated tyrosine hydroxylase (TTTH). Assays were carried out using the procedure of Kuczenski and Mandell (1972 a). The incubation mixture contained 0.11 M Tris acetate buffer to give a final pH of 6.1; 15 μM tyrosine-3,5-^{3}H; 221 μM DMPH$_4$; 0.05 M 2-mercaptoethanol; 435 μM ferrous ammonium sulfate; water and enzyme to a final volume of 0.1 ml. The concentration of heparin was 300 μg/ml and that of ammonium sulfate was 0.2 M, pH 6.1. All components of the assay were added to tubes kept in ice. The reaction was started by placing each sample in a 37°C water bath. The incubation was carried out for 20 min at 37°C and the reaction was stopped with the addition of 0.4 ml 3% trichloroacetic acid. Product was determined by measuring the amount of tritiated water released during the reaction and expressed as nmoles of product in 20 min. Ordinate represents the ratio between samples containing heparin, ammonium sulfate or both (V) and the corresponding control sample (Vo). C-enzyme alone; H-enzyme with heparin; A-enzyme with ammonium sulfate; H + A-enzyme with heparin and ammonium sulfate.

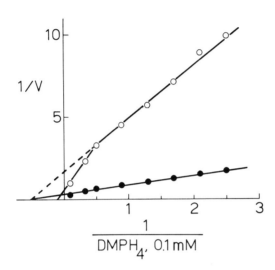

Figure 7. Double reciprocal plot of DMPH$_4$ concentration against the activity of rat brain tyrosine hydroxylase in the presence and absence of heparin. Soluble rat brain tyrosine hydroxylase was assayed as described for Figure 4. DMPH$_4$ concentrations were 40-1000 μM; the concentration of heparin was 1000 μg/ml. Ferrous ammonium sulfate was not included in the assay. Product was determined by measuring the amount of tritiated water released during the reaction and expressed as nmoles of product in 6 min.

TABLE 2

CHANGES IN $DMPH_4$ Km OF RAT BRAIN TYROSINE HYDROXYLASE

$DMPH_4$ μM	Fe^{2+} M	Control Km x 10^{-4}M	Heparin Km x 10^{-4}M	
13-200	--	2.2	2.2	(300 μg)
"	87.5	2.2	2.2	"
"	--	1.8	1.4	(1000 μg)
"	87.5	2.2	2.0	"
"	435	1.5	1.25	"
100-1000	435	5.0	1.47	"
"	--	9.5	2.6	"

Soluble rat brain tyrosine hydroxylase was assayed as described for Figure 4. Concentrations of $DMPH_4$, Fe^{2+} (ferrous ammonium sulfate) and heparin as indicated in the Table.

300 μg of heparin per ml while the caudate enzyme requires only 80 μg/ml and is inhibited at higher concentrations of heparin.

It is not possible to assess at the present time the significance of the changes in the tyrosine hydroxylase Km for $DMPH_4$ produced by varying the concentration of the pteridine cofactor or by adding heparin. The enzyme fractions used in these experiments are rather crude, even though they have been partially purified by ammonium sulfate fractionation. This is particularly true for the tyrosine hydroxylase prepared from the whole brain after the exclusion of the cortex and the cerebellum. It is pertinent to remember here that protein binding in such crude systems may change the actual concentration of substrates, activators and inhibitors. It is conceivable that the binding capacity of different proteins may be altered by the addition of heparin or salts. We have recently observed that the incubation mixtures of brain tyrosine hydroxylase become turbid during the incubation and even during the preincubation period; the addition of heparin prevents, to a certain degree, the development of this turbidity. Whether or not this phenomenon is related to the stimulatory effects of heparin is not known at the present time.

SUMMARY

1. The evidence which indicates that tyrosine hydroxylse is
located in the cell cytoplasm has been reviewed. These findings
support the hypothesis that there is a cytoplasmic pool of catecholamines which, by feedback control of tyrosine hydroxylase,
adjusts catecholamine biosynthesis to rapid changes in physiological
demands.

2. Some of the physical characteristics of the different molecular
forms of adrenal tyrosine hydroxylase have also been reviewed.
Adrenal tyrosine hydroxylase subjected to trypsin digestion has
a molecular weight of 34,000; the native form of the enzyme is
about 4.4 fold larger.

3. The different molecular forms of tyrosine hydroxylase have
some different kinetic characteristics. The native enzyme has
a Km for tyrosine about two-fold and for oxygen about three-fold
larger than the Km's of the trypsin-treated enzyme. The double
reciprocal plots of the native enzyme in which oxygen was the
variable substrate are curved downward; this suggests that tyrosine
hydroxylase is an allosteric enzyme.

4. All the initial velocity double reciprocal plots of tyrosine
hydroxylase are intersecting in the absence of added products,
indicating a sequential rather than a ping-pong mechanism.

5. Ferrous ion stimulates both forms of tyrosine hydroxylase,
but the stimulation of the trypsin-treated form is much larger
than the stimulation of the native form. This stimulation of
both enzyme forms is independent of the catalase-like action of
ferrous ions.

6. We have confirmed the findings of Kuczenski and Mandell that
heparin has a stimulatory effect on native brain and adrenal
tyrosine hydroxylases. However, we have found that the stimulation may occur without a concomitant decrease in the Km for DMPH4.
In contrast, trypsin-treated tyrosine hydroxylase is not stimulated by heparin. These findings suggest, but do not demonstrate,
that the native form of tyrosine hydroxylase is an allosteric
enzyme.

ACKNOWLEDGEMENTS

This work was supported by grant AM HE 13128 and in part by
grant GM 01447 from the National Institute of Health. Jose M.
Musacchio is a Research Scientist Awardee of the Public Health
Service grant 5-K2-MH-17,885.

REFERENCES

Ackers, G.K. 1964. Molecular exclusion and restricted diffusion
    processes in molecular-sieve chromatography. Biochemistry
    3: 723.
Alousi, A. and Weiner, N. 1966. The regulation of norepinephrine
    synthesis in sympathetic nerves: effect of nerve stimulation,
    cocaine and catecholamine-releasing agents. Proc. Nat. Acad.
    Sci. USA 56: 1491.
Besson, M.J., Cheramy, A., Gauchy, C. and Musacchio, J.M. 1972.
    Effect of some psychotropic drugs on tyrsoine hydroxylase
    activity in different structures of the rat brain. Eur. J.
    Pharmacol. (in press).
Cleland, W.W. 1967. Enzyme kinetics. Ann. Rev. Biochem. 36: 77.
Cleland, W.W. 1970. Steady state kinetics. In: The Enzymes,
    (Ed. Boyer, P.) New York: Academic Press, Vol. II, pp. 1.
Coyle, J.T. 1972. Tyrosine hydroxylase in the rat brain - co-
    factor requirements, regional and subcellular distribution.
    Biochem. Pharmacol. 21: 1935.
Ellenbogen, L., Taylor, R.J., Jr. and Brundage, G.B. 1965. On
    the role of pteridines as cofactors for tyrosine hydroxylase.
    Biochem. Biophys. Res. Commun. 19: 708.
Goldstein, M., Ohi, Y. and Backstrom, T. 1970. The effect of
    ouabain on catecholamine biosynthesis in rat brain cortex
    slices. J. Pharmacol. Exp. Ther. 174: 77.
Ikeda, M., Fahien, L.A. and Udenfriend, S. 1966. A kinetic
    study of bovine adrenal tyrosine hydroxylase. J. Biol. Chem.
    241: 4452.
Joh, T.H., Kapit, R. and Goldstein, M. 1969. A kinetic study of
    particulate bovine adrenal tyrosine hydroxylase. Biochem.
    Biophys. Acta 171: 378.
Kopin, I.J., Weise, V.K. and Sedvall, G.C. 1969. Effect of false
    transmitters on norepinephrine synthesis. J. Pharmacol.
    Exp. Ther. 170: 246.
Kuczenski, R.T. and Mandell, A.J. 1972 a. Regulatory properties
    of soluble and particulate rat brain tyrosine hydroxylase.
    J. Biol. Chem. 247: 3114.
Kuczenski, R.T. and Mandell, A.J. 1972 b. Allosteric activation
    of hypothalmic tyrosine hydroxylase by ions and sulfated
    mucopolysaccharides. J. Neurochem. 19: 131.
Kuczenski, R.T. and Mandell, A.J. 1972 c. Brain tyrosine
    hydroxylase: Activation by trypsin incubation. Proc. Nat.
    Acad. Sci. USA (in press).
Laduron, P. and Belpaire, F. 1968. Tissue fractionation and
    catecholamines-II. Biochem. Pharmacol. 17: 1127.
Levitt, M., Spector, S., Sjoerdsma, A. and Udenfriend, S. 1965.
    Elucidation of the rate-limiting step in norepinephrine bio-
    synthesis in the perfused guinea-pig heart. J. Pharmacol.
    Exp. Ther. 148: 1.

Levitzki, A. and Koshland, D.E., Jr. (1969). Negative cooperativity
    in regulatory enzymes. Proc. Nat. Acad. Sci. USA 69: 1121.
Martin, R.G. and Ames, B.N. 1961. A method for determining the
    sedimentation behavior of enzymes: Application to protein
    mixtures. J. Biol. Chem. 236: 1372.
McQueen, C.A. 1972. A kinetic study of the molecular forms of
    bovine adrenal tyrosine hydroxylase. M.S. Thesis, New
    York University Graduate School of Arts and Sciences.
Musacchio, J.M. 1967. Subcellular distribution of adrenal
    tyrosine hydroxylase. Pharmacologist 9: 210.
Musacchio, J.M. 1968. Subcellular distribution of adrenal
    tyrosine hydroxylase. Biochem. Pharmacol. 17: 1470.
Musacchio, J.M. 1971. Regulation of catecholamine biosynthesis:
    Tyrosine hydroxylase and dihydropteridine reductase. In:
    Brain Chemistry and Mental Disease, (Eds. Ho, B.T. and
    McIsaac, W.M.) New York: Plenum Publishing Corp., pp. 21.
Musacchio, J.M., D'Angelo, G.L. and McQueen, C.A. (1971). Di-
    hydropteridine reductase: Implication on the regulation of
    catecholamine biosynthesis. Proc. Nat. Acad. Sci. USA
    68: 2087.
Musacchio, J.M., Wurzburger, R.J. and D'Angelo, G.L. (1971).
    Different molecular forms of bovine adrenal tyrosine
    hydroxylase. Molec. Pharmacol. 7: 136.
Nagatsu, T., Levitt, M. and Udenfriend, S. (1964 a). Conversion
    of L-tyrosine to 3,4-dihydroxyphenylalanine by cell-free
    preparation of brain and sympathetically innervated tissues.
    Biochem. Biophys. Res. Commun. 14: 543.
Nagatsu, T., Levitt, M. and Udenfriend, S. (1964 b). Tyrosine
    hydroxylase: The initial step in norepinephrine biosynthesis.
    J. Biol. Chem. 239: 2910.
Nagatsu, T., Levitt, M. and Udenfriend, S. (1964 c). A rapid and
    simple radioassay for tyrosine hydroxylase activity. Anal.
    Biochem. 9: 122.
Nagatsu, T., Mizutani, K., Nagatsu, I., Matsuura, S. and Sugimoto,
    T. 1972. Pteridines as cofactor or inhibitor of tyrosine
    hydroxylase. Biochem. Pharmacol. 21: 1945.
Petrack, B., Sheppy, F. and Fetzer, V. 1968. Studies on tyrosine
    hydroxylase from bovine adrenal medulla. J. Biol. Chem.
    243: 743.
Petrack, B., Sheppy, F., Fetzer, V., Manning, T., CEertock, H. and
    Ma, D. 1972 a. Effect of ferrous ion on tyrosine hydroxylase
    of bovine adrenal medulla. J. Biol. Chem., (in press).
Petrack, B., Sheppy, F., Fetzer, V. and Manning, T. 1972 b. Effect
    of Fe^{++} on tyrosine hydroxylase of bovine adrenal medulla.
    In: Fifth International Congress on Pharmacology – Abstracts
    of Volunteer Papers, p. 182.
Shiman, R., Akino, M. and Kaufman, S. 1971. Solubilization and
    partial purification of tyrosine hydroxylase from bovine
    adrenal medulla. J. Biol. Chem. 246: 1330.

Stjarne, L. and Lishajko, F. 1967. Localization of different steps in noradrenaline synthesis to different fractions of a bovine splenic nerve homogenate. Biochem. Pharmacol. 16: 1719.

Udenfriend, S., Zaltzman-Nirenberg, P. and Nagatsu, T. 1965. Inhibitors of purified beef adrenal tyrosine hydroxylase. Biochem. Pharmacol. 14: 837.

Weiner, N., Waymire, J.C. and Schneider, F.H. 1971. The localization and kinetics of tyrosine hydroxylase of the adrenals of several species and of human chromaffin tumors. Acta Cientifica Venezolana 22(2): 79.

Weiner, N. and Selvaratnam, I. 1968. The effect of tyramine on the synthesis of norepinephrine. J. Pharmacol. Exp. Ther. 161: 21.

Wurzburger, R.J. and Musacchio, J.M. 1971. Subcellular distribution and aggregation of bovine adrenal tyrosine hydroxylase. J. Pharmacol. Exp. Ther. 177: 155.

NOREPINEPHRINE BIOSYNTHESIS IN RELATIONSHIP TO NEURAL ACTIVATION[*]

Norman Weiner, Frank C. Bove, Richard Bjur,
Gilles Cloutier and Salomon Z. Langer[**]

University of Colorado School of Medicine
Department of Pharmacology, Denver Colorado   80220

INTRODUCTION

Adrenergic nerve stimulation, which is associated with increased release and turnover of the neurotransmitter norepinephrine, is accompanied by increased synthesis of norepineprhine from tyrosine (for detailed review, see Weiner, 1970). This has been demonstrated in vivo (Gordon et al., 1966 a,b; Dairman et al., 1968) and in vitro (Alousi and Weiner, 1966; Roth, Stjarne and Euler, 1967; Weiner and Rabadjija, 1968). In our laboratories we have used the isolated vas deferens-hypogastric nerve preparation of the guinea pig and have shown that there is approximately a 50 per cent increase in norepinephrine synthesis during intermittent supramaximal nerve stimulation, employing a program of 25 Hz, stimulus duration of 5 msec, for 5 seconds of each minute over a period of one hour. Increased norepinephrine synthesis is demonstrable when tyrosine is used as precursor but does not occur when norepinephrine synthesis from labelled dihydroxyphenylalanine (DOPA) is examined (Weiner and Rabadjija, 1968). The level of tyrosine hydroxylase found in homogenates prepared from stimulated preparations is not different from that in sham stimulated organs. The increased synthesis associated with nerve stimulation is at least partially abolished when 6×10^{-6} M norepinephrine is added to the medium (Alousi and Weiner, 1966; Weiner and Rabadjija, 1968). This observation, and the observations of Udenfriend and co-workers (Udenfriend, Zaltzman-Nirenberg and Nagatsu, 1965; Ikeda, Fahien and Udenfriend, 1966) that catecholamines inhibit soluble, partially purified bovine adrenal medulla tyrosine hydroxylase by competition with the pteridine cofactor, suggested that enhanced norepinephrine synthesis from tyrosine during nerve stimulation is the result of reduced end-product feedback inhibition. Since the

89

levels of total norepinephrine in stimulated and sham stimulated vas deferens preparations were identical, we proposed that a small pool of norepinephrine, presumably free intraneuronal norepinephrine, ordinarily suppresses to some degree tyrosine hydroxylase activity and that with nerve stimulation the concentration of this pool of free intraneuronal norepinephrine is reduced and tyrosine hydroxylase activity is thereby enhanced (Alousi and Weiner, 1966; Weiner and Rabadjija, 1968).

A variety of subsequent pharmacological studies supports the validity of this postulate. For example, monoamine oxidase inhibitors, which do not affect tyrosine hydroxylase activity in homogenized tissue preparations or in preparations of partially purified enzyme, inhibit tyrosine hydroxylase activity of intact tissue (Weiner and Bjur, 1972). Similarly, amphetamine, tyramine and other indirectly acting sympathomimetic amines, which presumably release norepinephrine from storage sites, inhibit tyrosine hydroxylase activity in intact tissue but fail to affect the partially purified enzyme except at extremely high concentrations (Weiner and Selvaratnam, 1968; Kopin, Weiss and Sedvall, 1969; Weiner and Bjur, 1972). Finally, during acute depletion of norepinephrine by reserpine, an agent which blocks the uptake of catecholamines into storage vesicles, there is inhibition of tyrosine hydroxylase in intact tissue, but no effect of this drug is apparent on tyrosine hydroxylase activity when the tissue is homogenized and the enzyme is optimally fortified with cofactors (Weiner, et al., 1972; Pfeffer and Weiner, in preparation). With each of these drug treatments, the inhibition of tyrosine hydroxylase activity in intact tissue can be competitively antagonized by addition of synthetic pteridine cofactor, 6,7-dimethyltetrahydropterin (DMPH$_4$), to the incubation medium (Weiner and Bjur, 1972; Weiner et al., 1972; Pfeffer and Weiner, in preparation).

Effect of Pterin Cofactor on Norepinephrine Synthesis During Nerve Stimulation

If enhanced norepinephrine synthesis from tyrosine during nerve stimulation is due to reduced end-product feedback inhibition, this effect should similarly be antagonized by addition of the pterin cofactor to the medium. Presumably, in the absence of pterin cofactor, norepinephrine synthesis during nerve stimulation should be enhanced because free intraneuronal norepinephrine is somehow diminished as a consequence of neural activity. However, in both control and stimulated preparations, if sufficiently high pterin cofactor is added to the medium and reaches the intraneuronal site (as would be predicted from the studies with MAO inhibitors, tyramine, amphetamine and reserpine), end-product feedback inhibition should be eliminated in both control and stimulated preparations and tyrosine hydroxylase activity in each of these tissues should increase. Since the inhibition of the enzyme in the stimulated preparation is already smaller than that in the control preparation, because of the presumed lower concentration of free intraneuronal norepinephrine, tyrosine hydroxylase activity in the control preparation should increase to a greater degree until the enzyme activities in control and stimulated preparations approximate each other (Figure 1).

In order to evaluate this hypothesis, isolated guinea-pig hypogastric nerve-vas deferens preparations were stimulated for one hour in the presence of different concentrations of $DMPH_4$ in Krebs-Ringer bicarbonate buffer, 0.01 mM disodium ethylenediamine tetra-acetate, (Na_2EDTA) and 1×10^{-5} M L-tyrosine, containing 25-30 µCi $3,5-^3H$-L-tyrosine (43.8 Ci/mmole). Newly synthesized catecholamines were isolated by double column chromatography on alumina and Dowex-50-Na^+ and assayed by liquid scintillation spectrometry (Weiner and Rabadjija, 1968).

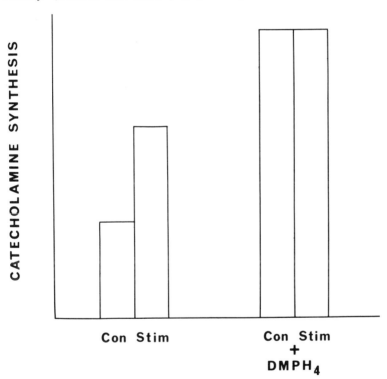

Figure 1. Postulated mechanism by which the pterin cofactor, $DMPH_4$, might abolish the increase in norepinephrine synthesis during nerve stimulation, if the effect of nerve stimulation is related to reduced end-product feedback inhibitions. Con = control preparation. Stim = stimulated preparation. For discussion, see text.

In contrast to the predicted result, based on end-product feedback inhibition which is competitive with the pterin cofactor, the addition of $DMPH_4$ was associated with a greater increase in tyrosine hydroxylase activity in the stimulated preparation than was observed in the control preparation, whether the experiments were performed in the absence (Figure 2) or in the presence (Figure 3) of 10^{-5} M norepinephrine. If one assumes that the concentration of the pterin cofactor, which is presumably tetra-hydrobiopterin (Lloyd and Weiner, 1971), is equivalent to 0.1 mM 6,7-dimethyltetrahydropterin ($DMPH_4$), a Lineweaver-Burk kinetic analysis of the effect of the exogenous cofactor on norepinephrine synthesis during nerve stimulation may be performed. This estimate of the amount of endogenous cofactor is justified by: (1) extrapolation of the substrate-velocity curve for catecholamine synthesis vs. $DMPH_4$ concentration to zero velocity (Figure 2), and (2) determination of the apparent Km of the enzyme for $DMPH_4$ in intact preparations and in homogenates prepared from vasa deferentia. If the endogenous pterin cofactor concentration is assumed to be equivalent to 0.1 mM $DMPH_4$, the Km for the tyrosine hydroxylase in intact preparations is 0.22 mM, a value which is identical to that obtained for the homogenate or soluble super-natant prepared from guinea-pig vas deferens tissues (Waymire and Weiner, unpublished).

Lineweaver-Burk analysis of the results obtained during nerve stimulation in the presence of different concentrations of pterin cofactor reveals that the Km for $DMPH_4$ was essentially unchanged with nerve stimulation, but the maximal tyrosine hydroxylase activity in the stimulated intact preparation was approximately double that observed in the corresponding control preparation (Figure 4, Table 1). Similarly, when kinetic analysis of tyrosine hydroxylase activity in intact tissue was performed with varying concentrations of tyrosine, the Km for tyrosine was unchanged, but the maximal velocity of the tyrosine hydroxylase reaction in the stimulated preparations was approximately double that found in the control vasa deferentia, indicating that the mechanism of enhanced norepinephrine synthesis during nerve stimulation does not involve an alteration in the affinity of the enzyme for tyrosine (Table 1). In contrast, when norepinephrine is added to the medium of either control or stimulated preparations, tyrosine hydroxylase activity is reduced and kinetic analysis with different concentrations of $DMPH_4$ indicates that the effect of norepinephrine is competitive with the pterin cofactor (Figure 4, Table 1).

Mandell and co-workers have demonstrated that heparin markedly increases the activity of brain tyrosine hydroxylase (Kuczenski and Mandell, 1972 a,b). It is unlikely that heparin is the mediator of the enhanced tyrosine hydroxylase activity during nerve stimulation since this large polyvalent anion probably does

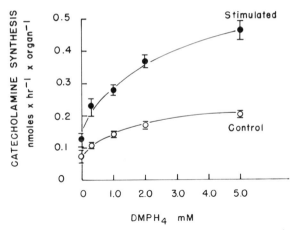

Figure 2. The effect of exogenous pterin cofactor (DMPH$_4$) on synthesis of catecholamines from tyrosine in stimulated and control hypogastric nerve vas deferens preparations of the guinea pig. Each value is the mean $\pm$ standard error of 4-6 determinations.

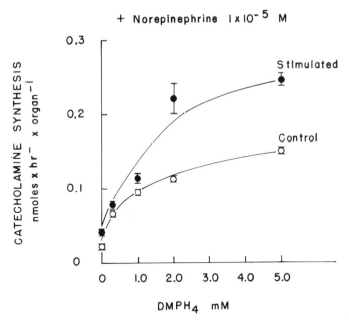

Figure 3. The effect of exogenous pterin cofactor (DMPH$_4$) on synthesis of catecholamines from tyrosine in stimulated and control vas deferens preparations of the guinea pig in the presence of 10^{-5} M norepinephrine. Each value is the mean $\pm$ standard error of 4 determinations.

TABLE 1

KINETIC CONSTANTS* OF TYROSINE HYDROXYLASE IN
INTACT VAS DEFERENS PREPARATIONS OF GUINEA PIG

	Effect of Nerve Stimulation and Norepinephrine			
	No Added Norepinephrine		10^{-5} M Norepinephrine	
	Control	Stimulated	Control	Stimulated
Km DMPH$_4$, mM	0.22	0.30	0.72‡	0.94‡
Vmax DMPH$_4$**	0.19	0.42†	0.17	0.29†
Km Tyrosine, mM	0.061	0.065	0.064	0.078
Vmax Tyrosine**	0.47	0.97†	0.33	0.46‡

*   Calculated according to the method of Wilkinson (1961).
** pmoles x hr^{-1} x vasa^{-1}
†   p <.05 vs. corresponding control values for Vmax.
‡   p <.05 norepinephrine vs. corresponding values without added
        norepinephrine

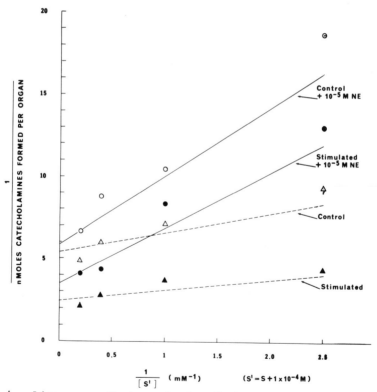

Figure 4. Lineweaver-Burk analysis of the results plotted in
Figures 2 and 3. The Km and Vmax values, shown in Table 1, were
calculated according to Wilkinson (1961).

not enter the nerve terminal. Furthermore, the effect of heparin appears to be in part competitively antagonized by pterin cofactor (Kuczenski and Mandell, 1972 b), whereas the increased tyrosine hydroxylase activity observed during nerve stimulation is not competitively overcome by pterin cofactor. Mandell and co-workers have suggested that enhanced tyrosine hydroxylase activity may be associated with a shift in the physical properties of tyrosine hydroxylase involving attachment to membranes with a concomitant reduction in the Km for DMPH4. Again, our DMPH4 studies would suggest that this is not the mechanism by which nerve stimulation produces increased tyrosine hydroxylase activity in the guinea-pig vas deferens preparation. Virtually all of the tyrosine hydroxylase in the non-stimulated guinea-pig vas deferens-hypogastric nerve preparation is located in the soluble fraction of isotonic sucrose homogenates and there is no change in this distribution in preparations which have been subjected to intermittent nerve stimulation for a period of one hour (Waymire and Weiner, unpublished).

It would thus appear that enhanced synthesis of norepinephrine during nerve stimulation is not the result of reduced end-product feedback inhibition involving a mechanism which is competitive with the pterin cofactor. It is still probable that the enhanced tyrosine hydroxylase activity associated with nerve stimulation is the result of reduced interaction with catecholamine, but this interaction may be at some allosteric site on the enzyme which is not the site of cofactor interaction. Alternatively, nerve stimulation and nerve terminal depolarization, which is accompanied by multiple biochemical events including sodium uptake, potassium exit and enhanced oxidative metabolism, may result in the production or activation of a positive allosteric effector or a diminution in the amount of a negative allosteric effector which does not compete with either tyrosine or the pterin cofactor for a site on the enzyme.

In order to evaluate further the mechanisms by which nerve stimulation leads to increased synthesis of norepinephrine from tyrosine, we have initiated studies on a preparation in which the intraneuronal dynamics of norepinephrine metabolism can be studied more precisely; namely, the isolated cat spleen which is prelabelled in vivo with ^{3}H-norepinephrine.

The Uptake and Metabolism of Norepinephrine in Perfused Organs

^{3}H-Norepinephrine, when injected into the intact animal or perfused through an isolated organ in low concentrations, is rapidly taken up by the tissue and is only slowly released over several hours, especially if the nerves are not stimulated (Hertting and Axelrod, 1961). The material is taken up into and retained in the tissues largely as intact norepinephrine. In the presence of cocaine or in the chronically denervated organ the uptake and retention of labelled norepinephrine is markedly impaired (Hertting et al., 1961). Hertting and Axelrod (1961) demonstrated that ^{3}H-norepinephrine which is taken up is localized in adrenergic nerve endings, since the ^{3}H-norepinephrine can be released by nerve stimulation but is not released when the isolated, perfused spleen is stimulated to contract with administered norepinephrine. The axonal membrane uptake system appears to be common for a variety of phenylethylamine derivatives. It is sodium dependent and probably involves a carrier mediated transport process (Iversen and Kravitz, 1966; Bogdanski and Brodie, 1969). It is selectively blocked by cocaine and a variety of tricyclic antidepressants including imipramine and desmethylimipramine. The storage vesicle uptake process is distinct from the axonal membrane uptake process in that the former is not blocked by either cocaine or the tricyclic anti-depressants. It appears to be selectively blocked by reserpine and related alkaloids. Brown and Gillespie (1957) have shown that the efficiency of the reuptake mechanism into the nerve terminal of the isolated perfused spleen is inversely related to the frequency of stimulation of the nerve. At low rates of stimulation virtually all of the released norepinephrine is taken up by the nerve ending; little or none spills over into the circulation. If the rate of nerve stimulation is increased the fraction of norepinephrine which is taken up falls rapidly and a greater proportion enters the circulation. If the uptake process is blocked, for example by phenoxybenzamine, virtually all of the norepinephrine which is released during stimulation enters the circulation and can be collected in the perfusate. It is of considerable interest that α-adrenergic receptor blockers are also potent inhibitors of the neuronal uptake mechanism. For example, phenoxybenzamine, hydergine and phentolamine block neuronal uptake of norepinephrine (Gillespie and Kirpekar, 1965; Iversen and Langer, 1969). Thoenen, Huerlimann and Haefely (1964) demonstrated that several α-blockers also block the neuronal uptake of norepinephrine but they could not demonstrate a close correlation between these two phenomena.

Kirpekar and Wakade (1968) demonstrated that, in the isolated perfused spleen from normal cats, approximately 66 per cent of the catecholamines are taken up by the spleen in one perfusion. Calcium has no influence on the uptake of norepinephrine perfused through the spleen. However, sodium appears to be required for the uptake process since removal of sodium from the perfusion fluid almost totally abolishes norepinephrine uptake. The uptake process appears to be energy dependent since iodoacetate and dinitrophenol together block the uptake of norepinephrine to a considerable degree. In addition, the uptake process is markedly temperature dependent. Both ouabain and the local anesthetic, tetracaine, block the uptake of norepinephrine to a considerable extent.

Mechanism of Norepinephrine Release from Neurons

A considerable amount of information has accumulated in recent
years about the physiological process of neurotransmitter release
from adrenergic tissues. Extensive studies by Douglas and co-
workers have demonstrated that secretion from the adrenal medulla
probably involves a process analogous to exocytosis wherein the
entire soluble contents of the adrenal chromaffin granules are
released on nerve stimulation (Douglas, 1966 a,b). Douglas and
Poisner (1966) demonstrated a stoichiometric secretion of adenine
nucleotides and catecholamines from the isolated perfused adrenal
gland. Using an immunological assay for the soluble proteins of the
chromaffin granule, Banks and Helle (1965), Blaschko and co-
workers (1967) and Kirshner et al. (1966) demonstrated that the
soluble granule protein is also secreted with the amines and ATP.
Insoluble membranous protein does not seem to leave the cell nor
do extragranular macromolecules (Schneider et al., 1967). These
results suggest that the catecholamines are released by a process
of exocytosis wherein fusion of the granule membrane to that of the
cell presumably occurs, followed by ejection of the contents of
the granule and return of the empty granule to the cytoplasm either
for reconstitution of its contents or for ultimate degradation.

Although the results are by no means wholly definitive, in
sympathetic nerve terminals analogous biochemical relationships
have been demonstrated. In the perfused rabbit heart and the
perfused cat spleen there is a direct relationship between the amount
of amine released and the calcium concentration of the perfusion
fluid (Huković and Muscholl, 1962; Kirpekar and Misu, 1967). It
has been shown recently that both dopamine-β-hydroxylase and
chromogranins are released from the isolated perfused spleen during
the process of nerve stimulation (Smith et al., 1970). Further
studies have suggested that the amount of macromolecules; notably,
chromogranins and dopamine-β-hydroxylase, secreted during stimulation of adrenergic neurons is low compared to the amount of norepinephrine secreted, suggesting that only partial exocytosis,
largely of the small molecules, occurs during sympathetic nerve
stimulation (DePotter et al., 1969; Smith et al., 1970). However,
Weinshilboum et al. (1971) claim that the proportion of catecholamines to dopamine-β-hydroxylase secreted from the isolated hypogastric nerve-vas deferens preparation during nerve stimulation is
similar to the relative amounts of catecholamines and soluble dopamine-β-hydroxylase which are readily extractable from the tissue by
freezing and homogenization. These workers therefore suggest that
the process of exocytosis may be involved in the secretion of the
adrenergic neurotransmitter, analogous to the process which appears
to occur in the adrenal medulla.

However, stoichiometric release of chromogranins, dopamine-β-hydroxylase and catecholamines from adrenergic neurons is difficult to reconcile with our current understanding of synthesis and turn-over of catecholamines relative to the synthesis and turnover of synaptic vesicles. Synaptic vesicles are believed to have a half-life in excess of 40 days (Dahlström and Häggendal, 1966; Dahlström, 1967), whereas norepinephrine turnover in adrenergic neurons in a variety of tissues is believed to occur in less than 24 hours. At the present time there is no evidence that synaptic vesicles are able to synthesize either chromogranins, dopamine-β-hydroxylase or ATP once they have migrated down the axon and have entered the preterminal and terminal regions of the neuron. Thus, if the process of complete exocytosis occurs, it is difficult to under-stand how synaptic vesicles lacking soluble dopamine-β-hydroxylase, chromogranins and ATP, in addition to catecholamine, could continue to be functional. On the other hand, most of the turnover of norepinephrine may represent spontaneous leakage of catecholamine from the synaptic vesicles and subsequent metabolism. If this is the explanation for the discrepancy between the turnover time of norepinephrine and that of synaptic vesicles it would suggest that over 90 per cent of norepinephrine synthesized is metabolized intraneuronally in what would appear to be a wasteful fashion.

The Contribution of Newly Synthesized
Norepinephrine to Neurotransmitter Release

Many studies during the past several years have emphasized the importance of norepinephrine synthesis in the maintenance of neuro-transmitter stores. Recent investigations by Kopin and co-workers suggest that newly synthesized norepinephrine may be especially important as a functional pool which is released preferentially during nerve stimulation (Kopin et al., 1968; Sedvall, Weise and Kopin, 1968; Gewirtz and Kopin, 1970). These conclusions are based in part upon results obtained from experiments involving the isolated perfused cat spleen in which labelled tyrosine is perfused briefly through the spleen prior to nerve stimulation. Kopin and co-workers found that the specific activity of the norepinephrine present in the splenic effluent exceeded that of the amine which remained in the spleen and they concluded that newly synthesized norepinephrine is preferentially released. This conclusion is based upon the assumption that labelled tyrosine is uniformly distributed throughout the adrenergic neurons. It is quite possible, however, that the norepinephrine synthesizing machinery closest to the axonal membrane may be preferentially exposed to the labelled tyrosine which is being perfused. Because of the non-uniform distribution of labelled precursor, the pool of norepineph-rine in this region may contain greater quantities of newly synthe-sized amine which is radiolabelled. It is equally likely that the pool of catecholamine which is proximal to the synaptic cleft and the axonal membrane will be preferentially released during nerve

stimulation. Under these conditions stimulation of the adrenergic
nerve would release peripheral stores of norepinephrine which have
a higher specific activity than that throughout the rest of the
organ.

On the other hand, it is conceivable that under normal circumstances tyrosine enters adrenergic neurons via the nerve terminals
and that norepinephrine synthesis occurs in this region of the
neuron largely because of the easy availability of precursor. If
this circumstance is correct, studies employing short-term labelling
of norepinephrine stores with ^{14}C-tyrosine may be quite appropriate
although it remains likely that synthesis in deeper stores in the
neuron, because of nonuniform labelling, is probably underestimated.

In analogous experiments Blakeley et al (1969) perfused the
spleen with labelled ^{3}H-tyrosine for periods of up to 4 hours.
When the splenic nerve was stimulated they found that the specific
activity of ^{3}H-norepinephrine in the effluent was equal to that in
the spleen, suggesting that newly synthesized norepinephrine was
not preferentially released by nerve stimulation.

Kopin et al. (1968) also treated cats with ^{3}H-norepinephrine
16-20 hours before surgical removal and perfusion of the spleen.
They compared the nerve stimulated release of ^{3}H-norepinephrine
and total norepinephrine in the presence of either tyrosine or
α-methyl-p-tyrosine and followed the specific activity of norepinephrine released. They found that the specific activity of
norepinephrine in the perfusate was considerably less in the
presence of tyrosine than in the presence of the inhibitor of
tyrosine hydroxylase, suggesting that newly synthesized norepinephrine was being released at a considerable rate.

Norepinephrine Dynamics in the Perfused Spleen
During Nerve Stimulation

In our studies, cats were anesthetized with ether, spinal
transsection and evisceration were performed and the cats were
administered either 50 or 100 μCi/kg of DL-^{3}H-norepinephrine (5.76 Ci/
mmole) or 50 μCi/kg L-^{3}H-norepinephrine (6.5 Ci/mmole) 4-6 hours
prior to stimulation of the spleen. After isolation of the spleen,
the splenic artery was cannulated and perfusion was initiated with
Krebs-Ringer bicarbonate medium modified by the addition of
5×10^{-3} M glucose, 1×10^{-4} M ascorbic acid, and 5×10^{-5} M L-
tyrosine. When inhibition of tyrosine hydroxylase was desired,
1×10^{-3} M DL-α-methyl-p-tyrosine was added to the perfusion fluid.
The perfusion fluid was maintained at 37°C and aerated with a
mixture of 95% O_2: 5% CO_2. Perfusion flow was maintained at
7.5 ml/minute. After a 30 minute equilibration period the splenic
nerves were stimulated at 20 Hz for 300 pulses at supramaximal

voltage. This train of stimulation was repeated every 15 minutes. Stimulation of the splenic nerve was by means of a Grass stimulator Model S-4E with needle electrodes which were placed around the splenic artery in which the splenic nerves are embedded. Optimal norepinephrine overflow was obtained with a stimulation frequency of 20 Hz (Figure 5). Splenic perfusion pressure was determined by means of a Statham P-23 transducer. Venous effluents from the spleen were collected and chilled in graduated centrifuge tubes to which were added 0.1 ml of 0.1 M Na_2EDTA in saline. Effluents were centrifuged to remove red cells and aliquots of the supernatant were assayed for total ^{3}H-content by liquid scintillation spectrometry. The remainder of the supernatants were adjusted to pH 2 with 1 N HCl and stored at 0°C. The acidified effluents were passed over Dowex-50 x 4 H$^+$ columns and the columns were washed with distilled water. The column effluents and the water wash which contained the ^{3}H-deaminated metabolites were assayed for total ^{3}H by liquid scintillation spectrometry. The amines were eluted from the Dowex column with 1 N HCl. Eluates were adjusted to pH 8.6, and norepinephrine was adsorbed on alumina and eluted with 0.2 N acetic acid. Aliquots of alumina eluates were assayed for ^{3}H-norepinephrine by liquid scintillation spectrometry and for total norepinephrine by the trihydroxyindole procedure. ^{3}H-Normetanephrine

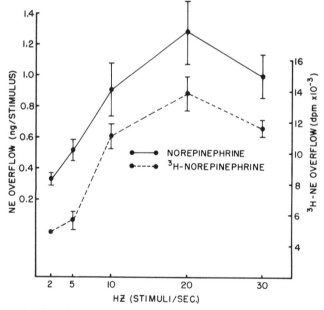

Figure 5. Relationship between frequency of stimulation (Hz) of the splenic nerves and the overflow of norepinephrine and ^{3}H-norepinephrine. Stimulus trains for each frequency consisted of 300 pulses; pulse width was 1 msec. Supramaximal voltage was employed. Each point represents the mean ± standard error of at least 4 values.

was determined as total ^{3}H minus (^{3}H-norepinephrine plus ^{3}H-deaminated catechols). At the end of the experiment, spleens were removed from the perfusion system and homogenized in 0.4 N perchloric acid and centrifuged. Supernatant aliquots were examined in a manner similar to that described for the splenic effluents.

In order to assess the uniformity of labelling of the spleen, spleens were stimulated for 15 seconds (20 Hz, 300 pulses) every 15 minutes for four hours either in the presence of: (1) tyrosine alone; (2) tyrosine plus α-methyl-p-tyrosine; or (3) tyrosine plus 1 x 10^{-5} M phenoxybenzamine (Figure 6). Splenic effluents were collected for 5 minutes from the beginning of the stimulation period. Thus, the fraction of the total 3H recovered in the overflow as ^{3}H-norepinephrine following nerve stimulation represents the mean ^{3}H-norepinephrine content of the perfusate collected for the 5 minute period beginning at the onset of stimulation. In addition, a 5 minute collection was made prior to each stimulation period.

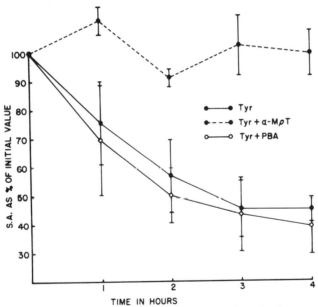

Figure 6. Specific activity (S.A.) of norepinephrine present in the splenic overflow during and following nerve stimulation. S.A. is presented as per cent of the value obtained after the first stimulation. Spleens were perfused with: (1) 5 x 10^{-5} M tyrosine (Tyr); (2) 5 x 10^{-5} M tyrosine + 1 x 10^{-3} M α-methyl-p-tyrosine (α-MpT); or (3) 5 x 10^{-5} M tyrosine + 1 x 10^{-5} M phenoxybenzamine HCl (PBA). Splenic nerves were stimulated every 15 min for 4 hr. All values represent the specific activity of norepinephrine, expressed as per cent of initial specific activity, in the overflow from the last stimulation period of each hour. PBA values represent the mean of two experiments and the vertical bars represent the range. All other points are the mean ± standard errors of at least 4 experiments.

Specific activity of norepinephrine in splenic effluents fell progressively with repeated stimulation in those experiments in which α-methyl-p-tyrosine was absent from the perfusion medium (Figure 6). In contrast, there was no significant alteration in the specific activity of norepinephrine released following nerve stimulation in the presence of the inhibitor of tyrosine hydroxylase. These results suggest that ^{3}H-norepinephrine perfused 4-6 hours prior to the experiment was uniformly distributed throughout those norepinephrine stores which are able to be released by nerve stimulation. In the presence of the inhibitor of tyrosine hydroxylase, approximately 55% of the ^{3}H released during and in the period immediately following nerve stimulation exits in the form of ^{3}H-norepinephrine. There is a tendency for the proportion of ^{3}H-norepinephrine in the splenic effluent after nerve stimulation to decline over several hours and this is associated with a modest increase in deaminated metabolites which appears in the splenic effluent (Figure 7). In contrast to stimulation mediated release

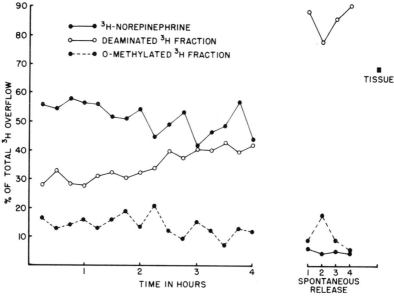

Figure 7. The overflow of ^{3}H-norepinephrine, ^{3}H-normetanephrine and ^{3}H-deaminated metabolites of norepinephrine from the perfused spleen during and immediately following nerve stimulation applied every 15 min for 4 hr. The spleen was perfused with Krebs-Ringer bicarbonate medium containing 5 x 10^{-5} M tyrosine and 1 x 10^{-3} M α-methyl-p-tyrosine and stimulated at 20 Hz (300 pulses) every 15 min. Spontaneously released ^{3}H-norepinephrine and metabolites were determined from prestimulation samples collected just prior to the last stimulation of each hour. Approximately 70% of the ^{3}H content of the spleen was recovered as ^{3}H-norepinephrine (solid square); the remainder of the ^{3}H in the spleen was in the form of deaminated metabolite.

of these substances, approximately 80-90% of the ^{3}H which is released spontaneously appears in the effluent as deaminated metabolite and less than 10% of the ^{3}H in the splenic effluent in the
absence of stimulation is in the form of ^{3}H-norepinephrine.

In order to evaluate the kinetics of ^{3}H-norepinephrine release
during and following nerve stimulation more precisely, in a few
experiments one-minute collections were made beginning with the
15-second stimulation period (Figure 8). Approximately 80% of the
[3]H which is collected in the minute following the initiation of
nerve stimulation is in the form of ^{3}H-norepinephrine. This
progressively declines in the ensuing minutes and is associated
with a progressive increase in the fraction of ^{3}H which appears
as deaminated metabolite. In the presence of phenoxybenzamine,
virtually all of the ^{3}H released from the spleen during nerve
stimulation and in the immediate post-stimulation period is in the
form of ^{3}H-norepinephrine, suggesting that, in the absence of

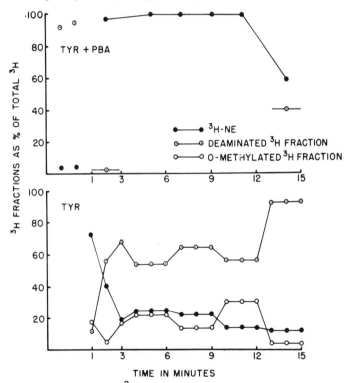

Figure 8. Time course of ^{3}H-overflow during a fifteen minute period
following stimulation of the isolated, perfused spleen at 20 Hz for
15 sec (300 pulses). Spleens were perfused with Krebs-Ringer bicarbonate medium containing 5×10^{-5} M tyrosine or 5×10^{-5} M tyrosine
+ 1×10^{-5} M phenoxybenzamine (PBA). ^{3}H-NE, ^{3}H-normetanephrine
(0-methylated ^{3}H-fraction) and ^{3}H-deaminated metabolites are
expressed as per cent of total ^{3}H in the splenic effluent.

phenoxybenzamine, approximately 1/3 of the ^{3}H-norepinephrine which
is released on nerve stimulation is taken up into the nerve ending
where it is deaminated prior to appearing in the perfusate.
However, both in control spleens and in spleens exposed to phenoxybenzamine, the ^{3}H which appears in the effluent during the intervals
when the nerves to the organ are not stimulated is almost wholly in
the form of deaminated metabolites. These results suggest that, in
the absence of nerve stimulation, norepinephrine is deaminated
within the nerve terminal and exits from the nerve terminal as
deaminated product.

The specific activity of the ^{3}H-norepinephrine released during
nerve stimulation was found to be much higher than that released
spontaneously (Figure 9). This marked discrepancy persisted
throughout 5 hours of intermittent stimulation and was apparent

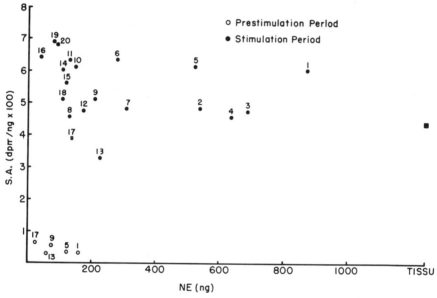

Figure 9. Relationship between specific activity of ^{3}H-norepineph-
rine and the norepinephrine content of the splenic effluent. The
spleen was perfused with Krebs-Ringer bicarbonate medium containing
5×10^{-5} M tyrosine + 1×10^{-3} M α-methyl-p-tyrosine and stimulated
at 20 Hz (300 pulses) every 15 min for 5 hr. The numbers corres-
pond to the values obtained during and immediately following each
successive stimulus period from the first to the twentieth stimulation. Prestimulation periods prior to the first stimulation of
each hour were selected for analysis (open circles). Similar results were obtained if α-methyl-p-tyrosine was omitted from the perfusion medium, except that there was a progressive fall in the
specific activity of the norepinephrine released during nerve
stimulation over time.

either in the presence or in the absence of α-methyl-p-tyrosine.
Even in the last hour of the experiment, when the amount of norepinephrine released during nerve stimulation was in the same range
as that released spontaneously in earlier stages of the experiment,
the specific activity differences were apparent. These results
suggest that, in contrast to the α-methyl-p-tyrosine studies described above (Figure 6), there is not homogeneous labelling of the
norepinephrine pools in the spleen with ^{3}H-norepinephrine. A possible explanation for the difference in specific activity between
these two pools of norepinephrine may relate to the greater lability
of newly synthesized norepinephrine (Figure 10). Thus, either
shortly prior to perfusion with the inhibitor of tyrosine hydroxylase, or during the perfusion in the absence of the inhibitor of
tyrosine hydroxylase, norepinephrine would be synthesized from
tyrosine and dilute a labile pool with non-radioactive amine. A
significant period of time may be required for the equilibration
of newly synthesized norepinephrine, formed in synaptic vesicles,
with bound norepinephrine which exists within the vesicles in a
storage complex with ATP and, perhaps, associated macromolecules.
During this period prior to equilibration, the newly synthesized
norepinephrine might leak from the storage vesicle and appear in
the axoplasm. In the axoplasm, it would be susceptible to deamina-
tion by mitochondrial monoamine oxidase. That which is not oxi-
datively deaminated either may be taken up again into the vesicles
or may, along with the deaminated metabolites, leak from the axon
and contribute to the pool of spontaneously released norepinephrine.
It would therefore be expected that this newly synthesized norepinephrine, released spontaneously, would have a lower specific
activity than the major, more stable pool of norepinephrine located
in a storage complex within the synaptic vesicles. In contrast,
during nerve stimulation, release of norepinephrine is presumably
by exocytosis and the bulk of the norepinephrine which exits from
the spleen would represent the more stable pool of norepinephrine
which had been bound in the storage complex prior to release. Since
the labelling of the spleen occurred several hours prior to nerve
stimulation, it would be anticipated that this pool of stable
norepinephrine would contain considerably more labelled amine than
the more labile pool of newly synthesized amine (Figure 10).

The Role of Newly Synthesized Norepinephrine
in Regulation of Norepinephrine Synthesis: Effect of Amphetamine

If it is assumed that the newly synthesized pool of norepinephrine is spontaneously released into the axoplasm at a considerably greater rate than the more stable pool of norepinephrine, one
might expect that newly synthesized norepinephrine or its deaminated
metabolites may constitute the critical pool of norepinephrine

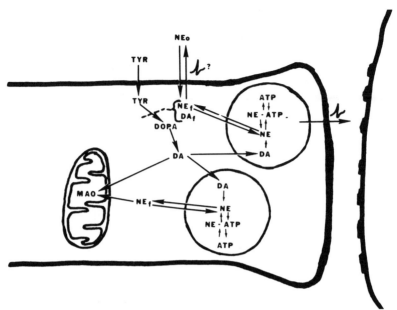

Figure 10.   Schematic diagram of the adrenergic nerve terminal.
Norepinephrine (NE) is present in the storage vesicle complexed to
ATP and perhaps macromolecular constituents of the vesicle.   Newly
synthesized dopamine (DA) is taken up into the vesicle where it is
converted to norepinephrine.   This norepinephrine may not be
incorporated into the storage complex immediately and may exit from
the vesicle, becoming the major source of extravesicular, intraneuronal norepinephrine.   This, along with small amounts of other
catechols, dopamine and 3,4-dihydroxyphenylalanine (DOPA), may be
the major inhibitor of tyrosine hydroxylase in the neuron.   Free
intraneuronal norepinephrine (NE_f) also: (1) may be metabolized
by mitochondrial monoamine oxidase (MAO); or (2) may directly leak
out of the neuron from the axoplasm (NE_o); or (3) may be taken up
into the storage vesicles where, ultimately, it may be incorporated
into the more stable storage complex.   Vesicle contents are released by exocytosis during nerve stimulation ($\checkmark$) and extravesicular norepinephrine also may be released when the axonal
membrane is depolarized ($\checkmark$?).

which regulates tyrosine hydroxylase activity by end-product
feedback inhibition.   Conversely, the stable norepinephrine
pool which is complexed to ATP and other vesicular constituents
would be expected to influence tyrosine hydroxylase activity
little (Figure 10).   Pharmacological studies using the intact
mouse vas deferens preparation appear to support this concept.
Thus, reserpine treatment for several days leads to a profound
depletion of the norepinephrine stores (greater than 95%),

but fails to affect tyrosine hydroxylase activity in the intact
preparation. When the activity of tyrosine hydroxylase in the
intact preparation is compared with total tyrosine hydroxylase as
determined by estimation of tyrosine hydroxylase activity in
fortified, supplemented homogenates of mouse vas deferens, the
relative activity in the intact tissue to the total activity,
assayed under optimal circumstances, is the same as that found in
preparations not treated with reserpine (Pfeffer and Weiner, in
preparation). Furthermore, the ability of 2×10^{-4} M amphetamine
to inhibit markedly tyrosine hydroxylase activity in incubated
mouse vas deferens preparations persists in preparations which
have been severely depleted of norepinephrine by reserpine treatment. Since the psychoactive effects of amphetamine persist, or
are even potentiated, after the administration of reserpine (Smith,
1963) but are antagonized by inhibition of tyrosine hydroxylase
(Weissman, Koe and Tenen, 1966), it would appear that amphetamine
preferentially releases newly synthesized norepinephrine from its
(presumably) more labile binding sites. We therefore decided to
determine whether inhibition of tyrosine hydroxylase, and therefore block of synthesis of norepinephrine, for several hours might
abolish the ability of amphetamine to inhibit norepinephrine
synthesis.

Mice were treated with 5 mg/kg reserpine, and 24 and 28 hours
later, with 100 mg/kg α-methyl-p-tyrosine. The animals were killed
at 31 hours and the vasa deferentia were removed and assayed for
tyrosine hydroxylase activity according to the coupled decarboxylase
assay (Waymire, Bjur and Weiner, 1971; Weiner and Bjur, 1972). In
the absence of amphetamine, the level of tyrosine hydroxylase
activity in intact vasa deferentia removed from mice which had been
treated with α-methyl-p-tyrosine was approximately 25 per cent of
control levels, presumably as a result of persistent inhibition
of tyrosine hydroxylase by α-methyl-p-tyrosine in the tissues.
Nevertheless, 2×10^{-4} M amphetamine failed to significantly depress
the tyrosine hydroxylase activity further (Table 2). These results
suggest that the labile pool of newly synthesized norepinephrine
may indeed be critical to regulation of tyrosine hydroxylase activity
and this pool, which is weakly bound to intracellular components
of unknown nature, is most susceptible to release by indirectly
acting sympathomimetic amines. One might speculate that in the
resting adrenergically innervated preparation, when the synaptic
vesicles are largely filled, newly synthesized catecholamine cannot be incorporated into the stable storage complex in the vesicle.
At least a portion of this newly synthesized amine accumulates in
the free form in the axoplasm and inhibits tyrosine hydroxylase
activity. In this regard, dopamine may be more important than
norepinephrine in regulating intraneuronal tyrosine hydroxylase
(Costa, 1970), since it is actually formed in the axoplasm
(Rutledge and Weiner, 1967; Weiner, 1970). We have observed that

TABLE 2

TYROSINE HYDROXYLASE ACTIVITY

IN THE INTACT MOUSE VAS DEFERENS

| | EFFECT OF 2 x 10^{-4} M AMPHETAMINE | | |
	- Amphetamine pmoles/hr/pair vasa	+ Amphetamine pmoles/hr/pair vasa	Percent Inhibition
Control	104.18 $\pm$ 8.01*	44.98 $\pm$ 1.98	57**
Reserpine[a]	84.38 $\pm$ 9.68	31.65 $\pm$ 1.88	62**
Reserpine[b]	64.22 $\pm$ 6.43	35.96 $\pm$ 1.52	44**
Reserpine + α-methyl-p-tyrosine[c]	27.12 $\pm$ 3.20	22.17 $\pm$ 2.78	18

[a] 5 mg/kg reserpine i.p. at 0 hour; sacrifice at 32 hours.

[b] 5 mg/kg reserpine i.p. at 0 hour and at 26 hours; sacrifice at 32 hours.

[c] 5 mg/kg reserpine i.p. at 0 hour and 100 mg/kg α-methyl-p-tyrosine i.p. at 24 hours and 28 hours; sacrifice at 31 hours.

* Each value is the mean $\pm$ S.E. of 4 separate determinations

** $p < .01$

dopamine is a more effective inhibitor of tyrosine hydroxylase than norepinephrine since the Ki of the former is approximately one-half that of the latter compound (Waymire and Weiner, unpublished).

CONCLUSION

Nerve stimulation of the vas deferens preparation of the guinea-pig is associated with increased synthesis of norepinephrine from tyrosine. The effect, which is due to increased conversion of tyrosine to dihydroxyphenylalanine, is not the result of increased levels of tyrosine hydroxylase enzyme protein, and is at least partially abolished by addition of norepinephrine to the medium. Kinetic studies indicate that the mechanism of increased norepinephrine synthesis from tyrosine during nerve stimulation is not related to reduced competitive antagonism between catecholamine and the pterin cofactor for tyrosine hydroxylase. Studies with isolated perfused spleens labelled with ^{3}H-norepinephrine indicate that a labile pool of newly synthesized norepinephrine is present in the adrenergic neuron and this pool does not rapidly equilibrate with the larger norepinephrine pool located in the vesicles. The inhibitory effect of amphetamine on tyrosine hydroxylase in intact tissue may result from the ability of amphetamine to release newly synthesized catecholamine into the axoplasmic pool. In this latter compartment the catecholamine has access to the enzyme and it is presumably this pool of catecholamine which is responsible for end-product feedback inhibition of the first step in norepinephrine synthesis.

FOOTNOTES

*   This work was supported by USPHS Grants NS-07927 and NS-07642
** Visiting Professor of Pharmacology. Present address: Instituto De Investigaciones Farmacologicas, Buenos Aires, Argentina

REFERENCES

Alousi, A. and Weiner, N. 1966. The regulation of norepinephrine synthesis in sympathetic nerves. Effect of nerve stimulation, cocaine and catecholamine releasing agents. Proc. Nat. Acad. Sci. 56: 1491-1496.

Banks, P. and Helle, K. 1965. The release of protein from the stimulated adrenal medulla. Biochem. J. 97: 40C-41C.

Blakeley, A.G.H., Brown, G.L., Dearnaley, D.P. and Harrison, V. 1969. The effect of nerve stimulation on the synthesis of ^{3}H-norepinephrine from ^{3}H-tyrosine in the isolated blood-perfused cat spleen. J. Physiol. (London) 200: 59p-60p.

Blaschko, H., Comline, R.L., Schneider, F.H. and Smith, A.D. 1967. Secretion of a chromaffin granule protein, chromogranin, from the adrenal gland after splanchnic stimulation. Nature 215: 58-59.

Bogdanski, D.F. and Brodie, B.B. 1969. The effects of inorganic ions on the storage and uptake of ^{3}H-norepinephrine by rat heart slices. J. Pharmacol. Exp. Therap. 165: 181-189.

Brown, G.L. and Gillespie, J.S. 1957. The output of sympathetic transmitter from the spleen of the cat. J. Physiol. 138: 81-102.

Costa, E. 1970. Simple neuronal models to estimate turnover rate of noradrenergic transmitters in vivo. In: Biochemical Psychopharmacology 2: 169-204.

Dahlström, A. 1967. The intraneuronal distribution of noradrenaline and transport and life span of amine storage granules in the sympathetic adrenergic neuron. Arch. Exp. Pathol. Pharmakol. 257: 93-115.

Dahlström, A. and Haggendal, J. 1966. Studies on the transport and life span of amine storage granules in a peripheral adrenergic neuron system. Acta. Physiol. Scand. 67: 278-288.

Dairman, W., Gordon, R. Spector, S., Sjoerdsma, A. and Udenfriend, S. 1968. Increased synthesis of catecholamines in the intact rat following administration of α-adrenergic blocking agents. Molec. Pharmacol. 4: 457-464.

DePotter, W.P., Schaepdryver, A.F., Moerman, E.J. and Smith, A.D. 1969. Evidence for the release of vesicle-proteins together with noradrenaline upon stimulation of the splenic nerve. J. Physiol. 204: 102-104.

Douglas, W.W. 1966 a. The mechanism of release of catecholamines from the adrenal medulla. Pharmacol. Rev. 18: 471-480.

Douglas, W.W. 1966 b. Calcium-dependent links in stimulus-secretion coupling in the adrenal medulla and neurohypophysis. In: Mechanisms of Release of Biogenic Amines. (Eds. Von Euler, U.S., Rosell, S. and Uvnas, B.) Oxford: Pergamon Press, pp. 267-289.

Douglas, W.W. and Poisner, A.M. 1966. On the relation between ATP splitting and secretion in the adrenal chromaffin cell:

extrusion of ATP (unhydrolyzed) during release of catecholamines. J. Physiol. 183: 249-256.

Gewirtz, G.P. and Kopin, I.J. 1970. Effect of intermittent nerve stimulation on norepinephrine synthesis and mobilization in the perfused cat spleen. J. Pharmacol. Exp. Ther. 175: 514-520.

Gillespie, J.S. and Kirpekar, S.M. 1965. The inactivation of infused noradrenaline by the cat spleen. J. Physiol. 176: 205-227.

Gordon, R., Reid, J.V.O., Sjoerdsma, A. and Udenfriend, S. 1966 a. Increased synthesis of norepinephrine in the cat heart on electrical stimulation of the stellate ganglion. Molec. Pharmacol. 2: 606-613.

Gordon, R., Spector, S., Sjoerdsma, A. and Udenfriend, S. 1966 b. Increased synthesis of norepinephrine in the intact rat during exercise and exposure to cold. J. Pharmacol. Exp. Therap. 153: 440-447.

Hertting, G. and Axelrod, J. 1961. Fate of tritiated noradrenaline at the sympathetic nerve endings. Nature 192: 172-173.

Hertting, G., Axelrod, J., Kopin, I.J. and Whitby, L.G. 1961. Lack of uptake of catecholamines after chronic denervation of sympathetic nerves. Nature 189: 66.

Huković, S. and Muscholl, E. 1962. Die Noradrenaline - Abgabe aus dem isolierten kaninchen - herzen bei sympatischer Nervenreizung und ihre pharmakologische beeinflussung. Arch. Exp. Pathol. Pharmakol. 244: 81-96.

Ikeda, M., Fahien, L.A. and Udenfriend, S. 1966. A kinetic study of bovine adrenal tyrosine hydroxylase. J. Biol. Chem. 241: 4452-4456.

Iversen, L.L. and Kravitz, E.A. 1966. Sodium dependence on transmitter uptake at adrenergic nerve terminals. Mol. Pharmacol. 2: 360-362.

Iversen, L.L. and Langer, S.Z. 1969. Effects of phenoxybenzamine on the uptake and metabolism of noradrenaline in the rat heart and vas deferens. Brit. J. Pharmacol. 37: 627-637.

Kirpekar, S.M. and Misu, Y. 1967. Release of noradrenaline by splenic nerve stimulation and its dependence on calcium. J. Physiol. 188: 219-234.

Kirpekar, S.M. and Wakade, A.R. 1968. Factors influencing noradrenaline uptake by the perfused spleen of the cat. J. Physiol. 194: 609-626.

Kirshner, N., Sage, H.J., Smith, W.J. and Kirshner, A.G. 1966. Release of catecholamines and specific protein from adrenal glands. Science 154: 529-531.

Kopin, I.J., Breese, G.R., Krauss, K.R. and Weise, V.K. 1968. Selective release of newly synthesized norepinephrine from the cat spleen during sympathetic nerve stimulation. J. Pharmacol. Exp. Therap. 161: 271-278.

Kopin, I.J., Weise, V.K. and Sedvall, G.C. 1969. Effect of false transmitters on norepinephrine synthesis. J. Pharmacol. Exp. Therap. 170: 246-252.

Kuczenski, R.T. and Mandell, A.J. 1972 a. Allosteric activation of hypothalamic tyrosine hydroxylase by ions and sulphated mucopolysaccharides. J. Neurochem. 19: 131-137.

Kuczenski, R.T. and Mandell, A.J. 1972 b. Regulatory properties of soluble and particulate rat brain tyrosine hydroxylase. J. Biol. Chem. 247: 3114-3122.

Lloyd, T. and Weiner, N. 1971. Isolation and characterization of a tyrosine hydroxylase cofactor from bovine adrenal medulla. Mol. Pharmacol. 7: 569-589.

Oliverio, A. and Stjarne, L. 1965. Acceleration of noradrenaline turnover in the mouse heart by cold exposure. Life. Sci. 4: 2339-2343.

Roth, R. H., Stjarne, L. and Euler, U.S. von. 1967. Factors influencing the rate of norepinephrine biosynthesis in nerve tissue. J. Pharmacol. Exp. Therap. 158: 373-377.

Rutledge, C.O. and Weiner, N. 1967. The effect of reserpine upon the synthesis of norepinephrine in the isolated rabbit heart. J. Pharmacol. Exp. Therap. 157: 290-302.

Schneider, F.H., Smith, A.D. and Winkler, H. 1967. Secretion from the adrenal medulla: biochemical evidence for exocytosis. Brit. J. Pharmacol. 31: 94-104.

Sedvall, G.C. and Kopin, I.J. 1967. Acceleration of norepinephrine synthesis in the rat submaxillary gland in vivo during sympathetic nerve stimulation. Life Sci. 6: 45-51.

Sedvall, G.C., Weise, V.K. and Kopin, I.J. 1968. The rate of norepinephrine synthesis measured in vivo during short intervals: influence of adrenergic nerve impulse activity. J. Pharmacol. Exp. Therap. 159: 274-282.

Smith, A.D., DePotter, W.P., Moerman, E.J. and De Schaepdryver, A.F. 1970. Release of dopamine-β-hydroxylase and chromogranin A upon stimulation of the splenic nerve. Tissue and Cell 2: 547-568.

Smith, C.B. 1963. Enhancement by reserpine and α-methyl-DOPA of the effects of d-amphetamine upon the locomotor activity of mice. J. Pharmacol. Exp. Ther. 142: 343-350.

Thoenen, H., Huerlimann, A. and Haefely, W. 1964. Wirkungen von Phenoxybenzamin, Phentolamin und Azapetin auf adrenergische Synapsen der Katzenmilz. Helv. Physiol. Acta. 22: 148-161.

Udenfriend, S., Zaltzman-Nirenberg, P. and Nagatsu, T. 1965. Inhibitors of purified beef adrenal tyrosine hydroxylase. Biochem. Pharmacol. 14: 837-845.

Waymire, J.C., Bjur, R. and Weiner, N. 1971. Assay of tyrosine hydroxylase by coupled decarboxylation of dopa formed from 1-^{14}C-L-tyrosine. Anal. Biochem. 43: 588-600.

Weiner, N. 1970. Regulation of norepinephrine biosynthesis. Ann. Rev. Pharmacol. 10: 372-390.

Weiner, N. and Bjur, R. 1972. The role of monoamine oxidase in the regulation of norepinephrine synthesis. In: Monoamines Oxidases: New Vistas. (Eds. Costa, E. and Sandler, M.), Vol. 5, Raven Press, pp. 409-419.

Weiner, N., Cloutier, G., Bjur, R. and Pfeffer, R.I. 1972. Modification of norepinephrine synthesis in intact tissue by drugs and during short-term adrenergic nerve stimulation. Pharmacol. Rev. 24: 203-221.

Weiner, N. and Rabadjija, M. 1968. The effect of nerve stimulation on the synthesis and metabolism of norepinephrine in the isolated guinea-pig hypogastric nerve-vas deferens preparation. J. Pharmacol. Exp. Therap. 160: 61-71.

Weiner, N. and Selvaratnam, I. 1968. The effect of tyramine on the synthesis of norepinephrine. J. Pharmacol. Exp. Therap. 161: 21-33.

Weinshilboum, R.M., Thoa, N.B., Johnson, D.G., Kopin, I.J. and Axelrod, J. 1971. Proportional release of norepinephrine and dopamine-β-hydroxylase from sympathetic nerves. Science 174: 1349-1351.

Weissman, A., Koe, B.K. and Tenen, S.S. 1966 Antiamphetamine effects following inhibition of tyrosine hydroxylase. J. Pharmacol. Exp. Therap. 151: 339-352.

Wilkinson, G.N. 1961. Statistical estimations in enzyme kinetics. Biochem. J. 80: 324-332.

USE OF SINGLE UNIT RECORDING IN CORRELATING TRANSMITTER

TURNOVER WITH IMPULSE FLOW IN MONOAMINE NEURONS

George K. Aghajanian, Benjamin S. Bunney and
Michael J. Kuhar

Departments of Psychiatry and Pharmacology
Yale University School of Medicine
New Haven, Connecticut   06519

In peripheral tissues there is clear evidence for a relationship between norepinephrine (NE) turnover and impulse activity in
adrenergic nerves (Alousi and Weiner, 1966; Gordon et al., 1966;
Stjarne et al., 1967; Sedvall et al., 1968). In the case of
monoamine neurons in the central nervous system the demonstration
of a correlation between impulse flow and turnover is inherently
more difficult. Initially, support for this concept came from
studies in which the metabolic effects of interrupting or stimulating known central monoamine pathways were determined. The first
experiments along these lines were carried out in spinal transected
animals by Andén and his coworkers. These studies were based on
the fact that the serotonin (5-hydroxytryptamine; 5-HT) and NE
nerve terminals of the spinal cord originate from 5-HT and NE-
containing perikarya of the lower brain stem (Carlsson et al.,
1964; Dahlström and Fuxe, 1965; Fuxe, 1965). Depletion caused by
inhibition at any step of NE or 5-HT biosynthesis was shown to be
highly dependent upon nervous impulse flow since depletion was much
more pronounced on the cranial than caudal side of a spinal transection (Andén et al., 1966 a,c, 1967 a). These studies implied
that the rate of turnover of 5-HT and NE within these two monoamine
pathways in the spinal cord was greater in the presence of a normal
flow of impulses. An effort was then made to determine whether
various drug-induced changes in monoamine metabolism were dependent
upon intact neuronal pathways. Amine depletion produced by agents
which displace or release 5-HT and NE from storage granules, was
found not to be prevented on the caudal side of a spinal transection (Andén et al., 1967 a, 1969). However, the increase in amines
obtained after monoamine oxidase inhibition was substantially
reduced caudal to the transection (Andén et al., 1967 a). Although

this specific result has apparently not been confirmed (Meek and
Fuxe, 1971), a general concept emerged from these studies to the
effect that drugs which increase or decrease central monoamine
turnover might do so by altering the rate of impulse flow within
monoaminergic pathways.

A similar approach (i.e., the analysis of the effects of
axotomy on monoamine turnover) has now been extended to studies
on the brain. Many antipsychotic drugs of the phenothiazine or
butyrophenone type have been shown to increase dopamine (DA)
turnover in the striatum (Carlsson and Lindqvist, 1963; Andén
et al., 1964 b; Juorio et al., 1966; Neff and Costa, 1966;
Nybäck et al., 1967; Corrodi et al., 1967; Gey and Pletscher,
1968). It has been hypothesized that a DA receptor blockade
produced by these drugs might lead to a compensatory increase in
the activity of dopaminergic cells via a neuronal feedback
mechanism (e.g., cf. Carlsson and Lindqvist, 1963). In support
of this hypothesis it has been shown that the increase in DA
turnover produced by these drugs is dependent upon the intactness
of the pathways arising from the DA-containing perikarya in the
substantia nigra and ventral tegmental area and projecting to the
dopaminergic terminals in the caudate-putamen and olfactory
tubercules (Andén et al., 1971; Nybäck and Sedvall, 1971; Cheramy
et al., 1970). These studies parallel the earlier ones in spinal
transected animals and extend the concept of impulse-flow dependent changes in brain monoamine turnover. The application of the
axotomy approach to the 5-HT system in the brain has yielded less
clear-cut results. It has been found that after acute unilateral
interruption of the fibers from 5-HT-containing neurons in the
midbrain raphe nuclei projecting to the forebrain (Dahlström and
Fuxe, 1965; Fuxe, 1965; Andén, 1966 b), the turnover of 5-HT on
the lesioned side does not differ markedly from that on the control
side (Bédard et al., 1972). In addition, the accumulation of
5-HT after inhibition of monoamine oxidase was not significantly
influenced by the hemisection. Thus, the relationship between
turnover and impulse flow as judged by the axotomy approach is
less clear for the 5-HT than DA system in brain. However, it has
been shown both in the spinal cord (Andén et al., 1964 a) and
brain (Aghajanian et al., 1967; Sheard and Aghajanian, 1968;
Gumulka et al., 1969; Kostowski et al., 1969; Shields and Eccleston,
1972) that stimulation of 5-HT pathways does result in an increased
turnover of this amine.

A new approach to the study of the relationship between monoamine turnover and impulse flow within monoaminergic systems is
the direct recording of the rate of firing of these neurons. The
effect upon firing rate of various drugs and other substances
which alter monoamine turnover can then be determined. The histochemical localization of certain monoamine neuronal perikarya to

well defined nuclei permits a high degree of assurance that the
recordings in such cases are from bona fide monoamine cells.
Specifically, there are three main clusters of monoamine neuronal
perikarya in the brain that lend themselves to recording purposes
as follows: 1) the locus coeruleus, a nucleus of NE-containing
cells located in the anterior pons, just beneath the ependyma of
the lateral aspect of the 4th ventricle; 2) the dorsal raphe
nucleus of the midbrain (as well as other raphe nuclei of the
brainstem) which are composed primarily of 5-HT-containing neurons;
and 3) the substantia nigra (zona compacta) and medial ventral
tegmentum, which are largely composed of DA-containing neurons
(Dahlström and Fuxe, 1965; Ungerstedt, 1971; Björklund et al.,
1971). By recording the electrical activity of these neurons
it is possible to test directly those hypotheses derived from
biochemical studies concerning the effects of drugs and other
treatments on the rate of firing of monoaminergic neurons. In
the following sections studies in which this approach is applied
to 5-HT and catecholamine (CA)-containing neurons in brain will
be described.

SINGLE CELL RECORDINGS: 5-HT-CONTAINING NEURONS

Psychotomimetic Drugs

It has been shown that administration of d-lysergic acid
diethylamide (LSD) produces a small but significant rise in the
concentration of 5-HT in brain (Freedman, 1961), a reduction in
the principal 5-HT metabolite, 5-hydroxyindoleacetic acid (Rosecrans
et al., 1967), a reduction in the formation of 5-HT from labelled
tryptophan precursor (Lin et al., 1969; Schubert et al., 1970),
and a reduced rate of depletion following inhibition of 5-HT
synthesis (Andén et al., 1968). Taken together, these studies
indicate that LSD causes a reduction in 5-HT turnover. Conversely,
stimulation of the raphe nuclei has been found to increase 5-HT
turnover (Aghajanian et al., 1967; Kostowski et al., 1969;
Gumulka et al., 1969; Shields and Eccelston, 1972). Since the
turnover of 5-HT is reduced by LSD it has been suggested that this
drug might depress the firing of 5-HT containing neurons of the
raphe (Aghajanian and Freedman, 1968; Andén et al., 1968). Direct
experimental examination of this hypothesis has demonstrated that
LSD and related psychotomimetic drugs have a powerful inhibitory
effect on the rate of firing of single raphe neurons in rats
(Aghajanian et al., 1968, 1970 a). The inhibition is seen at very
low doses of LSD (10-20 µg/kg) and is highly selective for raphe
neurons. N,N-dimethyltryptamine, a psychotomimetic related in
chemical structure to both LSD and 5-HT, is also effective in
inhibiting raphe neurons (Aghajanian et al., 1970 a).

The route of drug administration in these initial studies

was parenteral and therefore the precise site of action is uncertain.
To investigate the possibility that LSD might have a direct inhibitory action upon raphe neurons, the drug was applied locally by
microiontophoresis from multi-barreled micropipettes (Aghajanian
et al., 1972 a). Very dilute solutions of LSD (5 x 10^{-4} M in
5 x 10^{-2} M saline) were used to avoid nonspecific leakage effects
and excessive retaining currents. Under these conditions LSD
represents less than 1% of the cations in solution. The transport
number (Curtis, 1964) for LSD under these conditions was determined
to be 0.0028 (Haigler and Aghajanian, unpublished data). LSD in
this dilute solution at ejection currents which did not alter the
rate of firing of most non-raphe cells, had a powerful inhibitory
action on raphe neurons (Aghajanian et al., 1972 a). This inhibition was not accompanied by any decrease in action potential size
which might have indicated a non-specific, local anesthetic-like
effect. Interestingly, 5-HT applied by microiontophoresis was
also inhibitory. At submaximal ejection currents the inhibitory
effects of LSD and 5-HT given simultaneously were additive. The
fact that LSD has a direct depressant effect on raphe neurons does
not rule out the alternate possibility that LSD activates an
inhibitory feedback loop involving neurons postsynaptic to the
raphe. In any case, no matter whether the LSD-induced inhibition
of raphe neurons is through a direct effect, a feedback loop, or
perhaps some combination of the two, the inhibition of firing
correlates well with the observed reduction in 5-HT turnover seen
after systemic administration of LSD. On the other hand, mescaline,
which has variable effects on raphe cell firing rate (Aghajanian,
et al., 1970 a), does not appear to reduce 5-HT turnover (Freedman
et al., 1970).

Monoamine Oxidase Inhibitors

Monoamine oxidase inhibitors markedly increase 5-HT content
in brain by blocking its catabolism (Brodie et al., 1959).
Associated with this increase in concentration is a leakage of
5-HT into the ventricular fluid (Goodrich, 1969). In terms of
a neuronal feedback concept it might be expected that a leakage
of 5-HT onto postsynaptic receptor sites would lead to adjust-
ments in rate of firing of the presynaptic neurons. Therefore,
the possibility that monoamine oxidase inhibitors might alter the
rate of firing of raphe neurons was examined. All monoamine oxidase inhibitors tested, regardless of structural category (e.g.,
the hydrazines, iproniazid and nialamide, and the nonhydrazines,
pargyline and tranylcypromine) were found to depress the rate of
firing of raphe neurons (Aghajanian et al., 1970 b). With the
exception of iproniazid, an inhibitor with a slow onset of action,
this change was evident within 15-30 minutes after intraperitoneal
administration, a period during which there is rapid accumulation
of serotonin in brain (Tozer et al., 1966). This effect was

shown to be quite selective as is indicated by the fact that the
rate of firing of neurons in neighboring areas (e.g., pontine
nuclei, central grey, reticular formation, and interpeduncular
nucleus) was usually unaltered. While these results are consistent with a negative neuronal feedback mechanism, it is also
possible that the inhibition is caused by a local "leakage" of
5-HT from recurrent collaterals or the raphe cells themselves.
Also, the raphe depression after monoamine oxidase inhibitors
cannot necessarily be attributed solely to the increase in 5-HT,
since the concentration of catecholamines in brain also increases
after the administration of these drugs. Therefore, it is significant that p-chlorophenylalanine, a relatively selective inhibitor
of 5-HT synthesis (Koe and Weissman, 1966; Jéquier et al., 1967)
was effective in blocking the inhibition of raphe neurons by
monoamine oxidase inhibitors (Aghajanian, et al., 1970 b). This
suggests that the action of monoamine oxidase inhibitors upon
raphe neurons is mediated somehow through an accumulation of 5-HT.

5-HT Precursors

To test further the possibility of an inverse relationship
between raphe firing and 5-HT concentration the immediate precursor of 5-HT, 5-hydroxytryptophan, was given. 5-Hydroxy-
tryptophan has been shown to enter the brain and to induce an
increase in serotonin levels (Bogdanski, 1958). However, contrary
to expectations, high doses of L-5-hydroxytryptophan (up to 100 mg/
kg) had no significant effect on the firing of raphe units
(Aghajanian et al., 1970 b). This result seems inconsistent with
the hypothesis of a negative feedback or reciprocal relationship
between 5-HT level and firing rate. However, raphe cell fluorescence is not appreciably increased by the systemic administration
of 5-hydroxytryptophan even in the presence of a peripheral decarboxylase inhibitor (Dahlström and Fuxe, 1965; Fuxe et al., 1971).
Since endothelial cells throughout the brain become fluorescent
after administration of 5-hydroxytryptophan, it is possible that
5-hydroxytryptophan is metabolized in the latter cells before it
can reach raphe neurons. Consistent with this interpretation is
the fact that only a small fraction of brain aromatic amino acid
decarboxylase, the enzyme which converts 5-hydroxytryptophan to
5-HT is specifically located within the raphe system (Kuhar et al.,
1971). Moreover, there is an abnormal regional distribution of
5-HT following administration of this precursor (Moir and
Eccleston, 1968). Thus, the failure of 5-hydroxytryptophan to
depress the firing of raphe neurons does not provide firm negative
evidence against the notion of a reciprocal relationship between
5-HT levels and neuronal activity.

Loading doses of tryptophan, the initial precursor of 5-HT,
also increase brain 5-HT concentration (Hess and Doepfner, 1961;

Eccleston et al., 1965; Weber and Horita, 1965). The dependence
of brain 5-HT synthesis upon L-tryptophan levels is well within
the physiological range for this dietary amino acid (Fernstrom
and Wurtman, 1971). This finding can be explained by the fact
that tryptophan hydroxylase, the rate limiting enzyme responsible
for its conversion to 5-HT, has a high Km and the levels of
tryptophan normally present in brain would not saturate the enzyme
(Jéquier et al., 1967). There is evidence based on lesion studies
that brain tryptophan hydroxylase is located almost exclusively
within the raphe system (Kuhar et al., 1971). Therefore, 5-HT
synthesized from L-tryptophan should be selectively located within
raphe neurons. Consistent with this expectation is the finding
that there is a marked and selective increase in raphe cell fluorescence after the parenteral (Aghajanian and Asher, 1971) or
intraventricular administration of L-tryptophan (Aghajanian,
unpublished observations). This effect has a high degree of
specificity, as is evidenced by the fact that no neurons or other
cells outside the raphe show an increase in fluorescence after
the injection of tryptophan. The question thus arises as to whether
loading doses of L-tryptophan alter the rate of firing of raphe
neurons under the same conditions in which the fluorescence of
raphe cells is increased. Such studies have shown that the firing
of raphe neurons is depressed to the same extent as after treatment with monoamine oxidase inhibitors (Aghajanian, 1972). The
inhibition begins to appear within 15 minutes after L-tryptophan
administration at a time when the increase in raphe cell fluorescence is already evident. In contrast, D-tryptophan has no effect
on either rate of firing or fluorescence. Specificity is further
demonstrated by the fact that the catecholamine precursors, L-
tyrosine and L-3,4-dihydroxyphenylalanine, do not alter either
raphe cell fluorescence or firing rate.

The above results suggest that the depression of raphe
activity induced by L-tryptophan is associated with an increase
in the amount of serotonin within raphe cells. The selective
5-HT depletor, p-chlorophenylalanine (Koe and Weissman, 1966)
was used as a means of testing this hypothesis. This inhibitor
of tryptophan hydroxylase (Jéquier et al., 1967) has been shown
to prevent an increase in whole brain serotonin after the administration of L-tryptophan (Koe and Weissman, 1966; Aghajanian and
Asher, 1971). However, p-chlorophenylalanine does not prevent
the L-tryptophan-induced enhancement of raphe cell fluorescence
(Aghajanian and Asher, 1971). Furthermore, p-chlorophenylalanine
fails to block the usual depression of raphe unit firing by
L-tryptophan (Aghajanian, 1972). The possibility exists that
the fluorophore observed in raphe cells following the administration of L-tryptophan to p-chlorophenylalanine-pretreated animals
represents a different compound than in the absence of pretreatment. Björklund et al. (1971), using microspectrofluorometric

techniques, have suggested that some raphe neurons may in fact
contain a monoamine other than serotonin. However, it has
recently been shown that p-chlorophenylalanine is much more
effective in blocking 5-HT synthesis in the terminals than in the
perikarya of raphe neurons (Aghajanian et al., 1972 b). In fact,
despite p-chlorophenylalanine pretreatment, there is a marked
increase in raphe cell body 5-HT content after L-tryptophan loading. Since it has been shown that raphe cells can be inhibited
by the local, microiontophoretic application of 5-HT (see above)
it is possible that the local increase in 5-HT in raphe perikarya
after L-tryptophan loading results in a leakage of 5-HT onto
receptors which may be on the external surface of the cells.

Drugs that Block 5-HT Uptake

Certain tricyclic antidepressant drugs are also believed to
enhance the availability of brain indoleamines to receptors, but
by a different mechanism than do the monoamine oxidase inhibitors
or L-tryptophan. Tricyclic compounds with a tertiary side-
chain amine (e.g. imipramine, chlorimipramine, and amytriptyline)
have been shown to block the uptake of 5-HT into brain slices or
synaptosomes (Ross and Renyi, 1969; Carlsson, 1970; Shaskan and
Snyder, 1970). Since "reuptake" into nerve terminals by a high
affinity mechanism probably represents the major mechanisms by
which the action of 5-HT or other indoleamines would be terminated,
the tricyclic drugs can serve as an additional means for studying
interactions between indole "availability" and raphe firing.
The membrane uptake mechanism for 5-HT into synaptosomes under high
affinity conditions (i.e. at low concentrations) has been shown to
be specifically localized to nerve terminals of the raphe neurons
(Kuhar et al., 1972 a,b; Kuhar and Aghajanian, 1972). Selective
lesions of the midbrain raphe nuclei, which result in a loss of
5-HT-fluorescent terminals in the forebrain and large decreases
in forebrain 5-HT content and tryptophan hydroxylase activity,
lead to a marked loss of 5-HT uptake into forebrain synaptosomes.
(Figure 1). The uptake of amino acids, GABA, and catecholamines
in the same animals was unaffected. Thus, drugs which block 5-HT
uptake should have a selective action upon the raphe and 5-HT
receptive neurons. Consistent with the feedback hypothesis
(Corrodi and Fuxe, 1969), tricyclic drugs known to block serotonin
uptake, such as imipramine and chlorimipramine, were found to
markedly inhibit raphe firing (Sheard et al., 1972; Figure 2).
In contrast, their secondary amine analogues (e.g. desmethylimipramine), which are not highly effective in blocking serotonin
uptake, fail to alter the firing rate of raphe cells except at
much higher doses. As in the case of monoamine oxidase inhibitors,
the depression of raphe unit firing by the tricyclic drugs could
be partially or totally blocked by pretreatment with p-chlorophenylalanine, suggesting that the tricyclic drugs act indirectly in this

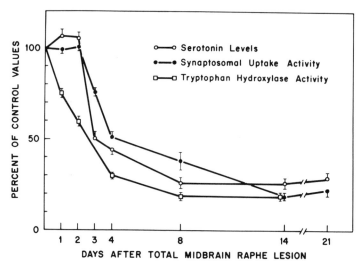

Figure 1. Time course of reduction of serotonin levels, synaptosomal uptake activity and tryptophan hydroxylase activity in forebrains of animals with total midbrain raphe lesions. Control values of synaptosomal uptake activity were 0.91 ± 0.11 µµmol of ^{3}H-5-HT per 4 min per 1.8 mg of protein (mean $\pm$ S.D., n=5), and of serotonin levels were 397 ± 50 ng/g of tissue (mean $\pm$ S.D., n=6). Tryptophan hydroxylase activity is included from a previous study. From Kuhar et al. (1972 b), reprinted with the permission of the Williams and Wilkins Co., Baltimore, Maryland.

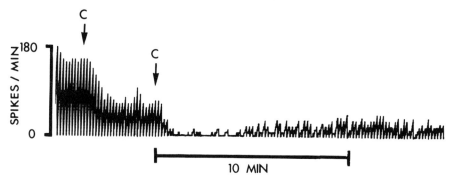

Figure 2. Effect of chlorimipramine (C) upon average discharge rate of a neuronal unit in the dorsal raphe nucleus of the midbrain. An initial dose of chlorimipramine HCl (0.25 mg/kg, i.v.) rapidly resulted in a 50% reduction in rate of firing. An additional 0.5 mg/kg caused a temporary cessation of firing. A slight recovery of gradual onset was seen within 15 min. For further details see Sheard et al. (1972).

system by preventing the termination of 5-HT action through the
reuptake mechanism. It is significant that there is a close
parallel between the ability of the tricyclic drugs to produce
a decrease in 5-HT turnover (Carlsson et al., 1969; Corrodi and
Fuxe, 1969) and a decrease in raphe cell firing.

SINGLE CELL RECORDINGS: CA NEURONS

CA Receptor Blockers

The clinically effective phenothiazines and the butyrophenone, haloperidol, have been shown to increase DA metabolite
concentration and turnover in the corpus striatum, requiring an
anatomically intact dopaminergic system to do so (Andén et al.,
1971; Nybäck and Sedvall, 1971; Cheramy et al., 1970). It has
been hypothesized that the phenothiazines and haloperidol, being
structurally related to dopamine (Horn and Snyder, 1971) have an
affinity for postsynaptic dopamine receptor sites. A receptor
blockade produced by these drugs might then lead to a compensatory
increase in activity of the dopaminergic cells via a neuronal
feedback mechanism (Carlsson and Lindqvist, 1963). Single unit
recordings from DA-containing cells in the rat substantia nigra
(zona compacta) and midbrain ventral tegmental area before and
after the administration of the antipsychotic drugs (e.g.
chlorpromazine, haloperidol, trifluoperazine, perphenazine and
fluphenazine) provide direct evidence in support of this hypothesis.
All of the above drugs markedly increase cell firing rate in very
small doses (Bunney et al., 1972 b). This effect was shown to be
selective in that the rate of firing of the great majority of cells
in other areas of the midbrain was either not affected or decreased
with administration of these drugs. Significantly, promethazine
and desimipramine, which have little antipsychotic activity
(Klein and Davis, 1969) and no effect on DA turnover (Nybäck et al.,
1968), had no effect on cell firing rate. Thus a direct correlation is established between the effect of these drugs on DA turnover and their effect on DA cell firing rate.

CA Release

Amphetamine has been shown to increase release of newly
synthesized NE and DA and block their reuptake (Glowinski
and Axelrod, 1966; Glowinski et al., 1966; Besson et al.,
1959, 1971 a,b). It has been suggested that amphetamine, by
increasing the concentration of CA postsynaptically, initiates
neuronal feedback inhibition of CA containing units (Corrodi
et al., 1967). By means of single unit recordings made from
the NE-containing cells of the locus coeruleus and dopaminergic cells of the rat midbrain (Dahlström and Fuxe, 1965; Ungerstedt, 1971) amphetamine has been shown to decrease greatly cell

firing rate in doses of 0.25 mg/kg to 1.50 mg/kg (Graham and
Aghajanian, 1971; Bunney et al., 1972 a; Figure 3). These
results are consistent with the neuronal feedback inhibition
theory proposed as an explanation of amphetamine effects on CA
metabolism. Alpha-methyl-p-tyrosine, which blocks the first
step in the synthesis of DA (Spector et al., 1965) blocks the

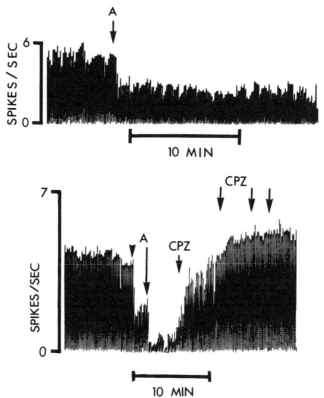

Figure 3.   (Upper) Effect of D-amphetamine (A) on the firing rate
of a dopaminergic cell.   Intravenous injection of D-amphetamine
(0.25 mg/kg) depressed unit activity approximately 40% with no
significant return toward baseline rate after 17 minutes. (Lower)
Reverse of D-amphetamine (A) induced depression of a dopaminergic
cell by chlorpromazine (CPZ). Two intravenous injections of D-
amphetamine (0.25; 0.50 mg/kg) resulted in a 75% decrease in the
activity of a dopamine-containing cell. Chlorpromazine (0.25 mg/kg)
intravenously, rapidly reversed the amphetamine induced depression
and returned firing rate almost to baseline levels. An additional
0.5 mg/kg of chlorpromazine increased firing rate beyond baseline
rate. Two further doses of chlorpromazine (0.5 mg/kg each) had
little additional effect on unit activity. Methods as described in
Bunney et al. (1972 a,b).

amphetamine induced DA cell depression (Bunney et al., 1972 a),
lending further support to the evidence that amphetamine exerts
its action mainly on the newly synthesized DA pools. Antipsychotic
phenothiazines and haloperidol also prevent and reverse the marked
slowing of unit activity seen with amphetamine (Bunney et al.,
1972 b; Figure 3).

Dopamine Receptor Stimulation

The first evidence that a drug might mimic the effect of the
putative neurotransmitter DA through direct stimulation of DA
receptor sites came from behavioral studies of apomorphine-induced
stereotyped behavior in rats (Ernst, 1967). Biochemically, apomorphine was found to retard depletion of brain DA produced by the
tyrosine hydroxylase inhibitor alpha-methyl-p-tyrosine--an effect
completely blocked by haloperidol (Andén et al., 1967 b; Persson
and Waldeck, 1970). In addition, apomorphine has been shown to
decrease the accumulation of H^3-DA when given i.p. 15 minutes
before H^3-tyrosine (Persson, 1970). It was suggested that these
findings could be explained by hypothesizing a decrease in neuronal
activity secondary to DA receptor stimulation by apomorphine
(Andén et al., 1967 b). Apomorphine has also been shown to inhibit
tyrosine hydroxylase activity directly, but only in doses higher
than those necessary to induce functional changes (Goldstein et al.,
1970). Again, by the use of single unit recording from dopaminergic units it has been possible to test directly hypotheses
derived from biochemical and, in this case, behavioral studies
concerning the effects of apomorphine on dopaminergic neurons.
Apomorphine given intravenously in the small dose of 0.1 mg/kg
temporarily inhibits DA unit activity (Bunney et al., 1972 a).
This effect is unaffected by pretreatment with alpha-methyl-p-tyrosine but is blocked by haloperidol. Thus the action of apomorphine on these cells, unlike that of amphetamine, was not
dependent on the presence of a newly synthesized pool of DA.

Dopamine Precursors

We have seen that amphetamine, possibly by increasing the
release of DA from dopaminergic terminals (and thus increasing
the concentration of DA available at postsynaptic receptors)
decreases DA cell firing rate. To test further the effect of
increased brain DA concentration on DA unit activity the
immediate precursor of DA, L-DOPA, was administered with high
and low doses of an aromatic amino acid decarboxylase inhibitor--
RO4-4602. In low doses RO4-4602 (50 mg/kg) does not cross the
blood brain barrier in appreciable amounts, thus selectively
preventing the peripheral decarboxylation of L-DOPA to DA. This
results in greater brain DOPA concentrations and ultimately
greater DA formation in the CNS (Butcher and Engel, 1969). At

high doses (800 mg/kg) enough RO4-4602 enters the brain to inhibit effectively the decarboxylation of DOPA to DA (Bédard et al., 1971) centrally, and thus lowers DA levels.

When conversion of L-DOPA to DA was prevented by high doses of RO4-4602, the systemic administration of L-DOPA had no effect on dopaminergic neuronal activity. However, after low doses of RO4-4602, L-DOPA markedly increases brain DA concentration and the rate of firing of DA neurons is decreased (Bunney et al., 1972 a). Again, these data suggest a correlation between increased transmitter availability and decreased impulse flow.

SUMMARY AND CONCLUSIONS

Direct unit recordings from both 5-HT and CA-containing neurons have indicated the existence of striking correlations between alterations in impulse flow and certain changes in monoamine metabolism. There appear to be two general mechanisms by which such a relationship can come about. First, there is a category of drug or precursor treatment which has a marked direct effect on monoamine synthesis or degradation. In such cases, changes in the rate of firing of monoamine neurons seem to be secondary to the biochemical changes. A clear example of this in the 5-HT system is the inhibition of raphe cell firing induced by monoamine oxidase inhibitors. The reduction in firing rate is associated with the accumulation of 5-HT, and when the synthesis of 5-HT is blocked by p-chlorophenylalanine no inhibition of raphe firing occurs. Another example would be the enhanced synthesis of 5-HT after L-tryptophan loading. The increase in synthesis resulting from precursor loading is presumably the cause and not the consequence of the associated decrease in the rate of firing of raphe neurons. Similar considerations can be applied to the CA neuronal systems. The depression of firing of DA-containing neurons by L-DOPA would seem to be secondary to an increased production of DA since the effect is blocked by the inhibition of central aromatic amino acid decarboxylase.

A second type of interaction between impulse flow and monoamine turnover can be postulated in which the metabolic change is secondary to an effect on neuronal firing rate. In the 5-HT system, LSD may be representative of this category. This drug does not appear to alter directly enzymes involved in the synthesis or degradation of 5-HT (Freedman et al., 1970; Schubert et al., 1970) yet it causes a reduction in turnover. Moreover, neither the depression of raphe firing nor certain behavioral effects of LSD (Appel and Freedman, 1970) are prevented by an inhibition of 5-HT synthesis. It has been suggested that LSD has a direct 5-HT receptor-stimulating action (Aghajanian and Freedman, 1968; Andén et al., 1968) which could result in a

compensatory neuronal feedback inhibition of raphe cell firing.
However, it may not be necessary to invoke the operation of such a
neuronal feedback loop in view of the fact that LSD has been shown
to inhibit raphe cells by direct, microiontophoretic application.
In either case, the decreased 5-HT turnover observed after LSD
may be secondary to a diminished rate of impulse flow in the raphe
system. A similar model could apply to the effect of apomorphine
or antipsychotic drugs upon DA neurons since these drugs have been
postulated respectively to directly stimulate or block DA receptors.

As for other drugs tested, a more complex relationship between
impulse flow and monoamine turnover must be considered. The
ability of the tertiary amine tricyclic compounds to depress raphe
unit firing is dependent upon the availability of 5-HT since this
effect is prevented by p-chlorophenylalanine. Presumably the
consequences of a block in reuptake of 5-HT produced by these
drugs is dependent upon an availability of 5-HT for release. In
any case, when the termination of 5-HT action at receptors is
blocked by tricyclic drugs this could lead to a diminished flow
of impulses in the raphe system. This, in turn, might explain the
diminished 5-HT turnover. However, a block in reuptake, by
reducing access to monoamine oxidase, could also account for the
diminished catabolism of 5-HT produced by these drugs. Similar
alternative explanations arise in attempting to relate alterations
in NE or DA metabolism induced by amphetamine to the depression
in firing rate of CA-containing neurons.

As is evident from the foregoing review, it has become cus-
tomary in recent years to invoke the concept of a compensatory
neuronal feedback loop. Such a "loop" would be activated in response to changing levels of "available" neurotransmitter at the
postsynaptic receptor site. In terms of this model, increasing
5-HT availability by administration of precursors, uptake inhibitors,
or monoamine oxidase inhibitors should result in a compensatory
feedback inhibition. Similarly, if LSD mimicked 5-HT at postsynaptic receptors, compensatory feedback inhibition would also
result. A comparable situation could exist for CA cells. Receptor
stimulation (e.g. by apomorphine) or an increase in CA availability
(e.g. by amphetamine or precursor administration) would result in
a compensatory inhibition, while on the other hand receptor
blockade (e.g. by antipsychotic drugs) would result in a compensatory activation.

An alternative to the above model can be constructed which
retains the notion of receptor effects, but does not involve a
postsynaptic neuronal feedback loop. If monoamine cell bodies
had inhibitory receptors, perhaps related to the presence of
inhibitory recurrent collaterals, an increase of monoamine availability at these receptors would result in inhibition. Conversely,

a decrease of monoamine availability or blockade of these receptors
would have the opposite effect. According to this model, it is
the 5-HT or CA receptor on its own cell which is important rather
than a postsynaptic receptor. In this context, it is significant
that 5-HT applied directly to raphe cell bodies has an inhibitory
action.

One or a combination of the above mechanisms may be involved
in mediating the interaction of biochemical events and change in
single cell activity. Some attempts at establishing a precise
cause and effect relationship between firing rate and turnover
have been attempted but much remains to be done in this area.
It is also evident from this review that there are many drugs or
manipulations not yet tested which potentially might affect the
activity of monoamine neurons. Nevertheless, the results to date
clearly show that drugs and amine precursors known to alter 5-HT
or CA metabolism have dramatic and selective effects on the
activity of central monoamine neurons.

REFERENCES

Aghajanian, G.K. 1972. Influence of drugs on the firing of
    serotonin-containing neurons in brain. Fed. Proc. 31:
    91-96.
Aghajanian, G.K. and Asher, I.M. 1971. Histochemical fluores-
    cence of raphe neurons: selective enhancement by tryptophan.
    Science 172: 1159-1161.
Aghajanian, G.K., Foote, W.E. and Sheard, M.H. 1968. Lysergic
    acid diethylamide: sensitive neuronal units in the midbrain
    raphe. Science 161: 706-708.
Aghajanian, G.K., Foote, W.E. and Sheard, M.H. 1970 a. Action
    of psychotogenic drugs on single midbrain raphe neurons.
    J. Pharmacol. Exp. Ther. 171: 178-187.
Aghajanian, G.K. and Freedman, D.X. 1968. Biochemical and
    morphological aspects of LSD pharmacology. In Psychopharma-
    cology: A Review of Progress, (Ed. Efron, E.H.) U.S.
    Government Printing Office, Washington, D.C., pp 1185-1193.
Aghajanian, G.K., Graham, A.W. and Sheard, M.H. 1970 b. Serotonin-
    containing neurons in brain: depression of firing by mono-
    amine oxidase inhibitors. Science 169: 1100-1102.
Aghajanian, G.K., Haigler, H.J. and Bloom, F.E. 1972 a. Lysergic
    acid diethylamide and serotonin: direct actions on serotonin-
    containing neurons. Life Sci. 11: 615-622.
Aghajanian, G.K., Kuhar, M.J. and Roth, R.H. 1972 b. Serotonin-
    containing neuronal perikarya and terminals: differential
    effects of p-chlorophenylalanine, (in preparation).
Aghajanian, G.K., Rosecrans, J.A. and Sheard, M.H. 1967.
    Serotonin: release in the forebrain by stimulation of
    midbrain raphe. Science 156: 402-403.

Alousi, A. and Weiner, N. 1966. The regulation of norepinephrine synthesis in sympathetic nerves: effect of nerve stimulation cocaine and catecholamine-releasing agents. Proc. Nat. Acad. Sci. (Washington) 56: 1491-1496.

Andén, N.-E., Carlsson, A., Hillarp, N.-A. and Magnusson, T. 1964 a. 5-Hydroxytryptamine release by nerve stimulation of the spinal cord. Life. Sci. 3: 473-478.

Andén, N.-E., Corrodi, H., Dahlström, A., Fuxe, K. and Hökfelt, T. 1966 a. Effects of tyrosine hydroxylase inhibition on the amine levels of central monoamine neurons. Life Sci. 5: 561-568.

Andén, N.-E., Corrodi, H., Fuxe, K. and Hökfelt, T. 1968. Evidence for a central 5-hydroxytryptamine receptor stimulation by lysergic acid diethylamide. Brit. J. Pharmacol. Chemother. 34: 1-7.

Andén, N.-E., Corrodi, H., Fuxe, K. and Ungerstedt, U. 1971. Importance of nervous impulse flow for the neuroleptic induced increase in amine turnover in central dopamine neurons. J. Pharmacol. 15: 193-199.

Andén, N.-E., Dahlström, A., Fuxe, K., Larsson, K., Olson, L. and Ungerstedt, U. 1966 b. Ascending monoamine neurons to telencephalon and diencephalon. Acta Physiol. Scand. 67: 313-326.

Andén, N.-E., Fuxe, K. and Henning, M. 1969. Mechanisms of noradrenaline and 5-hydroxytryptamine disappearance induced by alpha-methyl-DOPA and alpha-metatyrosine. Eur. J. Pharmacol. 8: 302-309.

Andén, N.-E., Fuxe, K. and Hökfelt, T. 1966 c. The importance of nervous impulse flow for the depletion of the monoamines from central neurons by some drugs. J. Pharm. Pharmacol. 18: 630-632.

Andén, N.-E., Fuxe, K. and Hökfelt, T. 1967 a. Effect of some drugs on central monoamine nerve terminals lacking nerve impulse flow. Eur. J. Pharmacol. 1: 226-232.

Andén, N.-E., Roos, B.-E. and Werdinius, B. 1964 b. Effects of chlorpromazine, haloperidol and reserpine on the levels of phenolic acids in rabbit corpus striatum. Life. Sci. 3: 149-158.

Andén, N.-E., Rubenson, A., Fuxe, K. and Hökfelt, T. 1967 b. Evidence for dopamine receptor stimulation by apomorphine. J. Pharm. Pharmacol. 19: 627-629.

Appel, J.B., Lovell, R.A. and Freedman, D.X. 1970. Alteration in the behavioral effects of LSD by pretreatment with p-chlorophenylalanine and alpha-methyl-p-tyrosine. Psychopharmacologia 18: 387-406.

Bédard, P., Carlsson, A., Fuxe, K. and Lindqvist, M. 1971. Origin of 5-hydroxytryptophan and L-DOPA accumulating in brain following decarboxylase inhibition. Naunyn-Scmeidebergs Arch. Pharmak. 269: 1-6.

Bédard, P., Carlsson, A. and Lindqvist, M. 1972. Effect of a transverse cerebral hemisection on 5-hydroxytryptamine metabo-

lism in the rat brain. Naunyn Schmeidebergs Arch. Pharmak.
      272: 1-15.
Besson, M.J., Cheramy, A., Feltz, P. and Glowinski, J. 1969.
      Release of newly synthesized dopamine from dopamine con-
      taining terminals in the striatum of the rat. Proc. Nat.
      Acad. Sci. 62: 741-748.
Besson, M.J., Cheramy, A., Feltz, P. and Glowinski, J. 1971 a.
      Dopamine: spontaneous and drug-induced release from the
      caudate nucleus in the cat. Brain Res. 32: 407-424.
Besson, J.M., Cheramy, A. and Glowinski, J. 1971 b. Effects of
      some psychotropic drugs on dopamine synthesis in the rat
      striatum. J. Pharmacol. Exp. Ther. 177: 196-205.
Björklund, A., Falck, B. and Stenevi, U. 1971. Classification
      of monoamine neurons in the rat mesencephalon: distribution
      of a new monoamine neuronal system. Brain Res. 32: 269-285.
Bogdanski, D.F., Weissbach, J. and Udenfriend, S. 1958.
      Pharmacological studies with the serotonin precursor,
      5-hydroxytryptophan. J. Pharmacol. Exp. Ther. 122: 182-191.
Brodie, B.B., Spector, S. and Shore, P.A. 1959. Interaction of
      monoamine oxidase inhibition with physiological and bio-
      chemical mechanisms in brain. Ann. N.Y. Acad. Sci. 80:
      609-614.
Bunney, B.S., Aghajanian, G.K. and Roth, R.H. 1972 a. L-DOPA,
      amphetamine and apomorphine: effects on firing rate of
      dopamine-containing neurons in the rat midbrain, (in
      preparation).
Bunney, B.S., Walters, J.R., Roth, R.H. and Aghajanian, G.K.
      1972 b. Dopaminergic neurons: effect of antipsychotic drugs
      and amphetamine on single cell activity (in preparation).
Butcher, L.L. and Engel, J. 1969. Behavioral and biochemical
      effects of L-DOPA after peripheral decarboxylase inhibition.
      Brain Res. 15: 233-242.
Carlsson, A. 1970. Structural specificity for inhibition of
      (^{14}C)-5-hydroxytryptamine uptake by cerebral slices. J.
      Pharm. Pharmac. 22: 729-732.
Carlsson, A., Corrodi, H., Fuxe, K. and Hökfelt, T. 1969.
      Effects of some antidepressant drugs on the depletion of
      intraneuronal brain catecholamine stores caused by 4,alpha-
      dimethyl-meta-tyramine. Eur.J. Pharmacol. 5: 367-373.
Carlsson, A., Falck, B., Fuxe, K. and Hillarp, N.-A. 1964.
      Cellular localization of monoamines in the spinal cord.
      Acta Physiol. Scand. 60: 112-119.
Carlsson, A. and Lindqvist, M. 1963. Effect of chlorpromazine
      and haloperidol on formation of 3-methoxytyramine and
      normetenephrine in mouse brain. Acta Pharmacol. Toxicol.
      20: 140-144.

Cheramy, A., Besson, M.J. and Glowinski, J. 1970. Increased
    release of dopamine from striatal dopaminergic terminals in
    the rat after treatment with a neuroleptic thioproperazine.
    Eur. J. Pharmacol. 10: 206-214.
Corrodi, H. and Fuxe, K. 1969. Decreased turnover in central 5-HT
    nerve terminals induced by antidepressant drugs of the
    imipramine type. Eur. J. Pharmacol. 7: 56-59.
Corrodi, H., Fuxe, K. and Hökfelt, T. 1967. The effect of some
    psychoactive drugs on central monoamine neurons. Eur. J.
    Pharmacol. 1: 363-368.
Curtis, D.R. 1964. Microiontophoresis. In: Physical Techniques in
    Biological Research V. Electrophysiological Methods Part A
    (Ed. Nastuk, W.L.) New York: Academic Press, pp. 144-190.
Dahlström, A. and Fuxe, K. 1965. Evidence for the existence of
    monoamine-containing neurons in the central nervous system.
    I. Demonstration of monoamines in the cell bodies of brain
    stem neurons. Acta Physiol. Scand. 62(232): 1-55.
Eccleston, D., Ashcroft, G.W. and Crawford, T.B.B. 1965. 5-
    Hydroxyindole metabolism in rat brain. A study of inter-
    mediate metabolism using the technique of tryptophan loading -
    II. Applications and drug studies. J. Neurochem. 12: 493-503.
Ernst, A.M. 1967. Mode of action of apomorphine and d-amphetamine
    on gnaw-compulsion in rats. Psychopharmacologia 10: 316.
Fernstrom, J.D. and Wurtman, R.J. 1971. Brain serotonin content:
    physiological dependence on plasma tryptophan levels.
    Science 173: 149-151.
Freedman, D.X. 1961. Effects of LSD-25 on brain serotonin. J.
    Pharmacol. Exp. Ther. 134: 160-166.
Freedman, D.X., Gottlieb, R. and Lovell, R.A. 1970. Psychotomimetic
    drugs and brain 5-hydroxyindole metabolism. Biochem. Pharmacol.
    19: 1181-1188.
Fuxe, K. 1965. Evidence for the existence of monoamine neurons
    in the central nervous system. IV. Distribution of monoamine
    nerve terminals in the central nervous system. Acta Physiol.
    Scand. 64(247): 41-85.
Fuxe, K., Butcher, L. and Engel, J. 1971. DL-5-hydroxytryptophan-
    induced change in central monoamine neurons after peripheral
    decarboxylase inhibition. J. Pharm. Pharmacol. 23: 420-424.
Gey, K.F. and Pletscher, A. 1968. Acceleration of turnover of ^{14}C-
    catecholamines in rat brain by chlorpromazine. Experientia
    24: 335-336.
Glowinski, J. and Axelrod, J. 1966. Effects of drugs on the
    disposition of H^3-norepinephrine in the rat brain. Pharmacol.
    Rev. 18: 775-785.
Glowinski, J., Axelrod, J. and Iversen, L.L. 1966. Regional studies
    of catecholamines in the rat brain. IV. Effects of drugs on
    the disposition and metabolism of H^3-norepinephrine and H^3
    dopamine. J. Pharmacol. Exp. Ther. 153: 30-41.

Goldstein, M., Freedman, L.S. and Backstrom, T. 1970. The inhibi-
    tion of catecholamine biosynthesis by apomorphine. J. Pharm.
    Pharmacol. 22 :715-717.
Goodrich, C.A. 1969. Effect of monoamine oxidase inhibitors on
    5-hydroxytryptamine output from perfused cerebral ventricles
    of anesthetized cats. Brit. J. Pharmacol. 37: 87-93.
Gordon, R., Reid, J.V.O., Sjoerdsma, A. and Udenfriend, S. 1966.
    Increased synthesis of norepinephrine in the rat heart on
    electrical stimulation of the stellate ganglia. Mol.
    Pharmacol. 2: 606-613.
Graham, A. and Aghajanian, G.K. 1971. Effects of amphetamine on
    single cell activity in a catecholamine nucleus, the
    Locus Coeruleus. Nature 234: 100-102.
Gumulka, W., Samanin, R., Garattini, S. and Valzelli, L. 1969.
    Effect of stimulation of midbrain raphe on serotonin (5-HT)
    levels and turnover in different areas of rat brain. Eur.
    J. Pharmacol. 8: 380-384.
Hess, S.M. and Doepfner, W. 1961. Behavioral effects and brain
    amine content in rats. Arch. Int. Pharmacodyn. 134 :89-99.
Horn, A.S. and Snyder, S.H. 1971. Chlorpromazine and dopamine :
    conformational similarities that correlate with the anti-
    schizophrenic activity of phenothiazine drugs. Proc. Nat.
    Acad. Sci. 68: 2325-2328.
Jéquier, E., Lovenberg, W. and Sjoerdsma, A. 1967. Tryptophan
    hydroxylase inhibition: the mechanism by which p-chloro-
    phenylalanine depletes rat brain serotonin. Mol. Pharmacol.
    3: 274-278.
Juorio, A.V., Sharman, D.F. and Trajkov, T. 1966. The effect
    of drugs on the homovanillic acid content of the corpus stri-
    atum of some rodents. Brit. J. Pharmacol. Chemother.
    26 :385-392.
Klein, D.F. and Davis, J.M. 1969. Diagnosis and drug treatment
    of psychiatric disorders. Baltimore: The Williams and
    Wilkins Company.
Koe, B.K. and Weissman, A. 1966. p-Chlorophenylalanine: a
    specific depletor of brain serotonin. J. Pharmacol. Exp.
    Ther. 154: 499-516.
Kostowski, W., Giacalone, E., Garattini, S. and Valzelli, L. 1969.
    Electrical stimulation of midbrain raphe: biochemical,
    behavioral and bioelectrical effects. Eur. J. Pharm. 7: 170-175.
Kuhar, M.J. and Aghajanian, G.K. 1972. Selective accumulation of
    H^3-serotonin by nerve terminals of raphe neurons: an auto-
    radiographic study (in preparation).
Kuhar, M.H., Aghajanian, G.K. and Roth, R.H. 1972 a. Tryptophan
    hydroxylase activity and synaptosomal uptake of serotonin in
    discrete brain regions after midbrain raphe lesions: correla-
    tions with serotonin levels and histochemical fluorescence.
    Brain Res. (in press).

Kuhar, M.J., Roth, R.H. and Aghajanian, G.K. 1971. Selective reduction of tryptophan hydroxylase activity in rat forebrain after midbrain raphe lesions. Brain Res. 35: 167-176.

Kuhar, M.J., Roth, R.H. and Aghajanian, G.K. 1972 b. Synaptosomes from forebrains of rats with midbrain raphe lesions: selective reduction of serotonin uptake. J. Pharmacol. Exp. Ther. 181: 36-45.

Lin, R.C., Ngai, S.H. and Costa, E. 1969. Lysergic acid diethylamide: role in conversion of plasma tryptophan to brain serotonin (5-hydroxytryptamine). Science 166: 237-239.

Meek, J.L. and Fuxe, K. 1971. Serotonin accumulation after monoamine-oxidase inhibition. Biochem. Pharmacol. 20: 693-706.

Moir, A.T.B. and Eccleston, D. 1968. The effects of precursor loading in the cerebral metabolism of 5-hydroxyindoles. J. Neurochem. 15: 1093-1108.

Neff, N.H. and Costa, E. 1966. Effect of tricyclic antidepressants and chlorpromazine on brain catecholamine synthesis. In: Proceedings of the First International Symposium on Antidepressant Drugs (Eds., Garattini, S. and Dukes, M.G.), Milan: Excerpta Medica International Congress Series No. 122: 28-34.

Nybäck, H., Borzecki, Z. and Sedvall, G. 1968. Accumulation and disappearance of catecholamine formed from tyrosine-^{14}C in mouse brain. Effect of some psychotropic drugs. Eur. J. Pharmacol. 4: 395-403.

Nybäck, H. and Sedvall, G. 1971. Effect of nigral lesion on chlorpromazine-induced acceleration of dopamine synthesis from (^{14}C) tyrosine. J. Pharm. Pharmacol. 23: 322-326.

Nybäck, H., Sedvall, G. and Kopin, I.J. 1967. Accelerated synthesis of dopamine-^{14}C from tyrosine-^{14}C in rat brain after chlorpromazine. Life Sci. 6: 2307-2312.

Persson, T. 1970. Drug induced changes in ^{3}H-catecholamine accumulation after ^{3}H-tyrosine. Acta Pharmacol. Toxicol. 28: 387-390.

Persson, T. and Waldeck, B. 1970. Further studies on the possible interaction between dopamine and noradrenaline containing neurons in the brain. Eur. J. Pharmacol. 11: 315-320.

Rosecrans, J.A., Lovell, R.A. and Freedman, D.X. 1967. Effects of lysergic acid diethylamide on the metabolism of brain 5-hydroxytryptamine. Biochem. Pharmacol. 16: 2011-2012.

Ross, S.B. and Renyi, A.L. 1969. Inhibition of the uptake of tritiated 5-hydroxytryptamine in brain tissue. Eur. J. Pharmacol. 7: 270-277.

Schubert, J., Nybäck, H. and Sedvall, G. 1970. Accumulation and disappearance of ^{3}H-5-hydroxytryptamine formed from ^{3}H-tryptophan in mouse brain: effect of LSD-25. Eur. J. Pharmacol. 10: 215-224.

Sedvall, G., Weise, W.K. and Kopin, I.J. 1968. The rate of norepinephrine synthesis measured in vivo during short

intervals: influence of adrenergic nerve impulse activity.
J. Pharmacol. Exp. Ther. 159: 274-282.

Shaskan, E. and Snyder, S.H. 1970. Kinetics of ^{3}H-5-hydroxy-
tryptamine uptake into synaptosomes from different regions
of rat brain. J. Pharmacol. Exp. Ther. 175: 404-418.

Sheard, M.H. and Aghajanian, G.K. 1968. Stimulation of the midbrain raphe: effect on serotonin metabolism. J. Pharmacol.
Exp. Ther. 163: 425-430.

Sheard, M.H., Zolovick, A. and Aghajanian, G.K. 1972. Raphe
neurons: effect of tricyclic antidepressant drugs (in
preparation).

Shields, P.J. and Eccleston, D. 1972. Effects of electrical
stimulation of rat midbrain on 5-hydroxytryptamine synthesis
as determined by sensitive radioisotopic method. J. Neurochem.
19: 265-272.

Spector, S., Sjoerdsma, A. and Udenfriend, S. 1965. Blockade of
endogenous norepinephrine synthesis by alpha-methyl-tyrosine
an inhibitor of tyrosine hydroxylase. J. Pharmacol. Exp.
Ther. 147: 86-95.

Stjarne, L.F., Lishajko, F. and Roth, R.H. 1967. Regulation of
noradrenaline biosynthesis in nerve tissue. Nature 215:
770-772.

Tozer, T.N., Neff, N.H. and Brodie, B.B. 1966. Application of
steady-state kinetics to the synthesis rate and turnover
time of serotonin in the brain of normal and reserpine
treated rats. J. Pharmacol. Exp. Ther. 153: 177-182.

Ungerstedt, U. 1971. Stereotaxic mapping of the monoamine
pathways in the rat brain. Acta Physiol. Scand. 267: 1-48.

Weber, L.J. and Horita, A. 1965. A study of 5-hydroxytryptamine
formation from L-tryptophan in the brain and other tissues.
Biochem. Pharmacol. 14: 1141-1149.

THE ROLE OF 3',5'-CYCLIC ADENOSINE MONOPHOSPHATE IN THE

REGULATION OF ADRENAL MEDULLARY FUNCTION

Ermino Costa and Alessandro Guidotti

Laboratory of Preclinical Pharmacology, NIMH

St. Elizabeths Hospital, Washington, D.C.   20032

Two main lines of evidence have contributed to our present understanding of the regulation of tyrosine hydroxylase activity in the adrenal medulla. One was provided by Axelrod (1971) by showing that tyrosine hydroxylase activity is regulated transynaptically, the other by Kvetnansky and collaborators (1971) by showing that the injection of dibutyryl cyclic AMP restores the activity of tyrosine hydroxylase in hypophysectomized animals.

The present report concerns experiments we carried out to ascertain whether in adrenal medulla the transynaptic control of tyrosine hydroxylase activity is related to changes of 3',5'-adenosine monophosphate (cyclic AMP) concentrations. If cyclic AMP were proved to function in the transynaptic regulation of tyrosine hydroxylase then, we would be able to assess whether and how protein kinases and histone kinases participate in the biochemical imprinting of synaptic events in the postsynaptic cell.

METHODS

Sprague Dawley rats (Zivic Miller Labs., Pa.) of about 180 g body weight were used in these experiments. In certain experiments we have used monolaterally splanchnicotomized rats. This surgery was performed five days before the experiment.

The dissection of adrenal medulla from the cortex was performed on a cold table (0-4°C) using a dissecting microscope. Following decapsulation of the gland, its further dissection was controlled by biochemical analyses and by fluorescent microscopy. The tissue termed medulla contained about 95% of the catecholamines present in the adrenal gland; in contrast, the cortex contained

135

about 99% of the corticosterone present in the adrenal. Corticosteroids were assayed by the method of Zenker and Bernstein
(1958); catecholamines and tyrosine concentrations in adrenals
were measured by the method of Neff et al (1971). This method
was also used to assay the specific radioactivity of dopamine,
epinephrine, and tyrosine in the adrenal gland of rats killed
at various times after an intravenous injection of $3',5'-^{3}H$
tyrosine (1.25 mc/kg; SA 30 c/mmole). The cyclic AMP concentration
was measured by a modification (Guidotti et al., 1972) of the
luciferin-luciferase method described by Ebadi et al. (1971).
Phosphodiesterase activity was assayed by the method of Weiss
et al. (1972) and adenylate cyclase activity by the method of
Krishna et al. (1969). Tyrosine hydroxylase activity was measured
by the method of Vaymire et al. (1971) using carboxyl labelled
tyrosine (S.A. 10 μCi/μmole).

RESULTS

A. Effect of Splanchnicotomy on Some Biochemical
Properties of Adrenal Glands

The results of some biochemical measurements performed in
intact and splanchnicotomized adrenal cortex, medulla and capsule

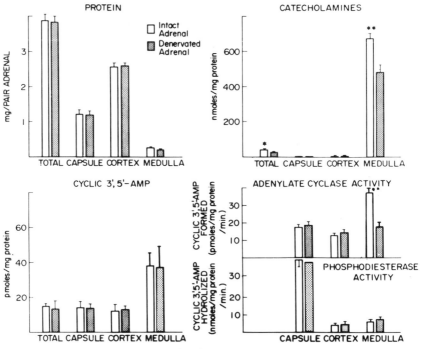

Figure 1. Proteins, cyclic 3',5'-AMP, and catecholamine content.
Adenylate cyclase and phosphodiesterase activity in various parts
of intact and splanchnicotomized adrenal gland of rat. Splanchnicotomy was performed 5 days before the assay. **p <0.01; *p <0.05

are reported in Figure 1. Splanchnicotomy neither changes the
protein content of adrenal cortex and medulla nor affects the
cyclic AMP concentrations and phosphodiesterase activities of both
tissues. However, the adenylate cyclase activity of medulla but
not that of cortex is significantly reduced by splanchnicotomy.
This deafferentation of the adrenal reduces the catecholamine concentration. Despite this reduction of medullary catecholamine
concentrations, splanchnicotomy fails to change the tyrosine
hydroxylase activity (see Table 2). The decrease of adenylate
cyclase activity elicited by splanchnicotomy is not due to the
formation of an inhibitory factor; when the homogenates of intact
and splanchnicotomized adrenal medulla were mixed, the adenylate
cyclase activity was equal to the sum of the enzyme activities
present in the two homogenates.

B. Effect of Cholinergic Drugs on Cyclic AMP
Concentrations and Tyrosine Hydroxylase Activity

The injection of 8.2 μmoles/kg i.p. of carbamylcholine elicits
a 14-fold increase of cyclic AMP concentrations of intact and
splanchnicotomized adrenal medulla (Table 1). The rate of this
increase is similar in intact and in the controlateral surgically
denervated medulla. The peak effect is reached in 24 minutes and
at 48 minutes the cyclic AMP concentrations are still 3-fold of
controls but are less elevated than at 24 minutes. The increase
of cyclic AMP concentrations elicited by carbamylcholine is also
similar in intact and denervated adrenal cortex. Although the
time course of the cyclic AMP accumulation is similar in cortex
and medulla, the molar rate of cyclic AMP accumulation elicited
by carbamylcholine in adrenal cortex is smaller than that recorded
in medulla (14 versus 25 pmoles/mg protein/min).

We then tested whether carbamylcholine was able to increase
the tyrosine hydroxylase activity of adrenal medulla. The results
of this experiment are reported in Table 2. These data show that
tyrosine hydroxylase activity is significantly increased 24 and
48 hours after the injection of 8.2 μmoles of carbamylcholine.
Splanchnicotomy fails to change the increase of tyrosine hydroxylase
activity elicited by carbamylcholine (Table 2).

C. Effect of Aminophylline Injections on Cyclic AMP
Concentration and Tyrosine Hydroxylase Activity of Adrenal

Aminophylline (200 μmoles/kg i.p.), an inhibitor of phosphodiesterase activity of adrenal medulla and cortex (Guidotti and
Costa, 1972) causes the cyclic AMP to accumulate in both adrenal
cortex and medulla (Table 3). While the maximal molar rate of
accumulation is slower in splanchnicotomized (6 pmoles/mg protein/
min) than in intact medulla (40 pmoles/mg protein/min) this rate is
similar in surgically denervated and intact cortex (50 pmoles/mg
protein/min). Not only does splanchnicotomy reduce the molar rate

TABLE 1

Cyclic 3',5'-AMP Concentrations in Intact and Splanchnicotomized Adrenal Cortex
and Medulla of Rats Receiving Carbamylcholine (8.2 μmoles/kg i.p.)

| TISSUE | SPLANCHNICOTOMY | CYCLIC 3',5'-AMP pmoles/mg protein (MEAN VALUES ± SEM) | | | | | |
| | | MINUTES AFTER CARBAMYLCHOLINE | | | | | |
		0	3	6	12	24	48
MEDULLA	NO	33 ± 3.0	30 ± 7.0	53* ± 2.6	200* ± 77	450* ± 7.0	110.1* ± 12
MEDULLA	YES	32 ± 2.3	37 ± 8.0	49* ± 5.6	200* ± 67	330* ± 54	100.2* ± 19
CORTEX	NO	5.6 ± 1.0	9.2 ± 2.1	26* ± 9.0	110* ± 30	190* ± 40	41* ± 6.0
CORTEX	YES	4.6 ± 0.8	12* ± 1.1	27* ± 6.3	88* ± 26	170* ± 33	37* ± 8.2

Each value represents the mean of at least four experiments. The concentrations of cyclic 3',
5'-AMP in adrenal medulla and cortex at various times after saline were not different from
those of rats not receiving saline.   * P <0.05

TABLE 2

Tyrosine Hydroxylase Activity in Intact and Splanchnicotomized Adrenal Gland
at Various Times After Carbamylcholine (8.2 μmoles/kg i.p.)

TYROSINE HYDROXYLASE ACTIVITY

nmoles DOPA Formed/Hr/Gland (Mean Value $\pm$ S.E.M.)

Hours After Carbamylcholine

SPLANCHNICOTOMY	0	24	48
NO	5.9 ± 0.5	$10 \pm 0.5^{*}$	$10.0 \pm 1.6^{*}$
YES	5.4 ± 0.6	$9 \pm 0.5^{*}$	

Each value is the mean of at least five experiments. Tyrosine
hydroxylase activity in adrenal glands at various times after
saline were not different from those of rats not receiving saline.
*P <0.05

TABLE 3

Cyclic 3',5'-AMP Concenbrations in Intact and Splanchnicotomized Adrenal Cortex and Medulla of Rats Receiving 200 µmoles/kg i.p. of Aminophylline

TISSUE	SPLANCHNICOTOMY	Cyclic 3',5'-AMP pmoles/mg protein (Mean Value ± SEM) Minutes After Aminophylline					
		0	3	6	12	24	48
MEDULLA	NO	42 ± 9.0	88 ± 25	190* ± 57	420* ± 80	380* ± 95	500* ± 60
MEDULLA	YES	38 ± 4.6	55 ± 12	75 ± 20	120 ± 75	200* ± 60	220* ± 40
CORTEX	NO	8.3 ± 2.4	40 ± 14	140* ± 44	460* ± 50	560* ± 100	320* ± 100
CORTEX	YES	12 ± 4	37 ± 11	160* ± 60	460* ± 95	580* ± 95	180* ± 20

Each value represents the mean of at least four experiments.   *P <0.05

of cyclic AMP accumulation in adrenal medulla but also the peak increase of cyclic AMP concentration is smaller in surgically denervated than in normal medulla. In contrast, splanchnicotomy does not change the time course and the extent of the cyclic AMP increase in adrenal cortex.

The data listed in Table 4 show that the tyrosine hydroxylase activity of the intact adrenal glands of rats receiving aminophylline is significantly greater than that of untreated rats. This increase endures for several days. In contrast, the tyrosine hydroxylase activity of splanchnicotomized adrenals of rats receiving aminophylline appears to be equal to that of splanchnicotomized rats not receiving aminophylline.

We assayed the in vivo turnover rate of catecholamines in normal rats and in rats injected with aminophylline (200 µmoles/kg i.p.) 24 hours earlier. Both groups of rats received a pulse injection of 3',5'-3H tyrosine and were killed 40 minutes later. All the rats used in these experiments were splanchnicotomized monolaterally. We found that the specific activity of adrenal gland tyrosine was changed neither by the surgery nor by the injection of aminophylline. In contrast, the aminophylline injection enhanced the specific activity of epinephrine in the intact, but not in the splanchnicotomized side (Figure 2). Splanchnicotomy reduced the specific activity of adrenal epinephrine.

D. Effect of Reserpine on Cyclic AMP Concentrations of Adrenal Cortex and Medulla

Reserpine increases tyrosine hydroxylase activity of adrenal gland and this effect is reduced by splanchnicotomy (Axelrod, 1971). We have studied whether reserpine (16 µmoles/kg i.p.) increases the concentration of cyclic AMP in adrenal cortex and medulla. The results of these experiments are reported in Table 5. The injection of reserpine elicited an increase of cyclic AMP concentrations in adrenal cortex and medulla lasting less than one hour. Splanchnicotomy almost abolishes the increase of cyclic AMP elicited by reserpine in adrenal medulla but not that in adrenal cortex. The rate of cyclic AMP accumulation in intact adrenal cortex is about 9 pmoles/mg protein/min and 6 pmoles/mg protein/min in the splanchnicotomized side. In contrast, the rate of accumulation of cyclic AMP in the intact adrenal medulla was about 11 pmoles/mg protein/min. This rate was reduced to about 3 pmoles/mg protein/min by splanchnicotomy.

E. Effect of ACTH on Cyclic AMP Concentrations and Tyrosine Hydroxylase Activity of Adrenal

Since carbamylcholine, aminophylline and reserpine in the dose

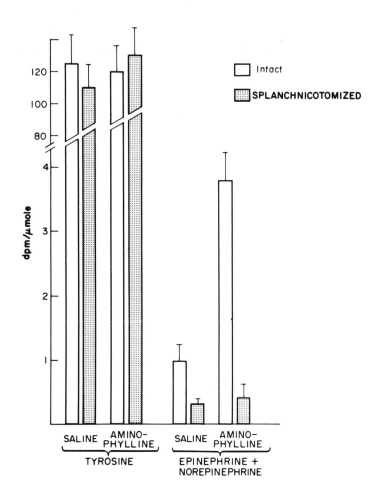

Figure 2. Specific activity of tyrosine and epinephrine in intact
and splanchnicotomized adrenal glands of rats receiving ^{3}H-L-
tyrosine 24 hours after aminophylline or saline. Aminophylline
was injected intraperitoneally in doses of 200 μmoles/kg.
3,5-^{3}H-tyrosine (31 Ci/mmole) 1.25 mCi/kg was injected into 5
controls and 5 aminophylline treated animals 40 minutes before
death.

TABLE 4

Tyrosine Hydroxylase Activity in Intact and Splanchnicotomized Adrenal
Gland at Various Times After Aminophylline (200 μmoles/kg i.p.)

SPLANCHNICOTOMY	Tyrosine Hydroxylase Activity nmoles/Dopa Formed/Hr/Gland (Mean Value ± S.E.M.) Hours After Aminophylline					
	0	6	14	24	48	72
NO	5.8 ± 0.3	7.7 ± 0.6	11 ± 1.2*	12 ± 1.2*	11 ± 1.8*	11 ± 0.9*
YES	5.8 ± 0.6	--	6.6 ± 0.3	7.7 ± 0.4	7.5 ± 0.8	--

Each value in the mean of at least 5 experiments.   *P <0.05

TABLE 5

Cyclic 3',5'-AMP Concentrations in Intact and Splanchnicotomized
Adrenal Cortex and Medulla of Rats Receiving 16 μmoles/kg i.p. of Reserpine

TISSUE	SPLANCHNICOTOMY	Cyclic 3',5'-AMP pmoles/mg protein (Mean Value ± SEM)				
		Minutes After Reserpine				
		0	5	15	30	60
MEDULLA	NO	43 ± 9.0	54 ± 6.1	160* ± 30	130* ± 35	55 ± 12
MEDULLA	YES	37 ± 7.2	42 ± 5.0	76 ± 19	48 ± 8	49 ± 7
CORTEX	NO	12 ± 1.2	22 ± 4	110* ± 40	86* ± 23	16 ± 6.1
CORTEX	YES	13 ± 3.5	25 ± 9.3	75* ± 6	90* ± 30	20 ± 5.2

Each value is the mean of at least four experiments.   * $P < 0.05$

range used are stressors they can release ACTH. We tested whether
ACTH could cause an accumulation of cyclic AMP in adrenal cortex
and medulla and whether this accumulation was associated with an
increase of tyrosine hydroxylase activity in the adrenal gland.
The data reported in Table 6 are the results of these experiments.
An injection of 50 mU/kg i.v. of ACTH can increase the cyclic AMP
concentrations of the intact adrenal medulla by 6-fold in 10 minutes; a similar increase in the concentration of cyclic AMP of
adrenal medulla of splanchnicotomized gland occurs only after an
injection of 500 mU i.p. of ACTH. Denervation fails to change the
increase of cyclic AMP elicited by ACTH in the adrenal cortex. The
initial rate of cyclic AMP accumulation (Table 6) after 50 mU/kg
i.v. of ACTH is 15 pmoles/mg protein/min in the intact adrenal
medulla but only 1.5 pmoles/mg protein/min in the intact adrenal
cortex. The data in Table 6 show that after 5 U/kg i.v. of ACTH
the cyclic AMP accumulates at a rate of 57 pmoles/mg protein/min
in the intact medulla and at a rate of 27 pmole/mg protein/min in
the intact cortex. When the tyrosine hydroxylase activity is
measured at various times after 5 U/kg i.v. of ACTH, the enzyme
activity (Table 7) is increased 48 hours after the injection, but
not at 24 hours. The tyrosine hydroxylase activity of the
splanchnicotomized gland is increased neither 24 nor 48 hours
after the injection of ACTH.

DISCUSSION

The data presented show that only carbamylcholine (8.2 μmoles/
kg i.p.) can increase equally well the tyrosine hydroxylase and
the cyclic AMP concentration in the splanchnicotomized and intact
adrenal medulla. If the cyclic AMP increase is rated as a molar
accumulation per mg protein and per unit time, then the molar
rate of cyclic AMP accumulation elicited by carbamylcholine is not
changed by surgical denervation neither in medulla nor in cortex.
The action of carbamylcholine on cyclic AMP concentrations and
tyrosine hydroxylase activity of adrenal medulla differs from that
of reserpine, aminophylline and ACTH because it is not abolished
by surgical denervation. As shown in this paper, these three drugs
are much less active on deafferented adrenal medulla than on normal
glands. Therefore, the effect of carbamylcholine on tyrosine
hydroxylase appears to differ from that of these drugs for it does
not require the presence of intact innervation. The difference in
the response of adrenal to carbamylcholine and ACTH makes it very
unlikely that the increase of tyrosine hydroxylase activity and
cyclic AMP concentrations of adrenal medulla caused by carbamylcholine injections can be explained through the release of ACTH.
However, direct measurements of the blood concentrations of this
peptide should be carried out before excluding such an action
categorically. Since carbamylcholine activates tyrosine hydroxylase
after splanchnicotomy, one could exclude that this pharmacologically

TABLE 6

Effect of Various Doses of ACTH on the Concentrations of Cyclic 3',5'-AMP in the Adrenal Cortex and Medulla of Monolaterally Splanchnicotomized Rats

TISSUE	SPLANCHNICOTOMY	Cyclic 3',5'-AMP pmoles/mg/protein (Mean Value ± SEM) ACHT (m IU/kg i.v.)				
		Saline	50	250	500	5000
MEDULLA	NO	30 ± 3.6	185* ± 11	200* ± 65	265* ± 43	605* ± 28
MEDULLA	YES	22 ± 8.0	61 ± 30	67* ± 16	175* ± 16	---
CORTEX	NO	7.8 ± 1.9	19.6* ± 2.1	75* ± 17	140* ± 18	280* ± 35
CORTEX	YES	9.3 ± 3.4	15.0 ± 1.2	63* ± 4.9	180* ± 7.0	---

The animals were anesthetized with nembutal (40 mg/kg i.p.) and killed 10 min after administration of ACTH i.v. Each value is the mean of at least 4 experiments. * $P < 0.05$

TABLE 7

Tyrosine Hydroxylase Activity in Intact and Splanchnicotomized
Adrenal Gland at Various Times after 5 IU/kg i.v. of ACTH

SPLANCHNICOTOMY	Tyrosine Hydroxylase Activity (nmoles Dopa formed/hr/gland (Mean Value $\pm$ S.E.M.)		
	Hours After ACTH		
	0	24	48
NO	4.8 ± 0.6	5.2 ± 0.4	7.8 ± 1.1*
YES	4.3 ± 0.4	4.0 ± 0.5	5.0 ± 1.2

Each value is the mean of at least 5 experiments.   * $P < 0.05$

induced increase of tyrosine hydroxylase is mediated through a
spinal reflex mechanism triggered by the prolonged hypotension
ensuing the injection of carbamylcholine. Moreover it appears of
interest to note that adrenal medulla is the first tissue where an
activation of adenyl cyclase system is brought about by injections
of a cholinomimetic drug.

Another marked distinction can be made between the action of
ACTH on tyrosine hydroxylase and that of aminophylline, reserpine,
and carbamylcholine. The increase of tyrosine hydroxylase activity
elicited by ACTH (5 IU/kg i.v.) has a latency of two days whereas
the increase of tyrosine hydroxylase activity elicited by the other
three drugs is already established within 24 hours or less. We
have also tested smaller doses of ACTH and we found that the increase
of tyrosine hydroxylase was not always noted. However, when present,
the increase of tyrosine hydroxylase elicited by this small dose of
ACTH is also delayed. Perhaps other factors must be taken into
consideration to account for the delayed appearance of the increase
of tyrosine hydroxylase elicited by ACTH.

Do our experiments show a correlation between the early
increase of cyclic AMP concentrations of adrenal medulla elicited
by the various drugs tested and the delayed (24 hours or more)
increase of tyrosine hydroxylase activity? The answer to this
question can be obtained by the data listed in Table 8. The
cyclic AMP concentrations can be enhanced by 5-fold or more without
eliciting a delayed increase in the tyrosine hydroxylase activity.
However, if we consider how the molar rate of cyclic AMP accumulation relates to the changes of tyrosine hydroxylase activity then
the data listed in Table 8 appears to indicate that the increase
of tyrosine hydroxylase activity occurs when the accumulation rate
of cyclic AMP proceeds at a rate of at least 10 pmoles/mg protein/
min.

Perhaps the ACTH effects on the medullary concentrations of
cyclic AMP are one exception to this rule. This hormone causes
an accumulation of cyclic AMP at a rate of 18.5 pmoles/mg protein/
min without consistently increasing tyrosine hydroxylase activity
of adrenal medulla. We might offer an alternative explanation for
such a discrepancy, but we cannot substantiate it with supporting
data: ACTH releases corticosteroids and this release may set in
motion a number of pertinent biochemical changes, including perhaps
an inhibition of protein synthesis, which may delay or prevent
the onset of the increase of tyrosine hydroxylase activity.
Another consideration concerns our present understanding of the
functional significance of the increase of cyclic AMP concentrations in a given tissue. It is presently believed that cyclic AMP
catalyzes the action of kinases, hence the measurement of cyclic
AMP concentrations may not be equated to the activation of a

selective kinase. In fact, we are almost sure that various kinases may be simultaneously activated when cyclic AMP concentration increases. Moreover, an apparently similar increase of cyclic AMP may activate different kinase systems because this increase may be localized in different cell compartments. We have shown that the dynamics by which the cyclic AMP increases may be more revealing than the measurement of concentrations of cyclic AMP, but we cannot yet relate this kinetic parameter to the function of the nucleotide in a given cell population. Perhaps we should not be relating concentrations of cyclic AMP to increase of tyrosine hydroxylase but rather the incorporation of radioactive phosphate into a given protein may relate to the increase of tyrosine hydroxylase activity.

Our results have clearly shown that in adrenals the adenylate cyclase system of medulla is neuronally and hormonally controlled. In contrast, the adenylate cyclase system of adrenal cortex is only hormonally controlled. Moreover, we could not support the proposal made by Paul et al. (1971) that medullary cyclic AMP is not involved in responses to stress for we have seen that during cold exposure both medullary and cortical cyclic AMP are increased (Guidotti and Costa, 1972). Finally, splanchnicotomy curtails the increase of medullary cyclic AMP but not that of cortical cyclic AMP.

We would like to summarize the concepts emerged from the present report with the diagram depicted in Figure 3. Reserpine, carbamylcholine and aminophylline affect the adenylate cyclase system of the adrenal chromaffin cells by different mechanisms. Reserpine action seems to be indirect and requires innervation of the gland. We propose that the effect of reserpine is indirect, perhaps through an acceleration of neuronal impulse traffic traveling through the splanchnic nerves. That the cholinergic nerve transmitter can influence the adenylate cyclase system of chromaffin cells is documented by the effects of carbamylcholine on the cyclic AMP concentrations of adrenal glands of normal and splanchnicotomized rats. To understand the effect of aminophylline we must consider its site of action. Aminophylline inhibits phosphodiesterase and therefore its effect on cyclic AMP concentrations is dependent on the activity of adenyl cyclase. Since denervation reduces this enzyme's activity, the rates of cyclic AMP accumulation in medulla elicited by aminophylline (200 μmoles/kg i.p.) are reduced in the splanchnicotomized medulla. As we have shown in Table 8, the increase of medullary tyrosine hydroxylase activity elicited by three drugs mentioned in Figure 3 is related to the rate of accumulation of cyclic AMP in adrenal medulla. We are currently testing this correlation by other pharmacological experiments. After having proved the validity of such correlation we intend to investigate the biochemical pathways involved in the increase of tyrosine hydroxylase activity mediated by cyclic AMP.

TABLE 8

Drug Effects on Cyclic 3',5'-AMP and Tyrosine Hydroxylase
Activity of Intact and Splanchnicotomized (Splanchx) Adrenal Medulla

DRUG	SPLANCHX	CYCLIC 3',5'-AMP		Tyrosine Hydroxylase % of Control
		Max. Inc. Concentration % of Controls	Max. Accumulation Rate (pmoles/mg prot./min)	
RESERPINE (16 μmoles/kg i.p.)	NO	400	11	180[*]
	YES	150	3	107
CARBAMYLCHOLINE (8.2 μmoles/kg i.p.)	NO	1500	25	180[*]
	YES	1100	25	150[*]
AMINOPHYLLINE (200 μmoles/kg i.p.)	NO	1200	40	190[*]
	YES	500	6	130

* $P < 0.05$

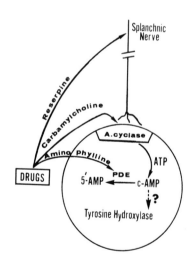

ADRENAL CHROMAFFIN CELLS

Figure 3. Diagrammatic representation of the effects of reserpine, aminophylline, and carbamylcholine on medullary adenylate cyclase and tyrosine hydroxylase.

In closing, we would like to mention that we believe that the increase of cyclic AMP concentration is not related to the release of catecholamines elicited by the three drugs tested. In fact, we have proved that the increase of cyclic AMP in medulla can be dissociated from catecholamine release. Maximal NE releasing doses of tyramine fail to increase the cyclic AMP concentrations in medulla. Moreover, the increase of tyrosine hydroxylase activity is not the consequence of the catecholamine release from medulla because tyramine fails to increase tyrosine hydroxylase activity although it releases catecholamines from adrenal medulla.

SUMMARY

Carbamylcholine (8.2 µmoles/kg i.p.) increase cyclic AMP concentrations in adrenal medulla and cortex: the extent of cyclic AMP increase elicited by carbamylcholine in cortex is much smaller than that caused by aminophylline (200 µmoles/kg i.p.) and ACTH (50 m IU/kg i.v.). Quantitatively the increase of cyclic AMP caused by carbamylcholine in medulla compares with the response elicited by aminophylline and massive doses of ACTH (5 IU/kg i.v.). Carbamylcholine can increase medullary cyclic AMP concentration after cholinergic nerves have been severed. Carbamylcholine increases tyrosine hydroxylase activity in both intact and denervated adrenal gland; ACTH, theophylline, and reserpine can increase tyrosine hydroxylase activity only if the splanchnic nerve is intact.

ACTH increases cyclic AMP in cortex and adrenal medulla: the threshold dose of ACTH to elicit such a response is lower for medulla than for adrenal cortex. ACTH increases also tyrosine hydroxylase activity but this effect occurs after a latency time of two days. In adrenal medulla, the rates of cyclic AMP accumulation elicited by reserpine, carbamylcholine and aminophylline correlate with the increase of tyrosine hydroxylase activity elicited by these drugs. In adrenal cortex, the extent of the increase of cyclic AMP concentrations elicited by the three drugs does not appear related to their ability of increasing tyrosine hydroxylase activity of the gland.

REFERENCES

Axelrod, J. 1971. Noradrenaline: fate and control of its biosynthesis. Science 173: 598.

Ebadi, M.S., Weiss, B. and Costa, E. 1971. Microassay of adenosine 3',5'-monophosphate (cyclic AMP) in brain and other tissues by luciferin luciferase system. J. Neurochem. 18: 183.

Guidotti, A. and Costa, E. 1972. In vivo estimation of 3',5'-adenosine monophosphate (c-AMP) turnover rate in rat adrenal medulla. Fed. Proc. 31: 555.

Guidotti, A., Weiss, B. and Costa, E. 1972. Adenosine 3',5'-mono-
phosphate concentrations and isoproterenol induced synthesis
of deoxyribonucleic acid in mouse parotid. Molec. Pharmac.
(in press).

Krishna, G., Weiss, B., Brodie, B.B. 1968. A simple sensitive
method for the assay of adenylcyclase. J. Pharm. Exp. Ther.
163: 379.

Kvetnansky, R., Gewirtz, G.P., Weise, V.K. and Kopin, I.J. 1971.
Effect of dibutyryl cyclic AMP on adrenal catecholamine synthesizing enzymes in repeatedly immobilized hypophysectomized
rats. Endocrinology 89: 50.

Neff, N.H., Spano, P.F., Groppetti, A., Wang, C.T. and Costa, E.
1971. A simple procedure for calculating the synthesis rate
of norepinephrine, dopamine and serotonin in rat brain. J.
Pharmacol. Exp. Ther. 146: 701.

Paul, M.I., Kvetnansky, R., Cramer, H., Silbergeld, S. and Kopin, I.J.
1971. Immobilization stress induced changes in adrenocortical
and medullary cyclic AMP content in the rat. Endocrinology
88: 338.

Vaymire, J.G., Jurr, B. and Weiner, N. 1971. Assay of tyrosine
hydroxylase by coupled decarboxylation of dopa formed from
L-^{14}C tyrosine. Anal. Biochem. 43: 588.

Weiss, B., Lehne, R., Strada, S. 1972. Rapid microassay of
adenosine 3',5'-monophosphate phosphodiesterase activity.
Anal. Biochem. 45: 222.

Zenker, N., and Bernstein, D.E. 1958. The estimation of small
amounts of corticosterone in rat plasma. J. Biol. Chem.
231: 695.

THE USE OF AUTORADIOGRAPHIC TECHNIQUES FOR THE IDENTIFICATION AND MAPPING OF TRANSMITTER-SPECIFIC NEURONES IN CNS

Leslie L. Iversen and Frederick E. Schon

MRC Neurochemical Pharmacology Unit, Department of
Pharmacology, University of Cambridge, and Physio-
logical Laboratory, University of Cambridge
Cambridge, England

INTRODUCTION

We now know of at least six different transmitter substances
used in synaptic transmission in the mammalian CNS. In most cases,
however, only fragmentary information is available on the distribution of the various categories of transmitter-specific neurone in
the CNS. Thus, for example, while gamma-aminobutyric acid (GABA)
is thought to be an important inhibitory transmitter substance in
many regions of the CNS (for reviews see Curtis and Johnston, 1970;
Hebb, 1970; Krnjević, 1970; Iversen, 1972), it is by no means clear
precisely which inhibitory neurones use GABA as transmitter, nor
indeed whether any inhibitory neurones using transmitters other
than GABA exist in various regions of the brain. Only in the case
of the monoamine transmitters, noradrenaline (NA), dopamine (DA)
and 5-hydroxytryptamine (5-HT) is there any detailed information
on the distribution of neuronal pathways involving specific transmitters. This information has become available during the past
ten years, following the development of histochemical techniques
which allow direct visualization of formaldehyde condensation
derivatives of the monoamines in the fluorescence microscope
(Carlsson, Falck and Hillarp, 1962; Dahlström and Fuxe, 1965;
Fuxe, 1965). The knowledge gained by the application of this
technique has acted as a potent stimulus in focussing attention on
the role of the monoamines in CNS function. In the case of cholinergic neurones in the CNS there is again a wealth of information
available from histochemical studies--in this case of the localization of the enzyme acetylcholinesterase (Lewis and Shute, 1966;
Krnjević and Silver, 1965). However, some controversy exists in
the interpretation of this information, since neurones containing
acetylcholinesterase activity are not necessarily cholinergic, but

153

may merely be cholinoceptive. For this reason, the development of
more direct histochemical techniques for visualizing acetylcholine
itself, or the more reliable marker enzyme choline acetyl transferase, are awaited (Kasa, 1971). No histochemical techniques are
available, however, which permit the identification and localization
of neurones using the amino acids GABA glycine or glutamate as
transmitters. Histochemical techniques which permit the localization of enzymes involved in the catabolism of GABA have been described; for GABA Glu. transaminase by van Gelder (1965) and for
succinic semialdehyde dehydrogenase by Sims, Weitsen and Bloom
(1971). Such techniques, however, suffer from the same disadvantage
as that used for acetylcholinesterase, i.e. the enzymes of GABA
catabolism are not known to be restricted to neurones using GABA
as transmitter.

The approach we will describe here represents an alternative
technique which may possibly have general application to the question of localizing transmitter specific neurones. This approach
derives from the knowledge which has recently been gained concerning
the existence of specific uptake systems for neurotransmitters in
nervous tissues. As Snyder will describe in more detail in another
chapter (Snyder, Chapt. 10) we now know that transport systems with
high specificity, and high affinity for their substrates, exist for
virtually all of the known transmitters. In the case of the monoamines there is good evidence that these special uptake systems
are specifically located in those neurones which use NA, DA or 5-HT
as transmitter, and that each of the different monoaminergic neurones
has its own particular uptake system (Iversen, 1967; 1971). The
work we shall describe here is an attempt to find out whether this
localization of special uptake process in transmitter-specific
neurones also applies to the amino acid transmitters. If it does,
then such neurones might be labelled selectively by exposure to the
appropriate radioactive amino acids, and could subsequently be
identified by autoradiographic techniques. This work is still in
an explorative phase, and we can do no more than present a progress
report at this stage. Before describing our own studies of the amino
acids, in which we have been particularly concerned with GABA, a
brief review will be given of the application of autoradiographic
techniques to the monoamines. Such studies form an important back-
ground to our own, since they illustrate the use of autoradiographic
techniques in systems which are more clearly defined than those
involving the amino acids.

MONOAMINES

The evidence that monoaminergic neurones have the specific
ability to accumulate exogenous amines is now considered so good
that the localization of labelled amines by autoradiographic

techniques can already be used as a method for identifying such
neurones. The availability of alternative techniques at both the
light microscope (fluorescence) and electron microscope (dense core
synaptic vesicles) levels means that the validity of the autoradiographic procedures can be checked against other procedures,
sometimes directly. Thus, by using freeze dried peripheral tissues
such as the iris after exposure to labelled NA and processing with
formaldehyde vapours Hökfelt and Ljungdahl (1971 b) reported that
the autoradiographic localization of labelled NA in sympathetic
terminals was very similar to the distribution of endogenous NA in
fluorescence microscopic examination of the same tissue. Similar
results were reported for various regions of brain after intraventricular injections of labelled NA or 5-HT by Fuxe et al.(1968).
Other studies using electron microscope autoradiography have shown
that labelled NA is localized in structures presumed to be adrenergic
nerve terminals in various peripheral tissues (Wolfe et al, 1962;
Devine and Simpson, 1968). Using the autoradiographic technique
to identify adrenergic terminals in spleen and other peripheral
tissues, Esterhuizen et al (1968) and Graham, Lever and Spriggs
(1968) were able to show that adrenergic nerve terminals in such
tissues did not contain acetylcholinesterase activity, detected
by histochemical staining in the same tissue sections. The latter
studies, at the electron microscopic level, illustrate the usefulness of the autoradiographic approach as a diagnostic tool for
identifying transmitter-specific structures. Although autoradiography may be redundant for localizing monoaminergic neurones at the
light microscope level, where the fluorescence histochemical approach
is already available, it may, nevertheless, have important uses in
identifying monoaminergic structures at the electron microscopic
level. Although NA-containing sympathetic nerve terminals can be
identified in the peripheral nervous system by their characteristic
content of dense-cored synaptic vesicles, such identification is
often much more difficult in the CNS (for review, see Hökfelt, 1965).
Labelled NA can be localized in nerve terminals and cell bodies of
adrenergic neurones in the CNS by autoradiographic techniques either
when the labelled catecholamine is injected into the CSF in vivo,
or when brain slices are incubated with labelled NA (Aghajanian and
Bloom, 1966, 1967 a; Descarries and Droz, 1970; Fuxe et al., 1968;
Ishii and Friede, 1967, 1968; Lenn, 1967; Hökfelt and Ljungdahl,
1971b).   In several of these studies an uptake of labelled NA
into dopaminergic neurones in the basal ganglia, arcuate nucleus
and median eminence was also demonstrated. This is not unexpected,
since the uptake mechanism in dopaminergic neurones has many
similarities to that in noradrenergic neurones, and can take up
NA with relatively high affinity (Snyder, Chapt. 10). Such lack
of selectivity could in principle be avoided, however, either by
the use of drugs known to inhibit the NA or DA uptake systems
selectively, or by using animals pretreated with the drug 6-
hydroxydopamine. Under appropriate treatment conditions it is

possible to achieve a selective destruction of noradrenergic
terminals in brain with this drug, leaving dopaminergic neurones
unaffected (Iversen and Uretsky, 1971). The uptake of labelled
dopamine by dopaminergic neurones in the retina has been studied
autoradiographically by Ehinger and Falck (1971) and by Kramer,
Potts and Mangnall (1971) but otherwise few studies appear to
have concentrated on dopaminergic systems elsewhere in the CNS.

Labelled 5-HT has been localized by light microscopy (Fuxe
et al., 1968) and by e.m. autoradiography (Aghajanian and Bloom,
1967 b) after injection of the labelled amine into rat CSF. The
amine appears to be localized primarily in 5-HT containing
structures, but 5-HT is also taken up with some avidity by adrenergic neurones (Shaskan and Snyder, 1970), and caution is thus
needed in the interpretation of such results. Bloom et al. (1972)
recommend prior treatment with 6-hydroxydopamine, to destroy
adrenergic terminals as a method of improving the selectivity of
5-HT labelling. Alternatively the simultaneous administration of
non-radioactive catecholamine might achieve the same end (Iversen,
1970).

In homogenates of various regions of rat brain the uptake of
labelled NA appears to take place predominantly into synaptosome
particles (Coyle and Snyder, 1969). This has been confirmed in
our laboratory by e.m. autoradiographic studies (Iversen, unpublished) of the localization of ^{3}H-NA in homogenates of rat cerebral
cortex and neostriatum. Statistical analysis of these results,
furthermore, indicates that ^{3}H-NA is taken up in an "all or none"
fashion by certain synaptosomes and not by others (Table 1)--these
presumably represent noradrenergic terminals in the cerebral cortex,
and dopaminergic terminals in the neostriatum. About 5% of all
synaptosomes from cortex were noradrenergic, and about 16% of those
from neostriatum were dopaminergic by these criteria (Table 1).
The latter estimate is in close agreement with that given by
Hökfelt (1965) of 16.4% for the proportion of dopaminergic terminals
in rat caudate nucleus, estimated by the cytochemical criterion of
terminals containing dense-cored synaptic vesicles after loading
with NA or α-methyl-NA.

Apart from the direct localization of exogenously applied
catecholamines, labelled DA or NA may also be generated by the
administration of the labelled precursor L-DOPA. Descarries and
Havrankova (1970) using this method found autoradiographic
labelling in neurones in the locus coeruleus and hypothalamus,
but in general this approach seems to have no advantage over the
administration of the amines themselves, particularly since little
is known of the specificity of uptake mechanisms for L-DOPA in CNS
neurones. Autoradiography may also be used to localize radioactively labelled drugs such as 6-hydroxydopamine, which can be

TABLE 1

Electron microscope autoradiographic labelling of synaptosome
populations with ^{3}H-noradrenaline in rat brain homogenates

	Labelled synaptosomes as % total population
Cerebral cortex	
30 days exposure	5.7 ± 0.30
60 days exposure	6.3 ± 0.32
Neostriatum	
10 days exposure	14.5 ± 1.42
60 days exposure	16.1 ± 2.09

Proportion of labelled synaptosomes was estimated on low
power electron autoradiographs after different radio-
autographic exposure periods. Homogenates were labelled
by incubation in vitro with 5 μM ^{3}H-NA, by the method
of Coyle and Snyder (1969). Results are means and
S.E. Mean for 5-6 analyses.

shown in this way to be selectively accumulated by adrenergic nerve terminals (Ljungdahl et al., 1971).

In the various studies described above labelled amines have been studied autoradiographically either in freeze-dried tissues, or after fixation--usually with glutaraldehyde. The latter procedure has been shown by Descarries and Droz (1970) to lead to retention of a substantial proportion of labelled NA in brain tissue and was the best of several fixatives tested. Since glutaraldehyde fixed tissues exhibit a much better preservation of morphological structure than can be obtained after freeze-drying, this seems to be the method of choice. It is, of course, essential when studying the autoradiographic localization of small diffusible substances such as the transmitters that methods be used which either fix the labelled substance covalently into the tissue--as occurs when amino compounds are exposed to polyaldehyde fixatives-- or which allow the use of frozen or freeze-dried preparations.

In summary, autoradiographic procedures have already proved useful in identifying monoaminergic structures--and are likely to have further applications in this respect, particularly in the CNS. Our extensive knowledge of the properties of uptake systems for NA, DA and 5-HT, should allow a sophisticated manipulation of the conditions for such experiments in future, to allow a more or less completely specific labelling of one or other of the three types of aminergic neurone.

AMINO ACIDS

The discovery of specific high affinity uptake processes for those amino acids (GABA, glycine and glutamate) thought to be neurotransmitters has prompted several groups independently to initiate autoradiographic studies with these amino acids. Thus, in addition to our own studies (Bloom and Iversen, 1971; Iversen and Bloom, 1972; Neal and Iversen, 1972; Schon and Iversen, 1972) similar work has been undertaken by Hökfelt and Ljungdahl (1970, 1971 a, 1971 b, 1972) by Ehinger (1970) and Ehinger and Falck (1971), by Lam and Steinman (1971) and by Matus and Denison (1971). The aim of all these studies has been to use the autoradiographic localization of the labelled amino acid as a means for identifying transmitter-specific neurones. The rationale of such an approach is dependent on the existence of uptake processes for the putative transmitter amino acids with affinities for their substrate which are far higher than the transport processes for amino acids present in all other tissues. Provided that relatively low concentrations of labelled amino acid are used for loading, the existence of these high affinity systems means that a preferential labelling of the high affinity sites in comparison with the low affinity sites generally distributed in tissues may be achieved.

A. GABA

(i) Introduction

There are only very few specific neuronal pathways in which there is evidence that this amino acid occurs and acts as an inhibitory transmitter. There is little doubt that the Purkinje cells in the cerebellum, and their axon terminals in the cerebellar and vestibular nuclei constitute one of the best defined systems of this type. There is good neurophysiological evidence that GABA is the inhibitory transmitter released at Purkinje axon terminals in the cerebellar nuclei (Ito, Yoshida, 1966; Obata et al., 1967) and a release of GABA has been demonstrated in response to cerebellar stimulation (Obata and Takeda, 1969). Furthermore, GABA and the biosynthetic enzyme glutamic acid decarboxylase disappear from cerebellar nuclei and Deiter's neurones when the Purkinje axons degenerate after cerebellar lesions (Fonnum, Storm-Mathisen and Walberg, 1970; Otsuka et al., 1971). From micro-analysis of the layers of tissue obtained by micro-dissection of hippocampus, Storm-Mathisen and Fonnum (1971) presented evidence for a localization of GABA within inhibitory neurones of the pyramidal cell layer of this structure. McGeer et al.(1971) have recently demonstrated a loss of GAD from substantia nigra following surgical lesions in the globus pallidus in the rat, suggesting the possible existence of GABA-containing neurones in a pallido-nigral pathway. Subcellular distribution studies of GABA and GAD have yielded somewhat confusing results: the biosynthetic enzyme GAD shows a clear synaptosomal localization (Fonnum, 1968) but the endogenous amino acid and radioactively labelled GABA show far less distinct synaptosomal localizations, perhaps because they are more easily lost from such particles during the subcellular fractionation procedures (Neal and Iversen, 1969). In the latter study, however, evidence was obtained that GAD, endogenous GABA and radioactively labelled GABA were all localized in a single population of synaptosomes. In other words the labelled amino acid appeared to be taken up by the same nerve terminals which contained endogenous GABA and GAD--a crucial assumption for the present purposes. This evidence is strengthened by the finding that synaptosomes containing labelled GABA could be partially separated from those containing labelled catecholamines or labelled glycine on density gradient centrifugation (Iversen and Snyder, 1968; Green, Snyder and Iversen, 1969; Iversen and Johnston, 1971). Csillik and Knyihar (1970) have attempted to use the binding of ^{14}C-thiosemicarbazide to freeze sectioned rat brain as the basis of an autoradiographic procedure for localizing GAD and GABA, but the specificity of such binding is not known.

(ii) Methods used for autoradiography

In our own studies the following general procedure is used. Tissue samples are fixed in buffered glutaraldehyde solution.

This has been found to lead to the retention of approximately two thirds of the initial amount of ^{3}H-GABA present in the tissue. Samples are then post-fixed in osmic acid, dehydrated in alcohol and embedded in a low viscosity epoxy resin. In all experiments thick sections (1-2 μm) are first cut from the resin blocks, and these are mounted on glass slides and dipped in Ilford L4 emulsion and processed for light microscope autoradiography. If these sections show a positive autoradiographic reaction after a one or two week exposure, appropriate areas are then selected for the preparation of thin sections from the same tissue blocks for e.m. work. Thin sections (approximately 75 nm) are cut with a diamond knife and mounted on celloidin coated slides, stained with lead citrate, carbon coated and dipped in diluted L4 emulsion according to the procedure of Salpeter and Bachmann (1964) and Budd and Salpeter (1969). After exposure for one to twelve weeks the autoradiograms are developed in Kodak D19b for two minutes at 20° and examined in a Phillips EM300 electron microscope.

Hokfelt and Ljungdahl (1971 a,b; 1972) have used both glutaraldehyde fixed tissues, and also freeze-dried specimens to avoid translocation of ^{3}H-GABA during autoradiography. They have also used a "dry" autoradiographic procedure in which emulsion is applied as a thin layer instead of dipping the samples in liquid emulsion. Ehinger and Falck (1971) also used freeze-dried tissues and a "dry" emulsion technique. Lam and Steinman (1971) used glutaraldehyde fixed tissues and a dipping technique. Our own results (Iversen and Bloom, 1972) and those of Orkand and Kravitz (1971) using a model system with ^{3}H-GABA and serum albumin suggest that glutaraldehyde treatment leads to the covalent fixation of a substantial proportion of ^{3}H-GABA-- probably onto tissue proteins. Once the tissue is fixed, therefore, we believe there is little danger that further translocations or losses of the labelled amino acids will occur and hence we have not used the stripping film or other "dry" emulsion application techniques.

(iii) <u>Results obtained with brain slices and other isolated tissues</u>

Our first e.m. autoradiographic studies were performed with small slices of cerebral cortex incubated <u>in vitro</u> with labelled GABA. In these experiments we found (Bloom and Iversen, 1971) that ^{3}H-GABA was highly localized over small nerve terminals and preterminal axons (Figure 1, Table 2). Furthermore, the labelling of nerve terminals occurred in an all or none manner, i.e. the proportion of terminals showing autoradiographic activity remained constant at about 30% regardless of the duration of the auto- radiographic exposure period (Table 3). These results thus appeared to confirm our most optimistic expectations: namely that GABA uptake sites were restricted to one category of neurone

TABLE 2

Localization of ^{3}H–GABA in rat cortical slices

(Average % $\pm$ S.E.M. (n = 5))

	SURFACE AREA	SILVER GRAINS
GLIAL CELLS	13 $\pm$ 1	2 $\pm$ 0.1
NEURONE PERIKARYA + DENDRITES	39 $\pm$ 3	11 $\pm$ 2
MYELINATED AXONS	5 $\pm$ 2	1 $\pm$ 0.1
UNMYELINATED AXONS	14 $\pm$ 1	11 $\pm$ 1
NERVE TERMINALS	23 $\pm$ 4	71 $\pm$ 2
SPACE	5 $\pm$ 1	3 $\pm$ 1

Values are means $\pm$ S.E. for five randomly selected low power electron micrographs. The area of tissue in each micrograph was 275 μm^2. The percentage of total area occupied by various tissue components was estimated by application of a 220 point grid; the distribution of silver grains was analysed in the same pictures, results are expressed as the mean percentages of total grain population located over the various tissue components (Iversen and Bloom, 1972).

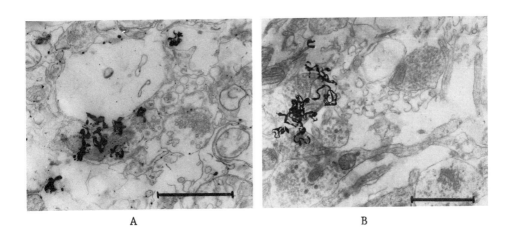

A   B

Figure 1. Electron microscope autoradiographs of slices of rat cerebral cortex (A) and substantia nigra (B) incubated with ^{3}H–GABA. Clusters of irregular electron dense silver grains are present over nerve terminals. The calibration lines represent 1 μm.

TABLE 3

Proportion of labelled terminals after different exposure times

Proportion of labelled terminals as %

Sample	Exposure time days =	10	20	30
Cerebral cortex slices – GABA		27.0 ± 2.4 (12)	27.2 ± 3.0 (5)	
Cerebral cortex homogenate – GABA		30.7 ± 2.38 (8)	33.7 ± 2.47 (12)	34.5 ± 2.52 (5
Striatum homogenate – GABA		35.4 ± 2.36 (5)	30.8 ± 3.23 (4)	34.0 ± 1.45 (5
Hippocampus homogenate – GABA		38.3 ± 2.84 (6)	45.4 ± 2.59 (6)	
Spinal cord homogenate – GABA		25.1 ± 2.00 (6)	24.0 ± 1.46 (5)	
Spinal cord homogenate – glycine		25.2 ± 2.32 (7)	29.4 ± 2.14 (7)	

(from Iversen and Bloom, 1972)

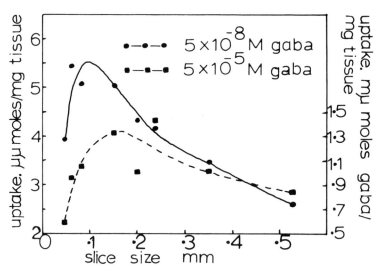

Figure 2. Effect of slice thickness on accumulation of ^{3}H–GABA by
rat cerebral cortex incubated with the labelled amino acid at
5×10^{-8} M and a 5×10^{-5} M for 10 minutes (Minchin and Iversen,
unpublished).

in the brain, and that these neurones, furthermore, constituted a
very important proportion of all the synaptic terminals in cerebral
cortex. We have subsequently studied the uptake of ^{3}H-GABA in
slices prepared from a variety of other regions of brain (Schon,
Hirsch and Iversen, unpublished). In slices of cerebellum and
substantia nigra the labelling was again localized to nerve
terminals (Table 4) although in the s. nigra labelling was also
seen over astrocytes and oligodendroglia. About half of all the
synaptic terminals in the s. nigra and in the granular layer of
the cerebellum were labelled with ^{3}H-GABA (Table 4). This high
proportion of labelling with ^{3}H-GABA is in good agreement with the
high GABA and glutamic decarboxylase activity in these brain regions
(Iversen, 1972). In our studies with slices we have failed to
observe any conspicuous accumulation of ^{3}H-GABA over nerve cell
bodies in any of the regions examined. In this respect our results
differ from the light microscope autoradiographic results reported
by Hökfelt and Ljungdahl (1971 a,b) who found accumulations of
^{3}H-GABA over stellate cells in the rat cerebellum, and over large
cells presumed to be neurones in the cerebral cortex and in the
hippocampus after incubation of slices of these tissues in vitro.
They also observed prominent accumulations of ^{3}H-GABA over what
appeared to be Bergmann glial cells in the granular layers of the
cerebellar cortex, which we have not observed. These differences
are probably attributable to differences in the techniques used to
prepare and label the slices of brain. We have been concerned to
achieve a complete penetration of the tissue slices with ^{3}H-GABA
in order to obtain a homogeneous labelling of all available uptake
sites. Previous studies (Iversen and Neal, 1968) and more recent
in this laboratory (Figure 2) have indicated that the optimum
thickness of slice to achieve a maximum uptake of ^{3}H-GABA in
cerebral cortex is not more than 100-200 μm. Consequently our
studies have used mechanically chopped tissue cut at 100 μm
intervals, or "Vibratome" sections cut at 200-300 μm from the
cerebellum or s. nigra. Hökfelt and Ljungdahl (1971 a,b), however,
have used somewhat thicker slices and have also added dextran to
the incubation medium to avoid the considerable swelling and
deterioration of morphological structure which otherwise occurs
in thin slices during incubation. This deterioration of structure
is particularly marked in large nerve cell bodies and in glial
elements, and may account for our failure to observe ^{3}H-GABA
uptake in such structures in slice experiments. The deterioration
of structure also means that tissue incubated in the form of slices
is not very suitable for fine structural studies at the e.m. level
(cf. Figure 1 and Figure 7). On the other hand slices have certain
advantages in that they can be labelled homogeneously, and large
amounts of ^{3}H-GABA can be introduced into them with ease. Such
preparations can be used, for example, to illustrate the gross
morphological distribution of nerve terminals capable of ^{3}H-GABA
uptake in various brain regions.

TABLE 4

Localization of ^{3}H-GABA uptake in nerve terminals of rat brain after incubation of slices in vitro and after injection in vivo.

BRAIN REGION	Nerve terminals as percentage of total surface area	Silver grains over nerve terminals as percentage of total grains	Labelled nerve terminals as percentage of total no. of terminals
	A	B	
IN VITRO			
Cerebral cortex	23.5 $\pm$ 3.6	70.7 $\pm$ 2.3	27
Cerebellum - Molecular layer	10.3 $\pm$ 0.9	50.2 $\pm$ 5.6	14
Cerebellum - Granular layer	10.6 $\pm$ 1.5	67.8 $\pm$ 2.9	46
Substantia nigra	6.8 $\pm$ 1.3	25.5 $\pm$ 3.9	51
IN VIVO			
Locus coeruleus	16.5 $\pm$ 2.4	43.3 $\pm$ 8.5	44
Periventricular grey of hypothalamus	13.3 $\pm$ 1.2	33.9 $\pm$ 2.9	39
Caudate nucleus	18.3 $\pm$ 1.9	35.6 $\pm$ 3.3	27

A. Percentage of total area occupied by nerve terminals was estimated by application of a multi-point grid to randomly selected low power electron micrographs of the various tissue. B. The distribution of silver grains over nerve terminals was analyzed in the same electron micrographs, and the results expressed as a percentage of the total grain population in each micrograph. Results are means $\pm$ S.E. Mean for 4-6 analyses in each case. Note that if radioactivity were randomly distributed over the tissue samples the values in B should approximately equal those in A. The results instead indicate a localization of ^{3}H-GABA over nerve terminals, which is even more marked if one considers that the labelling is restricted to one type of nerve terminal. Thus, for example, in cerebral cortex slices 71% of the total ^{3}H-GABA was localized over terminals which occupied only about 6% of the total surface area.

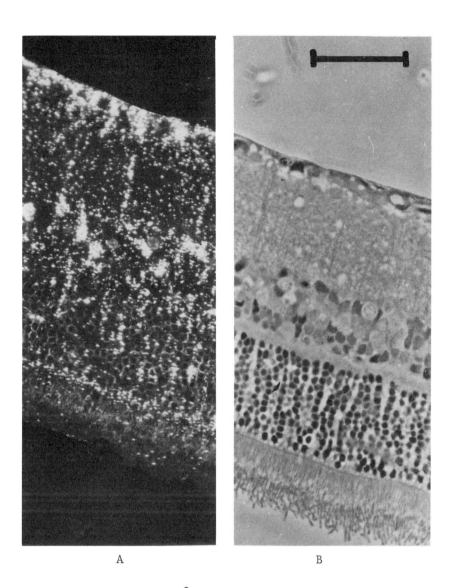

A   B

Figure 3.   Localization of ^{3}H-GABA in rat retina after incubation
in vitro. Dark field autoradiogram (A) with silver grains as
white dots is compared with a phase contrast micrograph of an
adjacent portion of the same tissue section (B).   The calibration
line represents 50 μm.

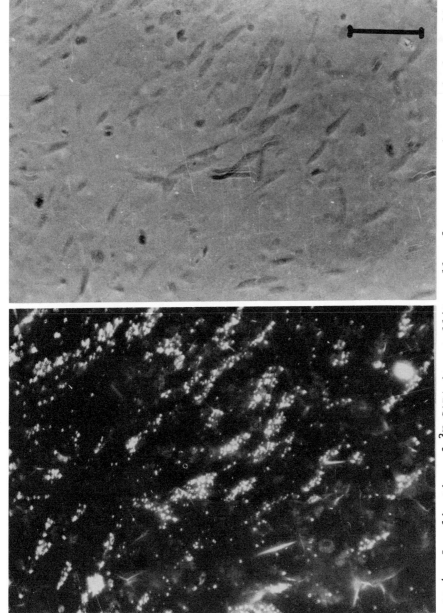

Figure 4. Localization of ³H-GABA in satellite cells of mouse superior cervical ganglion in tissue culture. Autoradiogram (to left) is compared with phase contrast micrograph of the same field (to right). Calibration bar represents 10 μm.

We have also studied ^{3}H-GABA localization after incubation of other isolated tissues with the labelled amino acid. Isolated rat retina shows an uptake of ^{3}H-GABA which has properties similar in many respects to those observed in slices of cerebral cortex or other regions of brain (Neal, 1972). We were, however, surprised to find on autoradiographic examination that ^{3}H-GABA in the isolated retina was predominantly localized over the glial elements—in Müller cells and fibers (Figure 3), (Neal and Iversen, 1972). This has since been observed also in similar experiments with isolated retinae from rabbit and monkey (Neal and Iversen, unpublished). The glial uptake of ^{3}H-GABA in the retina is so prominent that it is quite possible that a small additional neuronal component in the labelling may have been obscured by it. We find the retinal results particularly interesting because: a) the fine structure of the tissue is well preserved after incubations (unlike the situation in brain slices) and hence the result does not appear likely to be due to a damage artifact, and b) rather different results are obtained when ^{3}H-GABA is introduced into the eye in vivo (see paragraph (v) below). Lam and Steinman (1971) obtained different results in studies of the localization of ^{3}H-GABA in the goldfish retina. They incubated retinae in situ in isolated eye cups, and found a predominantly neuronal localization of ^{3}H-GABA, particularly in horizontal cells. Interestingly the accumulation of ^{3}H-GABA in these cells was much greater in tissue subjected to light stimulation.

A preliminary report (Bowery and Brown, 1972) that cells in sympathetic ganglia were also capable of ^{3}H-GABA uptake prompted us to examine ^{3}H-GABA uptake in this tissue also. We have used mouse sympathetic ganglia maintained in organ culture conditions for 14 days. Under the culture conditions used the ganglion neurones degenerated almost completely, but an outgrowth of satellite cells occurred around the explanted ganglion. When such preparations were exposed to ^{3}H-GABA, autoradiography demonstrated an accumulation of the labelled amino acid in the outgrowing glial elements (Figure 4) (Mackay and Iversen, unpublished data). Orkand and Kravitz (1971) have also reported a localization of ^{3}H-GABA over Schwann cell and connective tissue elements in crustacean nerve muscle preparations incubated with ^{3}H-GABA in vitro.

In summary, our own results and those of others with slices or other isolated tissues allowed several conclusions to be drawn: 1) the uptake of ^{3}H-GABA can occur into neurones, and especially into nerve terminals, 2) not all neurones or terminals are labelled by ^{3}H-GABA, 3) certain glial cells and their processes can also accumulate ^{3}H-GABA, 4) the exact result obtained, especially with regard to the occurrence of labelling in glia and nerve cell bodies appears to be highly dependent on the

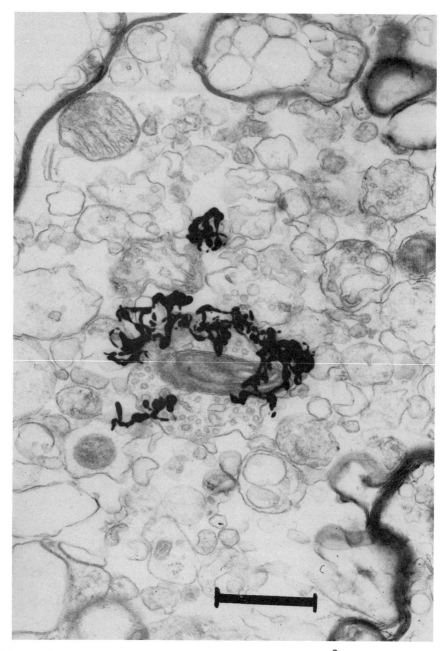

Figure 5. Electron microscopic localization of ^{3}H-GABA over a
synaptosome in homogenate of rat caudate nucleus, after incubation in vitro. Calibration bar represents 0.5 µm.

experimental conditions used and on the degree of preservation of
tissue structure which can be maintained in sliced tissue.

(iv) Results obtained after labelling brain homogenates with ^{3}H-GABA in vitro

^{3}H-GABA uptake occurs into particles with sedimentation
properties of synaptosomes when brain homogenates are incubated
in vitro (Weinstein et al., 1965; Iversen and Johnston, 1971).
We have examined the localization of ^{3}H-GABA in particulate
fractions after labelling homogenates of various regions of rat
CNS in this way (Bloom and Iversen, 1971; Iversen and Bloom, 1972).
In such samples ^{3}H-GABA was found to be highly localized over
synaptosomes, confirming our previous conclusions (Table 5,
Figure 5). As in brain slices, the labelling of synaptosomes
with ^{3}H-GABA was again of an "all or none" type, and it was
possible to obtain estimates of the proportion of GABA-containing
synaptosomes in the populations from various regions of the CNS
(Table 6). The use of homogenates has several advantages for such
studies: it removes other possible sites of ^{3}H-GABA uptake, since
glial cells and nerve cell bodies are largely destroyed by the
homogenization process, and for statistical analysis of the
proportion of terminals labelled with ^{3}H-GABA, sampling problems
are also considerably less than with tissue slices. The synaptosomes labelled with ^{3}H-GABA did not have any obvious morphological
features which distinguished them from those not labelled in this
way. They had similar dimensions and contained synaptic vesicles
of an average diameter of 46 nm, characteristic of those in most
other presynaptic terminals. We have not observed any relationship between the presence of ^{3}H-GABA in terminals and the occurrence of synaptic vesicles with elliptical or "flattened"
appearance (Uchizono, 1965). It should be pointed out, however,
that the occurrence of such flattened vesicles is highly dependent
on the precise conditions used in fixation and subsequent pre-
parative procedures (Bodian, 1970).

The results with brain homogenates thus confirmed the existence
of ^{3}H-GABA uptake sites in certain nerve terminals in CNS, and
indicated that such terminals--which we believe represent those
normally containing and releasing GABA--account for about one
third of all synaptic terminals in many regions of the CNS.

(v) Results obtained after labelling with ^{3}H-GABA in vivo

Because of the difficulties associated with the use of brain
slices, particularly the degeneration of fine structure which
occurs in such preparations, we have sought more recently to use
an alternative approach which allows labelling with ^{3}H-GABA
in vivo. This method then allows perfusion fixation of the brain
in situ, with a consequent improvement in the preservation of fine
structure for e.m. studies. A short report of this work has

TABLE 5

Localization of H^3-GABA in homogenate of hypothalamus

	Proportion of total surface area – per cent	Proportion of total silver grains – per cent
Synaptosomes	15.3 $\pm$ 1.42	71.9 $\pm$ 1.90
Free mitochondria	3.1 $\pm$ 0.88	1.5 $\pm$ 0.84
Myelin fragments	12.6 $\pm$ 2.58	4.3 $\pm$ 2.08
Unidentified membrane fragments	41.3 $\pm$ 1.23	21.7 $\pm$ 2.46
Space between particles	27.8 $\pm$ 1.51	0.8 $\pm$ 0.8

Values are means $\pm$ S.E. Mean for 5 low power micrograms (total area of each = $17\overline{5}$ μm^2); other details as for Table 2 (data from Iversen and Bloom, 1972).

TABLE 6

Proportion of nerve terminals labelled
with H^3-GABA in homogenate samples

BRAIN REGION	% LABELLED TERMINALS	NO. OF ANALYSES	TOTAL NO. TERMINALS
Cerebellum	12.9 $\pm$ 1.5	7	295
Medulla/Pons	25.4 $\pm$ 1.9	15	677
Cerebral Cortex	32.2 $\pm$ 1.7	20	1411
Striatum	34.2 $\pm$ 1.3	16	1039
Hypothalamus	35.1 $\pm$ 2.4	10	528
Hippocampus	41.9 $\pm$ 2.1	12	743

(from Iversen and Bloom, 1972)

appeared (Schon and Iversen, 1972). In preliminary biochemical studies we first tackled what we consider to be the two most important technical problems in such studies. Firstly, it is important that ^{3}H-GABA should penetrate to the brain as uniformly as possible. Because of the existence of an effective blood-brain barrier, systemic administration of labelled GABA is not practicable (Hespe, Roberts and Prims, 1969). We have, therefore, injected ^{3}H-GABA into the CSF, and have found that a combination of two injections, one into the lateral ventricle of the brain, followed 10-20 minutes later by an injection via the cisterna magna gives the most uniform distribution and the greatest retention of labelled GABA. As shown by Clark, Vivonia and Baxter (1968), however, in autoradiographic studies with ^{14}C-GABA, penetration of labelled GABA occurs for only a relatively short distance from the surface of the ventricular system--this is a problem which we have not so far found any solution to. A second problem, which has proved more readily soluble, is that the metabolism of the injected ^{3}H-GABA must be blocked--so that only the unchanged amino acid is present in the tissue samples used for autoradiographic analysis. Pretreatment of rats 30 minutes before ^{3}H-GABA injections with a large dose (80 mg/kg i.per) of amino-oxyacetic acid--a known inhibitor of GABA catabolism--completely prevented the formation of any labelled metabolites of ^{3}H-GABA in the brain for up to 40 minutes after an injection of labelled amino acid into the CSF. After such injections as much as 50% of the injected dose of ^{3}H-GABA remained in the brain 10 minutes after injection, and there was only a negligible further disappearance of the label during the next 30 minutes. On the other hand, in animals not treated with AOAA there was a rapid metabolism and disappearance of labelled GABA from the brain after injections into the CSF. This problem was less important in brain slices or homogenates, in which unchanged ^{3}H-GABA accumulated without significant metabolism even when AOAA was not present (Bloom and Iversen, 1971). For autoradiographic experiments we have used AOAA treated animals, and these were killed 10 minutes or 40 minutes after the last injection of ^{3}H-GABA and the brains fixed <u>in situ</u> by aortic perfusion with buffered glutaraldehyde solution (Schon and Iversen, 1972). Various regions of brain were then removed, post-fixed and treated as described before for autoradiographic analysis. The results obtained in such studies are as follows.

    a) <u>There was clear evidence of neuronal accumulations</u> of ^{3}H-GABA in many regions of the brain, although the distribution of label was uneven. Thus certain regions such as the cerebral cortex or spinal cord were almost completely unlabelled. Among structures bordering the ventricular system, labelling was generally only sufficiently intense in those areas of neuropil

immediately adjacent to the ependyma to allow e.m. autoradiographic
analysis; all statistical analyses refer only to tissue in such
subependymal areas. There was a variable penetration of ^{3}H-GABA
into the various brain regions adjacent to the ventricles; for
example, penetration was good in the locus coeruleus, periventricular grey of hypothalamus and the habenular nucleus, but poor in
most areas of hippocampus, and in the cuneate nucleus--perhaps
because the superficial areas of myelinated axons in the latter
regions restricted ^{3}H-GABA entry to the underlying structures. In
the cerebellar cortex, particularly at the base of the cerebellum,
penetration of ^{3}H-GABA was often good. Light microscope and e.m.
autoradiography results showed that in the superficial layers of
the cerebellum there were heavy accumulations of ^{3}H-GABA over cells
which could be identified as stellate cells (Figures 6 and 7)--an
inhibitory neurone type in which GABA is thought to be transmitter.
All the stellate cells appeared to be equally labelled (Figure 8).
It was also possible to identify stellate cell axons in the superficial layers of the cerebellar cortex and these were also heavily
labelled. Stellate cells accounted for $56 \pm 2.9\%$ of all silver
grains in the superficial half of the molecular layer, but represented only $13 \pm 1.8\%$ of the surface area in this region (n = 4).
Labelling of synaptic terminals some of which may represent the
terminals of stellate cells onto Purkinje dendrites could occasionally be seen in the molecular and deeper layers. No labelling
was seen, however, over Purkinje cells themselves or over their
dendritic processes. This is a surprising finding in view of the
evidence which suggests that GABA is the transmitter in such
neurones. We do not have any explanation of this result; it
seems unlikely to be due simply to a failure of ^{3}H-GABA to penetrate to the Purkinje cell layers of the cerebellum, since we have
observed labelling in glial cells in this region (see below).
Hökfelt and Ljungdahl (1971 b, 1972) also failed to see Purkinje
cell labelling in cerebellar slices in which the surrounding
tissue was heavily labelled. It should be remembered, however,
that there is no direct evidence that Purkinje cell bodies or
their dendrites contain appreciable amounts of endogenous GABA.

In the subependymal neuropil of the caudate nucleus there was
again a clear labelling of nerve cell bodies (Figure 7) which were
similar in size and shape to the stellate cells in the cerebellar
cortex. These cells had elliptical profiles a large nucleus with
a distinct nuclear invagination, and had relatively little endo-
plasmic reticulum in their cytoplasm. Their appearance might
suggest that they are neurones with relatively short axons,
perhaps local inhibitory interneurones. In the caudate nucleus
there were also numerous labelled presynaptic terminals (Table 4),
mainly of an axodendritic type. Such labelled synapses were also
seen in abundance in periventricular grey matter of the hypothalamus, and in the locus coeruleus (Table 4, Figure 9). No

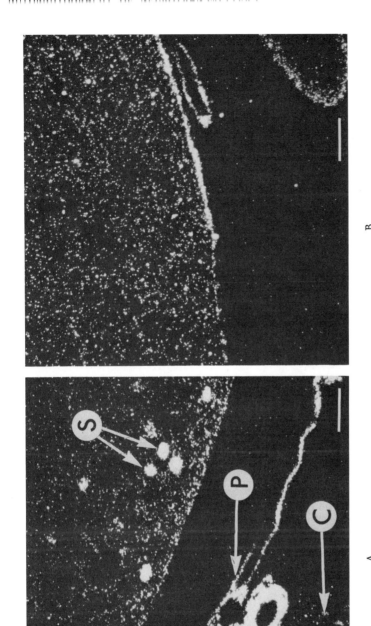

B

A

Figure 6. (A) = Dark field autoradiograph of the floor of the cerebellum after ³H-GABA administration in vivo. Heavy accumulations of silver grains are present over stellate cell bodies (S) and over the pia-arachnoid membrane (P). The choroid plexus (C) was relatively free of grains. In (B) the same region of the cerebellum after ³H-Glycine administration in vivo. Calibration bars represent 10 μm. (Schon and Iversen, 1972).

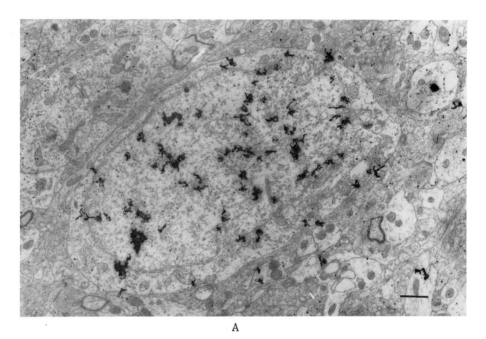

A

B

Figure 7. A neurone in the caudate nucleus (A) and a stellate
neurone in the cerebellar cortex (B), labelled with ^{3}H-GABA after
intraventricular injection of the labelled amino acid in vivo.
Calibration bar represents 1 μm.

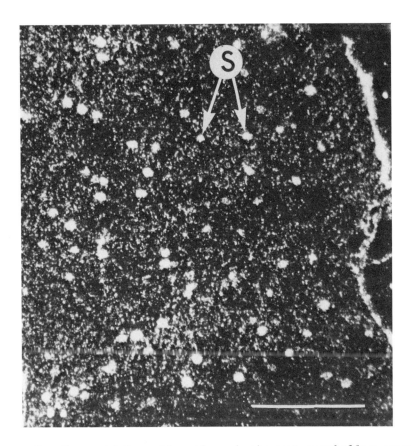

Figure 8. Tangential section through the rat cerebellar cortex
after labelling with ^{3}H-GABA <u>in vivo</u>. Note localization of
radioactivity over numerous stellate cells (S), (c.f. Figure 6).
Calibration bar represents 50 μm.

labelled nerve cell bodies, however, were seen in either of the
latter areas. In particular, there was a conspicuous absence of
labelling over the noradrenergic cells in the locus coeruleus.
Labelling over axosomatic synapses was also occasionally seen
particularly in the habenular nucleus and in the hypothalamus
(Figure 9). Preliminary results at a light microscope level
from the hippocampus indicated a localization of ^{3}H-GABA in the
region of the pyramidal cells (Figure 10), with labelled cell
bodies in this and surrounding layers of the tissue.

     The pattern of neuronal labelling seen after in vivo experi-
ments thus confirms that seen after in vitro studies, although
labelling of neuronal perikarya with ^{3}H-GABA was seen far more
clearly in the in vivo results presumably because of the better
preservation of their structure. As in the in vitro studies,
the labelling of neurones with ^{3}H-GABA in vivo was highly selective,
and in all probability represents a selective labelling of GABA-
containing structures. The failure of Purkinje cells or their
dendrites to show any accumulation of ^{3}H-GABA, however, suggests
either that not all GABA-containing neurones possess this uptake
ability, or alternatively that the GABA uptake sites in Purkinje
cells may be present only in the axon terminals and not in their
perikaryal or dendritic regions. It is interesting to note that
Csillik and Knyihar (1970) failed to observe binding of labelled
thiosemicarbazide over Purkinje cells in rat brain.

     b) In addition to neuronal accumulations of ^{3}H-GABA,
labelling was also evident over various extraneuronal structures,
after injection of the labelled amino acid in vivo. In all
regions of the ventricular system the ependymal cells showed a
heavy accumulation of ^{3}H-GABA. This labelling appeared to be
most pronounced at short time intervals after ^{3}H-GABA injection
(10 minutes) and become considerably less marked at 40 minutes
after injection--suggesting that ^{3}H-GABA was not firmly retained
at this site of accumulation. In animals not treated with AOAA
the accumulation of ^{3}H-GABA in the ependymal layers was much less
marked at all time intervals after injection (Figure 11) suggesting
that under such conditions GABA may be taken up and rapidly
metabolized in such extraneuronal sites. An intense labelling
of the ependymal cells was also seen when slices of brain from
AOAA treated rats were incubated with ^{3}H-GABA in vitro, indicating
that the labelling seen in vivo was not due simply to a preferential exposure of such sites to ^{3}H-GABA. Heavy labelling was
also seen in the pial membranes, particularly over the cerebellum
but also to some extent over the cerebral cortex, in which the
underlying neuropil remained almost completely devoid of labelling.
Little or no accumulation of ^{3}H-GABA was seen over the secretory
cells of the choroid plexus, however, after in vivo injections
(Figure 6). Blood vessels showed variable labelling with ^{3}H-GABA,

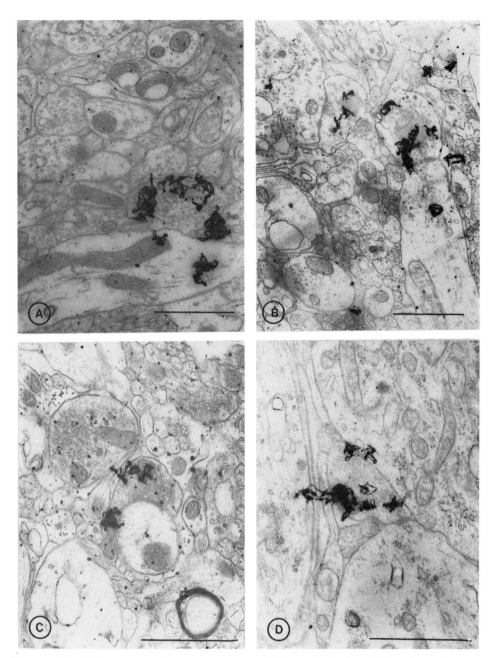

Figure 9. Electron microscope autoradiographic localization of ³H-GABA over presynaptic terminals in (A) caudate nucleus, (B) periventricular hypothalamus, (C) locus coeruleus, and (D) habenular nucleus of rat brain after labelling in vivo. Calibration bars represent 1 μm.

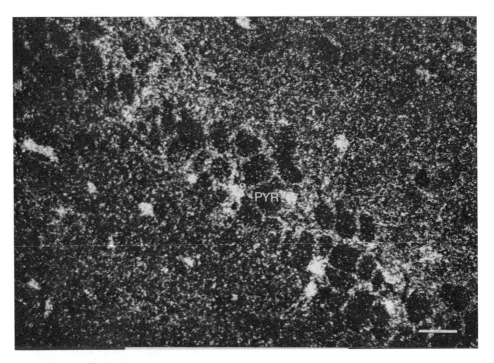

Figure 10. Dark field autoradiograph of rat hippocampus after
labelling with ³H-GABA in vivo. Note absence of label in large
neurones of the pyramidal cell layer (PYR), presence in small
cell bodies in all layers, and heavy neuropil labelling. The
ventricular surface is towards the upper right hand corner of
the field. Calibration bar represents 10 μm.

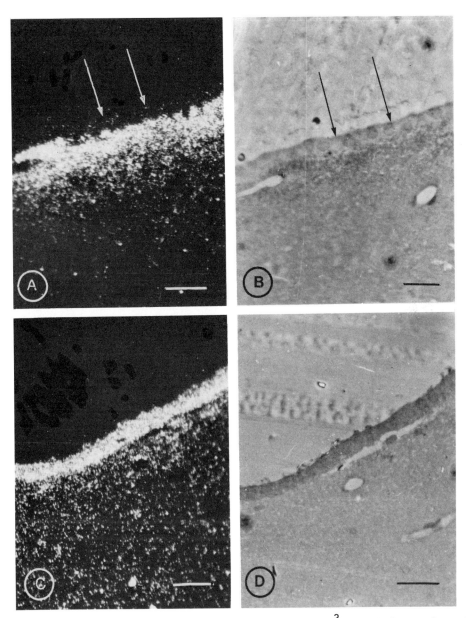

Figure 11. Labelling of ependymal tissue with ^{3}H-GABA in region of
the aqueduct after administration of label <u>in vivo</u>. (A) and (C) are
autoradiographs from animals killed 10 min after the intraventricular injection of ^{3}H-GABA; (A) being from an untreated animal, and
(C) from one treated 30 min previously with aminooxyacetic acid
(80 mg/kg, i.per.). The white arrows in (A) indicate the ventricular surface of the ependymal cells, which are largely unlabelled
in the absence of aminooxyacetic acid pre-treatment. (B) and (D) are
phase contrast micrographs of the same fields. Calibration bars
represent 10 μm.

with sometimes quite prominent accumulations of the labelled amino
acid. All of these sites of non-neuronal ^{3}H-GABA uptake--ependymal
cells, pial membranes and cerebral blood vessels are known to
represent regions with high GABA-Glu transaminase activity (van
Gelder, 1967). Such structures presumably accumulate ^{3}H-GABA only
when AOAA is present--the amino acid would otherwise be rapidly
metabolized in these sites.

        Another type of extraneuronal labelling was seen in all
regions of the brain, in which ^{3}H-GABA was accumulated by various
glial elements. This uptake of ^{3}H-GABA occurred mainly over
oligodendroglia, but was also seen occasionally over astrocytes,
which seemed to take up ^{3}H-GABA somewhat less avidly. In the
cuneate nucleus a particularly prominent glial labelling was
seen over oligodendroglia adjacent to the large neurones in this
nucleus (Figure 12). In this region 42 $\pm$ 3.3% of the ^{3}H-GABA was
found to occur over oligodendroglia, which accounted for only
15 $\pm$ 2.4% of the total surface area (n = 5). A similar pattern
of labelling was seen in the locus coeruleus, where in addition
to a clear labelling of axodendritic synapses, labelling was also
seen over oligodendroglia adjacent to the locus neurones (Figure 13).
In the caudate nucleus an unusual pattern of labelling was seen
over the three or four layers of glial cells underlying the ependyma, many of which were heavily labelled with ^{3}H-GABA. In regions
such as the habenular nucleus, cuneate nucleus and parts of the
hippocampus near the fimbria, where major fiber tracts underly the
ependyma, ^{3}H-GABA showed particularly prominent glial localization.
The labelling of glial cells by ^{3}H-GABA was far clearer in the
in vivo studies than in slices, presumably because of the poor
preservation of glial structure in slices after incubation in vitro.
The significance of such an uptake of ^{3}H-GABA by various glial cells
remains obscure; from our experience it does not appear to be a
universal property of glia but is restricted to certain categories
only.

        c) To complicate matters still further, results obtained by
Ehinger and Falck (1971) and confirmed by Neal and Iversen (unpublished) in the retina show a quite different pattern of GABA
labelling when in vitro results are compared with those obtained
from in vivo studies. In the latter studies ^{3}H-GABA was injected
into the occular fluid of the rabbit eye; after such injections,
^{3}H-GABA was found to be localized mainly over what appeared to be
amacrine cells in the inner nuclear layer (Figure 14), without any
obvious labelling of the glia (Müller cells) as seen after in vitro
labelling. Why such cells should accumulate ^{3}H-GABA so avidly in
in vitro experiments, but not after injection of labelled amino
acid into the eye remains mysterious. Lam and Steinman (1971), on
the other hand, failed to observe any significant difference in the
distribution of ^{3}H-GABA in goldfish retina incubated in vitro or

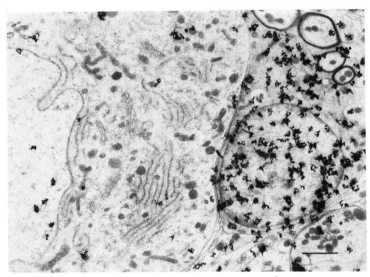

Figure 12. Prominent accumulation of ^{3}H–GABA over an oligodendro-
cyte adjacent to a large neurone showing sparse labelling in rat
cuneate nucleus 10 min after the intraventricular injection of
^{3}H–GABA. Calibration bar represents 1 µm.

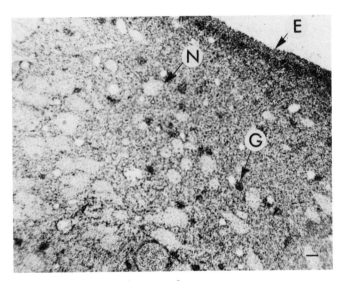

Figure 13. Localization of ^{3}H–GABA in the region of the locus
coeruleus in rat brain stem 40 min after the intracisternal injection of ^{3}H–GABA in vivo. Note absence of labelling over locus
neurones (N) and the prominent accumulation of radioactive amino
acid over glial cells (G) and the ependyma (E) and underlying
neuropil. Calibration bar represents 10 µm.

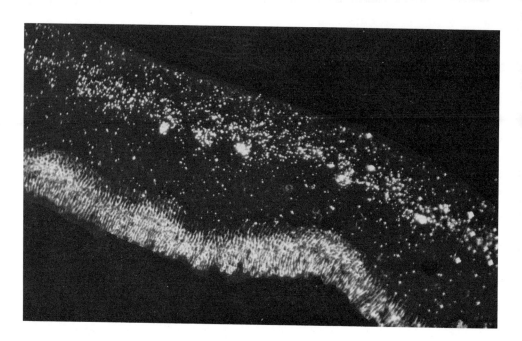

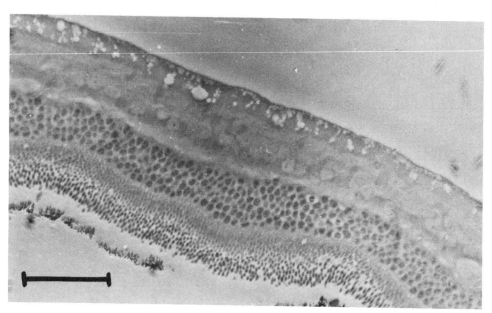

Figure 14.   Localization of ³H-GABA in rabbit retina after injection of the labelled amino acid into the ocular fluid <u>in vivo</u>. Dark field autoradiograph (above) is compared with phase contrast view of the same field (below).   Calibration bar represents 100 μm (c.f. Figure 3).

labelled by injection of ^{3}H-GABA into the vitreous humour.

To summarize, the preliminary results obtained from in vivo studies seem encouraging. The injection of ^{3}H-GABA into the CSF allows a clear labelling of certain neuronal cell bodies and processes, but this labelling is only present in tissue very close to the ventricular surface. This restricted penetration of the labelled amino acid may perhaps be overcome in future studies by local microinjections of ^{3}H-GABA into selected brain regions (Hökfelt and Ljungdahl, 1972). The results obtained after injections of ^{3}H-GABA in vivo, however, show quite clearly that ^{3}H-GABA uptake is not restricted to neurones in the CNS, but occurs also in several non-neuronal tissues, including various types of glial cell. Whether the accumulation of GABA by such structures is mediated by the same uptake process as that present in neurones remains to be determined; it may otherwise be possible to discover selective inhibitors for the neuronal and non-neuronal uptake systems which could be used to achieve a more selective pattern of labelling for autoradiographic studies.

B. Glycine

A specific, high affinity uptake system for glycine exists in the spinal cord, and brain stem but not in supraspinal areas of CNS (Neal and Pickles, 1969; Neal, 1971; Johnston and Iversen, 1971; Logan and Snyder, 1971). This uptake system may also exist in the retina (Brunn and Ehinger, 1972). The localization of uptake sites has been examined in autoradiographic studies at the light microscope and e.m. levels using ^{3}H-glycine and slices of rat and mouse spinal cord (Hökfelt and Ljungdahl, 1971 a; Matus and Dennison, 1971; Iversen, unpublished). At the light microscope level accumulations of ^{3}H-glycine were seen over the neuropil, particularly in ventral grey and around the large motor neurones (Figure 15); there was also labelling in small cells in most regions of spinal grey, and in fiber-like processes radiating out from the ventral grey matter (Figure 15). At the electron microscope level Hökfelt and Ljungdahl (1971 a) reported that there were accumulations of ^{3}H-glycine over nerve terminals, small myelinated axons and also over oligodendroglial cells--which probably represent the small labelled cells seen at the light microscope level. Matus and Dennison (1971) confirmed the localization of ^{3}H-glycine over certain nerve terminals in spinal cord, and in their experiments found a specific localization of label over synaptic terminals containing "flattened" synaptic vesicles. This relationship has not been consistently observed in our own studies, nor by Hökfelt and Ljungdahl (1971 a), but this may be due to differences in the techniques used in preparing the tissue samples for electron microscopy, and is clearly

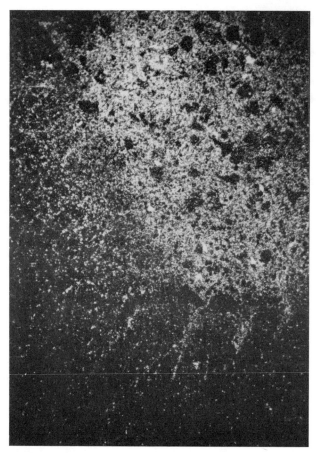

Figure 15. Dark field autoradiograph showing localization of
[3]H-glycine over ventral horn of mouse spinal cord, after incubation of sliced tissue with 5 μM ^{3}H-glycine in vitro. Note
absence of label over large motor neurones, presence of small
labelled cells and labelling in striations radiating into the
surrounding white matter.

TABLE 7

Proportion of labelled nerve terminals
in spinal cord homogenates

H[3]-GABA   (n = 11) - 24.6 ± 1.19%

H[3]-GLYCINE   (n = 14) - 27.9 ± 1.81%

H[3]-GABA +

H[3]-GLYCINE   (n = 10) - 50.8 ± 2.01%

(data from Iversen and Bloom, 1972)

a question which needs further examination.

In homogenates of spinal cord the high affinity uptake of ^{3}H-glycine is readily demonstrated (Johnston and Iversen, 1971), and as with ^{3}H-GABA this has also been studied by autoradiographic means (Iversen and Bloom, 1972). The ^{3}H-glycine taken up by homogenates or rat spinal cord was found to be highly localized over synaptosomes (Figure 16), and the labelling was again of an "all or none" type. We compared the labelling of synaptosomes in spinal cord homogenates after exposure to ^{3}H-GABA or ^{3}H-glycine alone and after exposure of homogenates to a mixture of the two amino acids. Each amino acid alone produced labelling of about 25% of the total synaptosomes population; the mixture gave an additive result, labelling about 50% of the total synaptosomes (Table 7). This result thus demonstrated that ^{3}H-GABA and ^{3}H-glycine were taken up by distinct sub-populations of the nerve terminals in spinal cord. We believe that these represent the terminals using the two inhibitory amino acid transmitters, which would thus together account for about half of all synaptic terminals in spinal cord.

We have not, so far been able to achieve an adequate labelling of spinal cord after glycine administration in vivo to allow autoradiographic studies. When ^{3}H-glycine was injected into the rat CSF, however, it served as a useful control for the specificity of ^{3}H-GABA uptake in supraspinal areas. For example, ^{3}H-glycine, unlike ^{3}H-GABA did not show any selective accumulation over stellate cells in the cerebellum (Figure 6) (Schon and Iversen, 1972). When ^{3}H-glycine was injected into the rabbit eye, however, Ehinger and Falck (1971) found it was selectively localized over neurones in the amacrine cell layers of the retina.

In summary, the preliminary autoradiographic results obtained with glycine in spinal cord and in retina suggest that this may be another suitable candidate for the application of such techniques. The high affinity uptake system for glycine exists only in those regions of CNS in which glycine acts as a transmitter. It seems likely from the results obtained so far that these glycine uptake sites may be associated primarily with the neurones using this transmitter. As with GABA, however, certain glial cells are also capable of selectively accumulating this amino acid (Hökfelt and Ljungdahl, 1971 a).

C. Glutamate and Other Amino Acids

There have been, so far, very few studies of the autoradiographic localization of glutamate or other putative transmitter amino acids in CNS tissue (Johnson, 1972). Apart from GABA and glycine, glutamate and aspartate are unique among amino acids in

exhibiting high affinity components in their uptake by synaptosomes
(Logan and Snyder, 1971). In slices of cerebellum incubated with
^{3}H-glutamate, however, Hökfelt and Ljungdahl (1972) reported that
the amino acid was localized largely over glial cells in this
tissue. Similar findings were reported by Ehinger and Falck
(1971) in rabbit retina, where ^{3}H-glutamate was localized over
Müller cells after in vivo injection into the eye. We have
confirmed this finding in rat retinae incubated with ^{3}H-glutamate
in vitro (Neal and Iversen, unpublished). In the rabbit retina
Ehinger (1972) has compared the autoradiographic localization of
19 of the common amino acids after in vivo injections. Of those
examined only five showed unusual localizations--the remaining
14 being localized over ganglion cells and diffusely distributed
in all other parts of the tissue. The five amino acids showing
different patterns of labelling were GABA, glycine and β-alanine,
which were localized mainly over neurones in the amacrine cell
layers, (whether β-alanine has its own specific uptake system, or
whether it is taken up by the GABA or glycine uptake systems in
retina is not, however, clear) and glutamate and aspartate which
were taken up almost exclusively by the glial cells (Müller fibers).
Salpeter and Faeder (1971) found that ^{3}H-glutamate was localized
over Schwann cells and other sheath and connective tissue elements
in insect nerve muscle preparations.

Thus, the results obtained so far suggest that glutamate
(and probably aspartate) are taken up mainly by glial elements
although in the absence of electron microscope studies, synaptic
uptake cannot be ruled out. An uptake of these amino acids by
glial cells might be important in terminating the actions after
their release as neurotransmitters.

CONCLUSIONS AND FUTURE PROSPECTS

Autoradiographic techniques seem likely to prove very useful
in providing information about the identity and distribution of
neurones using GABA or glycine as transmitters. The results
obtained so far are consistent with the assumption that the
neuronal uptake of these amino acids is specific to those neurones
using them as transmitters. It must be pointed out, however, that
there is not conclusive evidence to prove this assumption, and
far more needs to be learned of the validity of these novel
techniques before they can be used with confidence. For example,
we are exploring the possibility of combining autoradiographic
procedures with other cytochemical or histochemical procedures
for localizing catecholamines or acetylcholinesterase. In this
way it should be possible to examine the specificity of the
distribution of amino acid uptake sites in more detail. For
example, we would not expect ^{3}H-GABA to be taken up by presynaptic
nerve terminals which showed a positive reaction for acetylcholin-

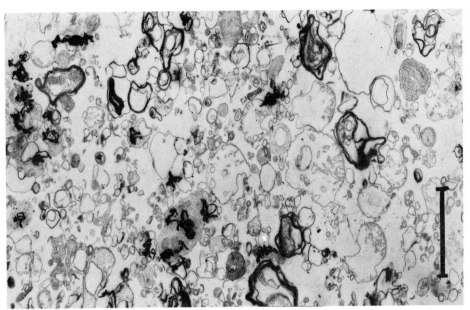

Figure 16. Electron microscope autoradiographic localization of
^{3}H-glycine over synaptosomes in a homogenate of rat spinal cord
labelled _in vitro_. Calibration bar represents 1 μm.

TABLE 8

Proportion of various transmitter-specific
terminals in homogenates of rat neostriatum

Transmitter	Method used to identify synaptosomes	% of total synaptosome population
DOPAMINE	autoradiographic (Table 1)	15
GABA	autoradiographic (Table 6)	34
ACETYLCHOLINE	cholinesterase staining*	12
UNIDENTIFIED	by difference	39

(*Iversen and Lewis, unpublished)

esterase, or which contain synaptic vesicles with dense cores after loading with monoamines. It may also be possible to begin drafting "balance sheets" for the various transmitters in certain areas of the CNS, with the help of autoradiographic techniques. As, for example, in Table 8 which shows such a balance sheet for the striatum of the rat. If all known and probable transmitters are added together we can account for only about 60% of the total synapses--indicating that unidentified transmitters (perhaps glutamate?) represent a very substantial proportion of the total. It should also be possible to combine autoradiographic methods with other well established techniques, such as the use of selective surgical lesions to provide terminal degeneration and axonal damming, in studies aimed at mapping the distribution of GABA or glycine containing pathways. Apart from making use of specific uptake processes to achieve a selective labelling of neurones with transmitter substances, autoradiographic procedures are also beginning to be used in other ways in neuroanatomical studies. For example, techniques have been described which are based on the autoradiographic demonstration of axoplasmically transported material synthesized from labelled precursors in the neuronal somata (Cowan et al., 1972). Such techniques promise to be valuable in determining the precise distribution of the cerebral projections of various neuronal pathways. Another approach which might be generally applicable is the identification and mapping of post-synaptic transmitter receptor sites by using radioactive receptor labels such as α-bungarotoxin in conjunction with auto-radiography (Barnard et al., 1971; Fanbrough and Hartzell, 1972). It is clear that the usefulness of these techniques for neuro-biology has only begun to be exploited.

REFERENCES

Aghajanian, G.K. and Bloom, F.E. 1966. Electron microscopic autoradiography of rat hypothalamus after intraventricular ^{3}H-norepinephrine. Science 153: 308-310.

Aghajanian, G.K. and Bloom, F.E. 1967 a. Electron microscopic localization of tritiated norepinephrine in rat brain: effect of drugs. J. Pharmac. Exp. Ther. 156: 407-416.

Aghajanian, G.K. and Bloom, F.E. 1967 b. Localization of tritiated serotonin in rat brain by electron microscopic autoradiography. J. Pharmacol. Exp. Ther. 156: 23-30.

Barnard, E.A., Wieckowski, J. and Chiu, T.H. 1971. Cholinergic receptor molecules and cholinesterase molecules at mouse skeletal muscle junctions. Nature 234: 207-209.

Bloom, F.E., Hoffer, B.J., Siggins, G.R., Barker, J.L. and Nicoll, R.A. 1972. Effects of serotonin on central neurones: micro-iontophoretic administration. Fed. Proc. 31: 97-106.

Bloom, F.E. and Iversen, L.L. 1971. Localizing ^{3}H-GABA in nerve terminals of rat cerebral cortex by electron microscopic autoradiography. Nature 229: 628-630.

Bodian, D. 1970. An electron microscopic characterization of classes of synaptic vesicles by means of controlled aldehyde fixation. J. Cell. Biol. 44: 115-124.

Bowery, N.G. and Brown, D.A. 1972. Observations on ^{3}H-γ-amino-butyric acid accumulation and efflux in isolated sympathetic ganglia. J. Physiol. (Lond.), 218: 32. (and Nature NB 238: 89-91)

Brunn, A. and Ehinger, R. 1972. Uptake of the putative neuro-transmitter, glycine into the rabbit retina. Invest. Ophthal. (in press).

Budd, G.C. and Salpeter, M.M. 1969. The distribution of labelled norepinephrine within sympathetic nerve terminals studied with electron microscope radioautography. J. Cell Biol. 41: 21-32.

Carlsson, A., Falck, B. and Hillarp, N.A. 1962. Cellular localiza-tion of brain monoamines. Acta physiol. scand. 56, Suppl. 196.

Clark, W.G., Vivonia, C.A. and Baxter, C.F. 1968. Accurate free-hand injection into the lateral ventricle of the conscious mouse. J. Appl. Physiol. 25:319-321.

Cowan, W.M., Gottlieb, D.I., Hendrickson, A.E., Price, J.L. and Woolsey, T.A. 1972. The autoradiographic demonstration of axonal connections in the central nervous system. Brain Res. 37: 21-51.

Coyle, J.T. and Snyder, S.H. 1969. Catecholamine uptake by synaptosomes in homogenates of rat brain: stereospecificity in different areas. J. Pharmac. Exp. Ther. 170: 221-231.

Csillik, B. and Knyihar, E. 1970. Distribution of ^{14}C-thiosemi-carbazide in the rat brain: an attempt to localize sites of γ-aminobutyric acid production. Nature 225: 562-563.

Curtis, D.R. and Johnston, G.A.R. 1970. Amino acid transmitters. In: Handbook of Neurochemistry, Vol. 4 (Ed. Lajtha, A.). New York: Plenum Press, pp. 115-134.

Dahlström, A. and Fuxe, K. 1965. Evidence for the existence of monoamine neurons in the central nervous system. Acta physiol. scand., 65, Suppl. 247.

Descarries, L. and Droz, B. 1970. Intraneuronal distribution of exogenous norepinephrine in the central nervous system of the rat. J. Cell. Biol. 44: 385-399.

Descarries, L. and Havrankova, J. 1970. Catécholamines endogènes marquées dans le systeme nerveux central. Etude radio-autographique.apprès L-3,4-dihydroxyphenylalanine tritée (DOPA-^{3}H). C.R. Acad. Sc. Paris 271: 2392-2395.

Devine, C.E. and Simpson, F.O. 1968. Localization of tritiated norepinephrine in vascular sympathetic axons of the rat intestine and mesentery by electron microscope radioautography. J. Cell. Biol. 38: 184-192.

Ehinger, B. 1970. Autoradiographic identification of rabbit retinal neurons that take up GABA. Experientia 26: 1063.

Ehinger, B. 1972. Cellular localization of the uptake of some amino acids into the rabbit retina (in press).

Ehinger, B. and Falck, B. 1971. Autoradiography of some suspected neurotransmitter substances: GABA, glycine, glutamic acid, histamine, dopamine and L-DOPA. Brain Res. 33: 157-172.

Esterhuizen, A.C., Graham, J.D.P., Lever, J.D. and Spriggs, T.L.B. 1968. Catecholamines and acetylcholinesterase distribution in relation to noradrenaline release. An enzyme histochemical and autoradiographic study on the innervation of the cat nictitating muscle. Brit. J. Pharmac. 32: 46-56.

Fambrough, D.M. and Hartzell, H.C. 1972. Acetylcholine receptors: number and distribution at neuromuscular junctions in rat diaphragm. Science 176: 189-191.

Fonnum, F. 1968. The distribution of glutamate decarboxylase and aspartate transaminase in subcellular fractions of rat and guinea-pig brain. Biochem. J. 106: 401-412.

Fonnum, F., Storm-Mathisen, J. and Walberg, F. 1970. Glutamate decarboxylase in inhibitory neurons. A study of the enzyme in Purkinje cell axons and boutons in the cat. Brain Res. 20: 259-275.

Fuxe, K. 1965. Evidence for the existence of monoamine neurons in the central nervous system. III. The monoamine nerve terminal. Z. Zellforsch. 65: 573-596.

Fuxe, K., Hökfelt, T., Ritzen, M. and Ungerstedt, U. 1968. Studies on uptake of intraventricularly administered tritiated noradrenaline and 5-hydroxytryptamine with combined fluorescence histochemical and autoradiographic techniques. Histochemie 16: 186-194.

Graham, J.D.P., Lever, J.D. and Spriggs, T.L.B. 1968. An examination of adrenergic axons around pancreatic arterioles of the cat for the presence of acetylcholinesterase by high resolution autoradiographic and histochemical methods. Brit. J. Pharmac. 33: 15-20.

Green, A.K., Snyder, S.H. and Iversen, L.L. 1969. Separation of catecholamine storing synaptosomes in different regions of rat brain. J. Pharmac. Exp. Ther. 168: 164-271.

Hebb, C. 1970. CNS at the cellular level: identity of transmitter agents. Ann. Rev. Physiol. 23: 165-192.

Hespe, W., Roberts, S.E. and Prins, H. 1969. Autoradiographic investigation of the distribution of ^{14}C-GABA in tissues of normal and amino-oxyacetic acid-treated mice. Brain Res. 14: 663-671.

Hökfelt, T. 1965. In vitro studies on central and peripheral monoamine neurons at the ultrastructural level. Z. Zellforsch. 91: 1-74.

Hökfelt, T. and Ljungdahl, A. 1970. Cellular localization of
   labelled gamma-aminobutyric acid (^{3}H-GABA) in rat cerebellar
   cortex: an autoradiographic study. Brain Res. 22: 391-396.
Hökfelt, T. and Ljungdahl, A. 1971 a. Light and electron microscopic autoradiography on spinal cord slices after incubation
   with labelled glycine. Brain Res. 23: 189-194.
Hökfelt, T. and Ljungdahl, A. 1971 b. Uptake of ^{3}H-noradrenaline
   and γ-^{3}H-aminobutyric acid in isolated tissues of rat:
   an autoradiographic and fluorescence microscopic study.
   Progress in Brain Res. 34: 87-102.
Hökfelt, T. and Ljungdahl, A. 1972. Autoradiographic identification of cerebral and cerebellar cortical neurons accumulating
   labeled gamma-aminobutyric acid (^{3}H-GABA). Exp. Brain Res.
   14: 354-362.
Ishii, T. and Friede, R.L. 1967. Distribution of a catecholamine-
   binding mechanism in rat brain. Histochemie 9: 126-135.
Ishii, T. and Friede, R.L. 1968. Tissue binding of tritiated
   norepinephrine in pigmented nuclei of human brain. Amer.
   J. Anat. 122: 139-144.
Ito, M. and Yoshida, M. 1966. The origin of cerebellar-induced
   inhibition of Deiter's neurones. I. Monosynaptic initiation
   of the inhibitory postsynaptic potentials. Exp. Brain Res.
   2: 330-349.
Iversen, L.L. 1967. The Uptake and Storage of Noradrenaline in
   Sympathetic Nerves. London: Cambridge University Press.
Iversen, L.L. 1970. Neuronal uptake processes for Amines and
   Amino Acid. In: Adv. Biochem. Psychopharmac. Vol. 2.
   New York: Raven Press, pp. 109-132.
Iversen, L.L. 1971. Role of transmitter uptake mechanisms in
   synaptic neurotransmission. Brit. J. Pharmac. 41: 571-591.
Iversen, L.L. 1972. The uptake, storage, release and metabolism
   of GABA in inhibitory nerves. In: Perspectives in
   Neuropharmacology (Ed.,Snyder, S.), New York: Oxford
   University Press, Inc., pp. 75-111.
Iversen, L.L. and Bloom, F.E. 1972. Studies of the uptake of ^{3}H-
   GABA and ^{3}H-glycine in slices and homogenates of rat brain
   and spinal cord by electron microscopic autoradiography.
   Brain Res. 41: 131-143.
Iversen, L.L. and Johnston, G.A.R. 1971. GABA uptake in rat central
   nervous system: comparison of uptake in slices and homogenates
   and the effects of some inhibitors. J. Neurochem. 18:1939-1950.
Iversen, L.L. and Neal, M.J. 1968. The uptake of ^{3}H-GABA by slices
   of rat cerebral cortex. J. Neurochem. 15: 1141-1149.
Iversen, L.L. and Snyder, S.H. 1968. Synaptosomes: different
   populations storing catecholamines and gamma-aminobutyric
   acid in homogenates of rat brain. Nature 220: 796-798.
Iversen, L.L. and Uretsky, N.J. 1971. Biochemical effects of 6-
   hydroxydopamine on catecholamine-containing neurones in the
   rat brain. In: 6-Hydroxydopamine and Catecholamine Neurones

(Eds., Malmfors, T. and Thoenen, H.), Amsterdam: North
   Holland Press.
Johnson, J.L. 1972. Glutamic acid as a synaptic transmitter in the
   nervous system, a review. Brain Res. 37: 1-19.
Johnston, G.A.R. and Iversen, L.L. 1971. Glycine uptake in rat
   central nervous system slices and homogenates: evidence for
   different uptake systems in spinal cord and cerebral cortex.
   J. Neurochem. 18: 1951-1961.
Kasa, P. 1971. Ultrastructural localization of choline acetyl-
   transferase and acetylcholinesterase in central and peripheral
   nervous tissue. Progr. Brain Res. 37: 337-344.
Kramer, S.G., Potts, A.M. and Mangnall, Y. 1971. Dopamine: a
   retinal neurotransmitter II. Autoradiographic localization of
   ^{3}H-DOPAMINE in the retina. Invest. Ophthalm. 10: 617-624.
Krnjević, K. 1970. Glutamate and γ-aminobutyric acid in brain.
   Nature 228: 119-124.
Krnjević, K and Silver, A. 1965. A histochemical study of
   cholinergic fibres in the cerebral cortex. J. Anat. 99: 711-759.
Lam, D.M.K. and Steinman, L. 1971. The uptake of γ-^{3}H-aminobutyric
   acid in the goldfish retina. Proc. Nat. Acad. Sci. USA
   68: 2777-2781.
Lenn, N.J. 1967. Localization of uptake of tritiated norepinephrine
   by rat brain in vivo and in vitro using electron microscopic
   autoradiography. Amer. J. Anat. 120: 377-390.
Lewis, P.R. and Shute, C.C.D. 1966. The distribution of cholinesterase in cholinergic neurons demonstrated with the electron
   microscope. J. Cell. Sci. 1: 381-390.
Ljungdahl, A., Hökfelt, T., Jonsson, G. and Sachs, C. 1971. Autoradiographic demonstration of uptake and accumulation of
   ^{3}H-6-hydroxydopamine in adrenergic nerves. Experientia
   27: 297-299.
Logan, W.J. and Snyder, S.H. 1971. Unique high affinity uptake
   systems for glycine, glutamic and aspartic acids in central
   nervous tissue of the rat. Nature 234: 297-299.
Matus, A.I. and Dennison, M.E. 1971. Autoradiographic localization
   of tritiated glycine at "flat-vesicle" synapses in spinal
   cord. Brain Res. 32: 196-197.
McGeer, P.L., McGeer, E.G., Wada, J.A. and Jung, E. 1971. Effects
   of globus pallidus lesions and Parkinson's disease on brain
   glutamic acid decarboxylase. Brain Res. 32: 425-431.
Neal, M.J. 1971. The uptake of ^{14}C-glycine by slices of mammalian
   spinal cord. J. Physiol. (Lond.), 215: 103-118.
Neal, M.J. 1972. The uptake of ^{3}H-γ-aminobutyric acid by the retina.
   J. Physiol. (Lond.) (in press).
Neal, M.J. and Iversen, L.L. 1969. Subcellular distribution of
   endogenous and ^{3}H-GABA in rat cortex. J. Neurochem. 16:
   1245-1252.

Neal, M.J. and Iversen, L.L. 1972. Autoradiographic localization of ^{3}H-GABA in rat retina. Nature, New Biology 235: 217-218.

Neal, M.J. and Pickles, H. 1969. Uptake of ^{14}C-glycine by rat spinal cord. Nature 223: 679-680.

Obata, K. and Takeda, K. 1969. Release of γ-aminobutyric acid into the fourth ventricle induced by stimulation of the cat's cerebellum. J. Neurochem. 16: 1043-1047.

Obata, K., Ito, M., Ochi, R. and Sato, N. 1967. Pharmacological properties of the postsynaptic inhibition by Purkinje cells axons and the action of γ-aminobutyric acid on Deiter's neurones. Exp. Brain Res. 4: 43-57.

Orkand, P.M. and Kravitz, E.A. 1971. Localization of the sites of γ-aminobutyric acid (GABA) uptake in lobster nerve-muscle preparations. J. Cell. Biol. 49: 75-89.

Otsuka, M., Obata, K., Miyata, Y. and Tanaka, Y. 1971. Measurement of γ-aminobutyric acid in isolated nerve cells of cat central nervous system. J. Neurochem. 18: 287-295.

Salpeter, M.M. and Bachmann, L. 1964. Autoradiography with the electron microscope. J. Cell. Biol. 22: 469-482.

Salpeter, M.M. and Faeder, I.R. 1971. The role of sheath cells in glutamate uptake by insect nerve muscle preparations. Prog. Brain Res. 34: 104-114.

Schon, F. and Iversen, L.L. 1972. Selective accumulation of ^{3}H-GABA by stellate cells in rat cerebellar cortex in vivo. Brain Res. 42.

Shaskan, E.A. and Snyder, S.H. 1970. Kinetics of serotonin uptake into slices from different regions of rat brain. J. Pharmac. Exp. Ther. 175: 404-418.

Sims, K.L., Weitsen, H.A. and Bloom, F.E. 1971. Histochemical localization of brain succinic semialdehyde dehydrogenase-- a γ-aminobutyric acid degradative enzyme. J. Histochem. Cytochem. 19: 405-415.

Storm-Mathisen, J. and Fonnum, F. 1971. Quantitative histochemistry of glutamate decarboxylase in the rat hippocampal region. J. Neurochem. 18: 1105-1111.

Uchizono, K. 1965. Characteristics of excitatory and inhibitory synapses in the central nervous system of the cat. Nature 207: 642-643.

van Gelder, M.M. 1965. A comparison of γ-aminobutyric acid metabolism in rabbit and mouse nervous tissue. J. Neurochem. 12: 239-244.

van Gelder, M.M. 1967. A possible enzyme barrier for γ-aminobutyric acid in the central nervous system. Prog. Brain Res. 29: 259-268.

Weinstein, H., Varon, S., Muhlemann, D.R. and Roberts, E. 1965. A carrier-mediated transfer model for the accumulation of ^{14}C-γ-aminobutyric acid by subcellular brain particles. Biochem. Pharmac. 14: 273-288.

NEURONAL UPTAKE OF NEUROTRANSMITTERS AND THEIR PRECURSORS:

STUDIES WITH "TRANSMITTER" AMINO ACIDS AND CHOLINE

Solomon H. Snyder, Henry I. Yamamura, Candace B. Pert,

William J. Logan and James P. Bennett

Departments of Pharmacology and Experimental Therapeutics
and Psychiatry and the Behavioral Sciences, Johns
Hopkins University School of Medicine, Baltimore,
Maryland 21205

I. INTRODUCTION

Most neurotransmitters, except for acetylcholine, possess high affinity neuronal uptakes. With reasonably well established transmitter candidates such as catecholamines, serotonin and GABA, these uptake systems are studied with a view to characterizing the synaptic behavior of the transmitter in question. With more questionable transmitter candidates, such as the amino acids, before characterizing subtleties of their synaptic activities, it is crucial first to determine whether they are in fact neurotransmitters. In our laboratory, uptake studies have been employed to adduce evidence in support of certain amino acids as transmitters. Specifically, we have compared the synaptosomal accumulation of numerous amino acids and found that unlike most amino acids, glutamic and aspartic acids and glycine (in the spinal cord and brain stem) are transported by unique high affinity systems into distinct populations of synaptosomes. In this way neuronal uptake has provided powerful biochemical support for the proposition that these compounds are neurotransmitters in the mammalian central nervous system.

Less extensively studied but of no less potential importance are neuronal uptake systems for transmitter precursors. Precursor uptake might conceivable regulate transmitter synthesis. There is considerable evidence that levels of tryptophan in the brain regulate serotonin formation (Wurtman and Fernstrom, 1972; Tagliamonte et al., 1971). However, it is difficult to study such

195

precursor uptake systems directly. Amino acid precursors of neurotransmitters are accumulated by uptake systems which subserve the
many non-transmitter metabolic functions of these amino acids
(Blasberg et al., 1970). Such general uptake systems may mask
the transmitter-precursor transport. For example, in an attempt
to identify selective uptake of tryptophan into serotonin neurons,
Kuhar et al. (1972) measured synaptosomal uptake of a wide range
of tryptophan concentrations in areas of the brain rich in
serotonin terminals before and after destruction of the serotonin
neurons by raphe lesions. There was no fall in tryptophan uptake
after raphe lesion, indicating that tryptophan uptake into serotonin
neurons must constitute only a small portion of the uptake of
tryptophan into those brain areas for general metabolic needs.

For the cholinergic system one might speculate that choline
uptake regulates acetylcholine synthesis. Thus, the electrical
activity as well as acetylcholine output of the superior cervical
ganglion ceases quickly when the ganglion is deprived of exogenous
choline (Birks and Macintosh, 1961). Moreover, although acetylcholine turnover in the brain probably varies tremendously in the
presence of environmental or pharmacological manipulations, there
is little evidence of marked parallel changes in the activity of
choline acetyltransferase.

Despite the likelihood that choline uptake is a key regulatory
mechanism of cholinergic neuronal activity, numerous studies have
failed to demonstrate choline accumulation selectively by cholinergic neurons. There have been various reports of choline uptake
systems in kidney (Sung and Johnston, 1965), erythrocytes (Askari,
1966; Martin, 1968), brain slices (Schuberth et al., 1965) and
synaptosomes (Diamond and Kennedy, 1969; Marchbanks, 1969; Potter,
1968; Hemsworth et al., 1971) which have relatively low affinity
for choline and little associated acetylcholine formation so that
it is not clear whether the choline is accumulated selectively into
cholinergic neurons. As with amino acid precursors of neurotransmitters, choline has numerous metabolic roles besides serving as a
precursor of acetylcholine. Thus, it is quite possible that choline
uptake into the non-transmitter pools might mask uptake into
cholinergic neurons.

We will describe recent work in our laboratory showing that
there are indeed at least two kinetically distinct transport
systems for choline into brain synaptosomes and the guinea pig
ileum respectively. One of these uptake systems, which possesses
high affinity, an absolute dependence on sodium and is associated
with acetylcholine formation, appears to reflect choline uptake
selectively into cholinergic neurons.

II. AMINO ACID TRANSMITTER UPTAKE SYSTEMS

The well known and reasonably well established transmitters
such as acetylcholine, catecholamines and serotonin, probably
account for transmission at only a small percentage of brain
synapses. Thus, in the corpus striatum which is "loaded" with
dopamine, only about 15% of the nerve terminals appear to store
catecholamines, and in the hypothalamus, which contains the
highest levels of norepinephrine in the brain only 3% of the
nerve terminals accumulate catecholamine (Hökfelt, 1970). Since
the brain contains less serotonin than catecholamines, this compound may account for yet a lower percentage of synapses. Acetylcholine is physiologically active on only a portion of central
neurons and is thus probably associated only with a small percentage of nerve terminals (McLennan, 1970).

It is likely that amino acids are, quantitatively, more
prominent transmitters. Electron microscopic autoradiography
of accumulated GABA, thought to label all terminals which utilize
GABA as a transmitter, shows a labelling of 20-40% of nerve
terminals depending on the brain region examined (Bloom and
Iversen, 1972). Similar autoradiographic studies of glycine in
the spinal cord (Hökfelt and Ljundahl, 1971; Matus and Dennison,
1971) suggests that it is associated with about 30% of the
synapses (Hokfelt, personal communication). There is no comparable autoradiographic data for glutamic acid.

Neurophysiologically, fairly convincing evidence exists for
glycine as an inhibitory transmitter in the spinal cord (Curtis
et al., 1968; Werman et al., 1968). Though glutamic acid is well
known to excite almost all neurons, there is little if any ancil-
lary neurophysiologic data to support its candidacy as a neurotransmitter.

Some of the most impressive biochemical studies supporting
roles for amino acids as transmitters have been performed by
Aprison and co-workers (Aprison and Werman, 1965; Graham et al.,
1967) and Johnston and co-workers (Johnston, 1968; Johnston et al.,
1969). Much of this work involved determination of amino acid
concentrations in different parts of the spinal cord. The
relatively high levels in ventral grey of aspartic acid and
glycine suggest that these might serve as excitatory and inhibitory
transmitters, respectively, of spinal cord interneurons (Graham
et al., 1967; Johnston, 1968; Johnston et al., 1969). The high
concentration of glutamic acid in the dorsal grey on the other
hand is consistent with its being the excitatory transmitter of
afferent sensory nerves (Graham et al., 1967). There are parallel
decrements in number of interneurons and of glycine concentration
following anoxic damage to the spinal cord, further evidence

supporting a role for glycine as a transmitter in these interneurons. The failure of GABA levels to fall after such procedures
suggests that it is associated with a different group of neurons
(Davidoff et al., 1967). These experiments and the autoradiographic findings noted above imply that these amino acid putative
transmitters are associated with the major neuronal class—the
interneuron. Such interneurons would probably not form projections
similar to those shown for the catecholamines and serotonin. Their
identification would require different approaches.

Work in our laboratory over the past few years has been
addressed to the proposition that the transmitter pools of amino
acid transmitter candidates probably represent only a portion of
the endogenous levels of these substances. This assumption could
explain such findings as the failure to demonstrate a selective
localization of any amino acids to synaptosomal fractions (Mangan
and Whittaker, 1966). How might one examine selectively such transmitter pools? To secure this aim, we made another assumption. We
have postulated that nerve terminals which utilize certain amino
acids as transmitters may have selective transport systems of
relatively high affinity for accumulating these compounds.

One major problem in attempting to identify "transmitter"
uptake systems for amino acids into nerve terminals is that transport systems are well known for all amino acids in most mammalian
tissues including brain (Blasberg, 1968; Blasberg et al., 1970;
Christensen and Liang, 1965; Schultz et al., 1970; Winter and
Christensen, 1965). Because the generalized amino acid transports
are ubiquitous and because they have relatively low affinity for
their substrates (Blasberg, 1968), it is not likely that they
have a specific function in inactivating postulated transmitter
pools. Uptake systems for hypothetical amino acid transmitter
pools might be anticipated to have more affinity than do the
general amino acid transports, because such a high affinity would
probably be required to remove the compound from the synaptic
cleft efficiently.

Accordingly, we assessed the accumulation of a variety of
radiolabelled amino acids into crude synaptosomal preparations
in the brain and spinal cord. We employed a wide range of amino
acid concentrations in order to evaluate both low affinity and
postulated high affinity transports (Logan and Snyder, 1971).

In these studies of amino acid transport, either nuclei-free
homogenates of brain or spinal cord tissue or a crude mitochondrial
pellet were utilized. In all cases, it could be shown that under
our incubation conditions the accumulated amino acids were unmetab-
olized. Accumulated amino acids were localized to the synaptosomal
fraction of sucrose gradients within osmotically sensitive

particles which mimicked faithfully the behavior of synaptosomes
(Logan and Snyder, 1972) (Figure 1). These data, together with
the electron microscopic autoradiographic localization of accumulated glycine in the spinal cord to nerve terminals (Hökfelt and
and Ljundahl, 1971; Matus and Dennison, 1971), indicates that the
uptakes we have examined represent transport into nerve terminal
particles.

A.   Cerebral Cortical Uptake of Amino Acids

The accumulation of all amino acids examined in the cerebral
cortex was saturable. Double reciprocal plots for the accumulation of alanine, arginine, leucine, serine, lysine and glycine in
the cerebral cortex described straight lines with positive ordinate
intercepts (Figure 2). Moreover, least squares fitting of the
data by the method of Cleland (1967) also indicated that a single
transport system gave the best fit for these results. Km values
for these compounds were 0.2-3.3 x 10^{-3} M (Table I).

By contrast double reciprocal analysis of the uptake of
glutamic and aspartic acids in the cerebral cortex produced

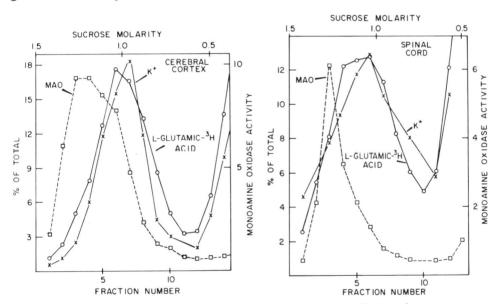

Figure 1. Continuous sucrose density gradient profiles for
accumulated L-^{3}H-glutamic acid, potassium (K$^+$), and monoamine
oxidase (MAO) activity in cerebral cortex and spinal cord
homogenates. Incubation media contained 2.1 x 10^{-5} M L-^{3}H-
glutamic acid. Radioactivity and K$^+$ content are plotted as percent of total in the gradient. MAO activity is expressed as moles
of indoleacetic acid formed per hour.

TABLE 1

KINETICS OF AMINO ACID UPTAKE INTO HOMOGENATES
OF RAT CENTRAL NERVOUS SYSTEM

Amino Acid	Km values x 10^4 M	
	Low Affinity Uptake	High Affinity Uptake
CEREBRAL CORTEX		
L-Aspartic acid	3.68 ± 1.94	0.169 ± 0.128
L-Glutamic acid	10.53 ± 4.58	0.201 ± 0.034
Glycine	7.63 ± 0.53	---
L-Alanine	4.53 ± 0.24	---
L-Arginine	6.24 ± 1.11	---
L-Leucine	3.51 ± 0.46	---
L-Lysine	33.28 ± 4.66	---
L-Serine	2.16 ± 0.35	---
SPINAL CORD		
L-Aspartic acid	37.62 ± 14.17	0.215 ± 0.777
L-Glutamic acid	49.02 ± 13.51	0.143 ± 0.037
Glycine	9.23 ± 6.38	0.265 ± 0.141
L-Alanine	10.58 ± 0.71	---
L-Arginine	26.79 ± 7.58	---
L-Leucine	91.36 ± 30.18	---
L-Lysine	57.07 ± 22.95	---
L-Serine	10.81 ± 2.06	---

A minimum of 6 concentrations of every amino acid were incubated
in quadruplicate with homogenates.

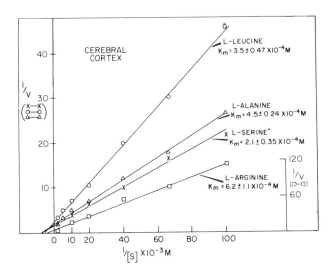

Figure 2. Double-reciprocal plot of uptake into cerebral cortex homogenates of representative large and small neutral and basic amino acids. All describe straight lines with positive ordinate intercepts. Km values and their standard errors were computed using least squares fit of the linear Michaelis-Menten equation to the data. Velocity (V) is expressed as micromoles of amino acid accumulated per gram/4 min.

curves (Figure 3) which could be resolved into two components graphically. Moreover, computer analysis of the least squares fitting of these data show that a single component uptake gave a poor fit, while a two component system described the data with much less variance (Figure 4). The Km values calculated by the least squares fit for the high affinity uptake of glutamic and aspartic acids were about $2-3 \times 10^{-5}$ M while the low affinity transport for these compounds had Km values of about $0.5-1.0 \times 10^{-3}$ M.

Because the Km value for the high affinity uptake of glutamic acid is similar to that reported earlier for GABA and because glutamic acid is the metabolic precursor of GABA, we wondered whether glutamic acid could be transported into GABA neurons. However, GABA in concentrations as high as 10^{-3} M failed to significantly reduce the accumulation of radioactive glutamic acid into cerebral cortical or spinal cord homogenates. Moreover, subcellular fractionation studies to be described below show that GABA and glutamic acid are localized in different populations of synaptosomes.

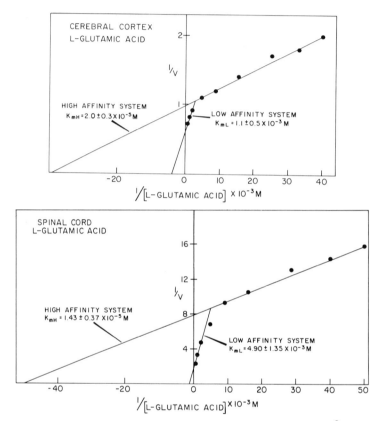

Figure 3.   Double-reciprocal plots of the uptake of L-^{3}H-glutamic acid into cerebral cortical and spinal cord homogenates. In both tissues the data describe curves which can be resolved into two straight line components.   Km values and their standard errors were determined using the computed least squares fit to the data of the quadratic kinetic equation for two systems.   Velocity (V) is expressed as micromoles of L-glutamic acid accumulated per gram/4 min.

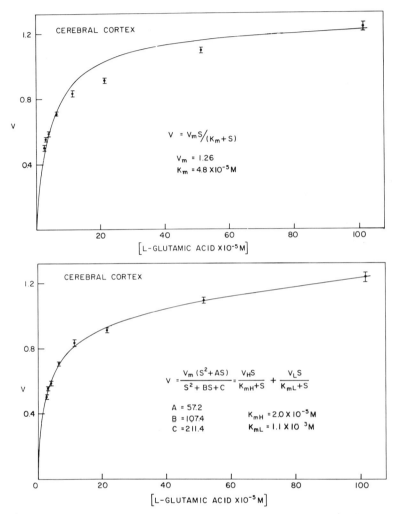

Figure 4. Velocity-substrate concentration plots of L-glutamic acid uptake in cerebral cortex homogenates. The lines represent the computed least squares fit to the data points. Velocity (V) is expressed as micromoles of L-glutamic acid accumulated per gram/ 4 min. Upper: Fit of linear Michaelis–Menten equation representing single transport system. Lower: Fit of quadratic kinetic equation representing two component system. Vertical bars indicate one standard deviation in each side of the mean value.

B. Spinal Cord Uptake of Amino Acids

As had been observed in the cerebral cortex, in the spinal cord all amino acids were accumulated by saturable mechanisms. Also like in the cerebral cortex double reciprocal plots for the uptake of alanine, arginine, leucine, lysine and serine in the spinal cord yielded single straight lines. Moreover, least squares analysis of these data show that they fit a single system with Km values of $1-9 \times 10^{-3}$ M (Logan and Snyder, 1972).

The kinetic behavior of glutamic and aspartic acids in the spinal cord were similar to what had been observed in the cerebral cortex (Figure 3), with readily distinguishable high and low affinity uptakes.

The behavior of glycine was strikingly different in the spinal cord than in the cerebral cortex. Whereas glycine had been accumulated via a single component low affinity uptake in the cerebral cortex, in the spinal cord double reciprocal plots for glycine uptake produced curves that could be resolved into two components graphically (Figure 5). The high affinity uptake for

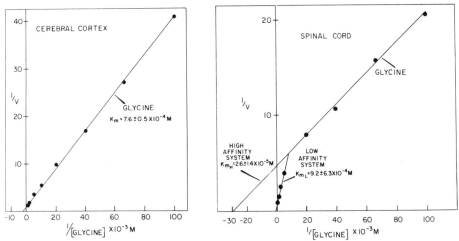

Figure 5. Double-reciprocal plots of glycine uptake into cerebral cortical and spinal cord homogenates. Data for the cerebral cortex describe a straight line with positive ordinate intercept typical of Michaelis-Menten single system kinetics. Spinal cord data are best described by 2 straight lines with positive ordinate intercepts indicating a two component system. A single system Michaelis-Menten equation gave the best fit to the cerebral cortex data whereas a two component equation gave the best fit to the spinal cord data. Km values and their standard errors were determined from the respective computed equations. Velocity (V) is expressed as micromoles of glycine accumulated per gram/4 min.

glycine in the spinal cord had a Km value of 2.6×10^{-5} M,
similar to results obtained independently by Johnston and Iversen
(1971), while the low affinity system had a Km of 0.9×10^{-3} M.
These authors also found high affinity uptake of glycine in the
brain stem.

C. Mutual Competition of Glutamic and Aspartic Acid
Uptake and Influence of Metabolic Inhibitors

Both in the cerebral cortex and spinal cord the uptakes of
glutamic and aspartic acids were kinetically similar, suggesting
that they might be accumulated by the same transport system. To
evaluate this possibility we studied the mutual inhibition of
glutamic and aspartic acid uptakes in cerebral cortex and spinal
cord by the kinetic techniques of Lineweaver and Burk (1934) and
Dixon (1953). In all cases the mutual inhibition of uptake was
competitive and the Ki values for inhibition by one amino acid
of the uptake of the other were the same as the Km values.

This strongly suggests that glutamic and aspartic acids can
be accumulated by the same or similar transport systems. Glutamic
and aspartic acids still might have quite different neuronal
localizations, but because of their structural similarity, serve
as substrates for each other's uptake systems. The localization
of these two amino acids to different neuronal systems is supported by the differing regional localizations of endogenous
aspartic and glutamic acid within the spinal cord (Johnston, 1968).

To assess the possible metabolic requirements of the high
and low affinity transports of glutamic acid, uptake at low
(2×10^{-5} M) and high (10^{-3} M) concentrations of glutamic acid
into cerebral cortical homogenates was studied in the presence
of a variety of metabolic inhibitors. Azide, cyanide and the
omission of glucose had minimal effects on glutamic acid uptake at
both concentrations. Dinitrophenol, iodoacetamide and ouabain
decreased glutamic acid uptake at both concentrations about
30-40%, while incubation at 4°C reduced uptake 90%. Thus, there
do not appear to be any marked differences in the metabolic
requirements for the two glutamic acid transport systems.

D. Ionic Requirements of High Affinity Amino Acid Transports

Although the gross energy requirements for the high affinity
amino acid transports were not markedly different from those of
the low affinity transports, we wondered whether there might be
other metabolic differences. While ouabain depressed somewhat
the accumulation of high concentrations of amino acids, previous
studies had indicated that amino acid uptake by brain slices was

not markedly sodium dependent. We examined the uptake of a
variety of amino acids into synaptosomal preparations of the
cerebral cortex and spinal cord at varying sodium concentrations
(Table II). At low concentrations (10^{-5} M) glutamic and aspartic
acid uptake in the cerebral cortex was markedly dependent on the
presence of sodium. Omitting sodium from the medum resulted in a
20-25-fold decrease in the uptake of glutamic and aspartic acids,
while glycine, alanine, leucine and arginine uptakes were much
less affected.

In the spinal cord, glutamic and aspartic acid transport
showed a sodium requirement similar to that observed in the
cerebral cortex. Strikingly, glycine, whose accumulation in
the cerebral cortex was only slightly influenced by sodium showed
a profound sodium requirement in the spinal cord.

By contrast, at high concentrations (10^{-3} M) none of the
amino acids examined in the cerebral cortex or spinal cord showed
as marked a sodium requirement as was seen with 10^{-5} M concentrations of glutamic and aspartic acids and glycine (in spinal cord).
At high concentrations glutamic and aspartic acid uptakes in the
cerebral cortex were reduced more by sodium omission than were
the accumulation of other amino acids. The continuing sodium
dependence at high glutamic acid concentrations might be explained
by our preliminary calculations; using the Michaelis-Menten
equation, even at 10^{-3} M considerable amounts of glutamic and
aspartic acids would enter the high affinity system.

The sodium requirement for uptake of low concentrations of
glutamic and aspartic acids and glycine could not be satisfied by
equimolar concentrations of Tris, choline or lithium. The fact
that the uptakes of glutamic and aspartic acids and glycine (in the
spinal cord) were affected by sodium deficiency differentially
at low and at high amino acid concentrations supports the observation that these compounds are transported to synaptosomes by two
distinct systems.

E. Localization of High Affinity Amino Acid
     Transports to Unique Synaptosomal Fractions

If the high affinity amino acid transports represent accumulation by a circumscribed population of amino-acidergic nerve
terminals, such neurons might differ in their physical properties
from other neuronal populations. By subcellular fractionation
studies we have obtained strong support that the high affinity
uptake systems for glutamic and aspartic acids and for glycine
do represent transport into neurons using them as transmitters.

TABLE 2

EFFECT OF Na OMMISSION ON THE UPTAKE OF VARIOUS AMINO ACIDS INTO SYNAPTOSOMAL FRACTIONS

	[Amino Acid] = 10^{-3} M			[Amino Acid] = 10^{-5} M		
	Uptake Rate = (mμmoles/gm/4 min) ± S.E.		Uptake Ratio	Uptake Rate = (mμmoles/gm/4 min) ± S.E.		Uptake Ratio
	[Na]=143 mM	[Na]=0 mM	$\frac{0 \text{ mM Na}}{143 \text{ mM Na}} \times 100$	[Na]=143 mM	[Na]=0 mM	$\frac{0 \text{ mM Na}}{143 \text{ mM Na}} \times 100$
CEREBRAL CORTEX						
L-Glutamic Acid	804 ± 90	365 ± 31	45*	200 ± 15	8.4 ± 1.0	4.2*
L-Aspartic Acid	652 ± 49	273 ± 28	42*	143 ± 12	8.9 ± 1.0	6.2*
Glycine	703 ± 55	651 ± 36	93	30.4 ± 4	25 ± 3	82
L-Alanine	776 ± 52	709 ± 50	91	39.6 ± 3	34 ± 2.6	86
L-Leucine	690 ± 130	592 ± 73	86	25.4 ± 2	23.4 ± 1.0	92
L-Arginine	110 ± 7	109 ± 10	99	12.0 ± 1.5	15.7 ± 1.7	131
SPINAL CORD						
L-Glutamic Acid	160 ± 18	63 ± 4	40*	7.2 ± 0.3	0.30 ± 0.05	4.0*
L-Aspartic Acid	137 ± 18	97 ± 16	71	12 ± 1.3	0.6 ± 0.08	5.0*
Glycine	220 ± 10	147 ± 11	67	20.2 ± 1.4	3.9 ± 0.3	19*
L-Alanine	151 ± 8	105 ± 13	70	4.7 ± 0.6	3.4 ± 0.4	72
L-Leucine	166 ± 11	163 ± 11	98	3.9 ± 0.1	3.9 ± 0.1	100
L-Arginine	130 ± 35	122 ± 7	94	2.3 ± 0.4	3.4 ± 0.4	148

Homogenates from rat cerebral cortex or lumbosacral spinal cord were incubated with 10^{-3} M and 10^{-5} M amino acids in Krebs-Ringer phosphate solutions for normal Na concentration (143 mM) or Krebs-Ringer Tris solutions for deficient Na concentration (0 mM). Isotonic sucrose (0.32 M) was used to replace Na ion in the Na-deficient media. After centrifugation, the pellets were analyzed for accumulated [³H]-amino acids as described in the text. Values for glutamic acid do not take into account the final concentration of endogenous glutamic acid released by homogenization (1.5 x 10^{-5} M). Data represent the mean values for 4 separate determinations. (Difference between 0 Na and 143 Na uptake rates: * P < 0.001)

By centrifugation of crude synaptosomal preparations on sucrose density gradients for brief intervals, "incomplete equilibrium sedimentation", one can partially resolve populations of synaptosomes storing different transmitters (Kuhar et al., 1970, 1971).

In these studies, slices of brain tissue were incubated in physiological media containing one amino acid labelled with carbon-14 and another with tritium. After incubation crude mitochondrial fractions containing synaptosomes were prepared and centrifuged for 15 minutes (100,000 x g) on linear continuous sucrose gradients (1.5-0.2 M or 1.5-0.5 M). This technique of incomplete equilibrium sedimentation resolves particles that store different neurotransmitters better than density equilibrium techniques (Kuhar et al., 1970, 1971), and by labelling one putative transmitter with tritium and another with carbon, subtle differences in sedimentation properties can be readily detected.

We were able to show that in the cerebral cortex glutamic and aspartic acids labelled a unique synaptosomal fraction differing from that which accumulated other amino acids (Wofsey et al., 1971). Even more strikingly, synaptosomes which accumulate glycine selectively could be separated from those accumulating other amino acids in the spinal cord and brain stem but not in the cerebral cortex (Arregui et al., 1972; Snyder et al., 1973). This regional distribution of unique glycine synaptosomes parallels nicely that of the high affinity glycine uptake system.

How might one demonstrate directly that the high affinity amino acid transport systems label the unique amino acid storing synaptosomes? We made use of the absolute sodium requirement for the high affinity transport systems for these amino acids as a tool to link the high affinity transports with the unique synaptosomes. Thus, low concentrations of glycine in the spinal cord and the acidic amino acids in spinal cord and cerebral cortex will enter the high affinity transports selectively in the presence of physiologic concentrations of sodium. But in sodium deficient media, these compounds should be transported predominantly by the low affinity systems which presumably label all synaptosomes homogeneously. Accordingly, homogenates of cerebral cortex or spinal cord were incubated with glutamic acid of one isotope in the presence of normal sodium concentrations and glutamic acid with the other label in the absence of sodium. In the presence of sodium the glutamic acid accumulating particles sedimented in a less dense region of the gradient than did those from preparations incubated in the absence of sodium (Figure 6). Similar results were obtained for glutamic acid in the cerebral cortex, and for the glycine synaptosomes in the spinal cord. These experiments demonstrate that the high affinity, sodium

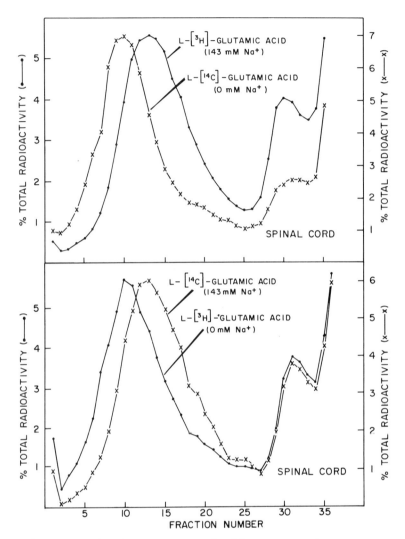

Figure 6. Distribution patterns in linear, continuous sucrose density gradients of synaptosomal fractions that accumulate ^{3}H- and ^{14}C-glutamic acid in the presence of normal Na$^+$ concentration (143 mM) or no added Na$^+$. Homogenates from rat spinal cord were incubated with 10^{-5} M 1-glutamic acid in Krebs-Ringer-Phosphate solution (143 mM Na$^+$) or Krebs-Ringer-Tris solution (0 mM Na$^+$) and subjected to subcellular fractionation as described in the text.

requiring uptakes of glutamic and aspartic acids and glycine (in the spinal cord) label the unique synaptosomal fractions which accumulate these compounds.

It is quite possible that the high affinity uptakes for these amino acids provide a major means for their inactivation after synaptic release. If this is so, a search for drugs which selectively influence these uptake processes might provide valuable tools with which to elucidate the synaptic pharmacology of the transmitter amino acids. Such drugs might conceivably possess therapeutic utility. With simpleminded notions of glutamic acid as a major excitatory and GABA as a major inhibitory transmitter, one might predict that inhibitors of glutamic acid uptake would be convulsant drugs, while agents which block GABA uptake might be useful anticonvulsants.

III. CHOLINE UPTAKE

Our studies with amino acids provided valuable experience in attempts to uncover choline transport selectively by cholinergic neurons. Just as with the amino acids, we were concerned that the choline transport systems described by numerous workers subserved the general metabolic functions of choline and was not related directly to cholinergic neuronal activity. Similarly we expected that the uptake into cholinergic neurons would not be as prominent quantitatively as the other uptake systems, simply because cholinergic neurons are only a small percentage of the cellular elements in any tissue. However, we suspected that, because of need for rapid and efficient supplies of choline into the cholinergic neurons, the "transmitter-linked" choline uptake would have a relatively high affinity. Some very recent reports did hint at cholinergic neuronal uptake of choline, since synaptosomal accumulation of low choline concentrations showed sodium dependence (Haga, 1971) and was associated with significant acetylcholine formation (Green et al., 1971).

Accordingly, our strategy involved incubating tissue preparations with a wide range of choline concentrations, hoping that at low concentrations, we might be able to demonstrate a high affinity uptake system, relatively uncontaminated by quantitatively greater systems with less affinity.

A. Studies with Brain Tissue

To maximize the likelihood of demonstrating choline uptake into cholinergic neurons, we utilized the corpus striatum, which is the area of the brain richest in acetylcholine content.

Male Sprague-Dawley rats (150-200 g) were decapitated. The

corpus striatum was rapidly dissected (Glowinski and Iversen, 1966) and homogenized in 30 volumes of ice-cold 0.32 M sucrose containing 10^{-7} M Soman in a Potter-Elvehjem glass homogenizer fitted with a Teflon pestle (0.004-0.006 inch clearance). We showed that Soman at the concentration employed completely inhibits acetylcholinesterase without influencing choline uptake. After centrifugation at 1,000 x g for 10 minutes the pellet was discarded and the supernatant fluid centrifuged at 17,000 x g for 60 minutes. The resultant pellet was reconstituted to the original volume with 0.32 M sucrose and 0.1 ml of the tissue suspension was added to 1.9 ml of a Krebs phosphate solution, pH 7.4, containing 11.1 mM glucose and varying concentrations of ^{3}H-choline (17 Ci/moles; Amersham-Searle). Under these incubation conditions, even if all the endogenous choline were to have leaked out of the particles and choline levels increased during incubation (Browning, 1971), the resultant concentration of choline in the medium would be only 1 x 10^{-7} M hence contribute much less than the exogenous ^{3}H-choline to the final concentration of choline in the medium. The mixture was incubated at 30°C for 4 minutes, the reaction was stopped by adding 50 µl each of choline (0.4 M) and neostigmine (0.04 M), and the mixture was centrifuged at 27,000 x g for 15 minutes. After the pellets were washed with ice-cold 0.9% NaCl containing 1.0 mM neostigmine, they were recentrifuged at 48,000 x g for 10 minutes and accumulated radioactivity was extracted into Triton X-100: toluene phosphor and assayed by liquid scintillation spectrometry.

The relative amounts of radiolabelled choline, acetylcholine, betaine and phosphorylcholine were determined by high voltage paper electrophoresis (Helbronn and Carlsson, 1960). The accumulation of radioactivity was linear at all ^{3}H-choline concentrations employed for at least 4 minutes and with varying concentrations of brain tissue. When pellets obtained from these incubations were layered on continuous sucrose density gradients (0.32-1.5 M) and centrifuged for 90 minutes (Coyle and Snyder, 1969) the accumulated radioactivity was localized to an area of the gradient enriched in synaptosomes and separable from the profile of monoamine oxidase activity, a mitochondrial marker. Hypotonic shock completely liberated the particulate radioactivity. These observations indicate that radioactivity accumulated after incubation with ^{3}H-choline was localized predominantly to the synaptosomal fraction. Kinetics of uptake were determined by double-reciprocal plots (Lineweaver and Burk, 1934) and by least squares fitting of a substrate velocity curve to the data with computer programs donated by W.W. Cleland, which provided Km values and their standard errors (Cleland, 1967).

Crude synaptosomal preparations of the corpus striatum were incubated with concentrations of ^{3}H-choline varying from 5 x 10^{-7} M

to 2 x 10^{-2} M. Double reciprocal plots of accumulated radioactivity
always resulted in curves (Figure 7) which could be resolved into
two components graphically as well as by computer analysis with
calculated Km values of 1.2 x 10^{-6} M and about 9.4 x 10^{-5} M for the
high and low affinity uptake systems respectively. We found a
similar dual affinity uptake system for ^{3}H-choline in synaptosomal
preparations of the rat cerebral cortex. Moreover, in other

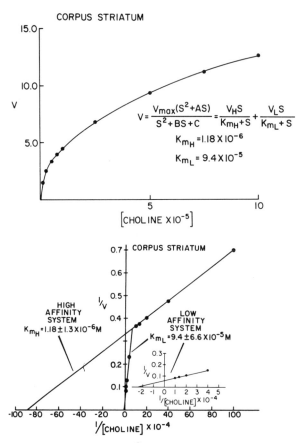

Figure 7. Kinetic analysis of ^{3}H-choline uptake by homogenates of
the rat corpus striatum. Upper: computed least squares fit of the
velocity (V) expressed as mμmol/^{3}H-choline/g/4 min accumulated into
homogenates of rat corpus striatum at different concentrations,
assuming transport by a two component system. Each point is the
mean of 4 determinations. Analysis of these data assuming a one
component system gave a poor fit. Lower: double reciprocal plot
of velocity (V) of ^{3}H-choline uptake into rat striatal homogenates
at different choline concentrations, using the same uptake data as
in the upper figure.

experiments the crude synaptosomal preparation was resolved by
discontinuous sucrose gradient centrifugation into synaptosomal
and mitochondrial fractions (Whittaker, 1965). The high affinity
choline transport system was localized to the synaptosomal
fraction.

Electrophoretic analysis of the accumulated radioactivity
showed that at 5×10^{-7} M ^{3}H-choline concentration, 70% of
accumulated radioactivity was present as acetylcholine. This
proportion decreased progressively to 61%, 47%, 23% and 16% at
^{3}H-choline concentrations of 1×10^{-6} M, 1×10^{-5} M, 5×10^{-5} M
and 1×10^{-4} M, respectively. Negligible amounts of ^{3}H-phosphoryl-
choline were present until medium concentrations of ^{3}H-choline
reached 5×10^{-5} M and 10^{-4} M, when phosphorylcholine accounted
for 8% and 10% respectively of the accumulated radioactivity.
No ^{3}H-betaine was detected until 10^{-4} M medium concentration of
^{3}H-choline when it accounted for 10% of the accumulated radioactivity.

Because the high affinity uptake of choline is associated with
a marked degree of acetylcholine formation, one might ask if the
apparent saturation kinetics of the high affinity choline uptake
are simply a reflection of a saturation of choline acetyltransferase. This does not seem likely, because the Km for choline
acetyltransferase preparations is about 2×10^{-5} M (Potter et al.,
1968), which is considerably higher than the Km for the high
affinity choline uptake. It is more probable that the high affinity
transport represents choline accumulation by subcellular components, presumably cholinergic synaptosomes, which synthesize
acetylcholine and that the low affinity system involves constituents which do not synthesize acetylcholine. Hence, with higher
concentrations of ^{3}H-choline, more would enter the compartments
which are not associated with acetylcholine formation.

The effects of drugs and varying metabolic conditions on the
two choline transport systems were examined by incubating preparations with low (5×10^{-7} M) and high (10^{-4} M) concentrations of
^{3}H-choline (Table 3). Replacement of sodium by lithium or sucrose
reduced the accumulation of low concentrations of choline more
than 95% but lowered the uptake of the high concentration of
choline only 45-60%. Ouabain (10^{-4} M), an inhibitor of the sodium
potassium ATPase, reduced the uptake of low concentrations of
choline 45%, but lowered the uptake of high choline concentrations
only 13%. Thus, the high affinity choline uptake appears to have
a marked dependence on sodium and the sodium-potassium ATPase
system, while the low affinity choline uptake is much less
sensitive to these ionic manipulations.

TABLE 3

INFLUENCE OF SODIUM OMISSION ON CHOLINE
UPTAKE BY STRIATAL SYNAPTOSOMES

Incubation Conditions*	^{3}H-Choline Accumulation (percent of control)	
	At 5 x 10^{-7} M	At 1 x 10^{-4} M
Sodium Replaced by Lithium (140 mM)	2.9	39.1
Sodium Replaced by Sucrose (320 mM)	5.3	55.8
Calcium Replaced by Sucrose (320 mM)	88.5	95.8
Ouabain (0.1 mM)	54.4	87.3

*Standard incubation medium contained Krebs-PO$_4$ buffer, at 30°C, Soman (0.1 μM) and either 0.5 μM or 100 μM ^{3}H-choline. Data are the mean values of triplicate determinations which varied by less than 10%.

A variety of drugs influenced the high and low affinity transports of choline. Hemicholinium-3 inhibited both the high and low affinity transports competitively (Lineweaver and Burk, 1953), with Ki values for the high and low affinity systems, respectively, of 8 x 10^{-7} M and 1 x 10^{-4} M. Acetylcholine, in the presence of Soman (0.1 μM), inhibited both uptake systems competitively with a Ki value of 9 x 10^{-6} M for the high affinity system and 1.7 x 10^{-4} M for the low affinity system. Atropine inhibited high and low affinity systems competitively with the same Ki value (2 x 10^{-4} M) for both transports, while scopolamine failed to affect either choline transport system at 10^{-3} M. The high and low affinity uptake systems were unaffected by 10^{-3} M concentrations of physostigmine, betaine, d-amphetamine, bicuculline, pentylenetetrazol, arecholine and mescaline.

Does the high affinity choline transport described here represent uptake into cholinergic nerve terminals? In support of this possibility is our finding that the high affinity choline uptake was associated with a marked degree of acetylcholine formation. Moreover, Kuhar et al. (1972 a) found that lesions in the medial septal nucleus and nucleus of the diagonal band of the rat reduce sharply the uptake of low concentrations of ^{3}H-choline into synaptosomal preparations from the hippocampus. By contrast the uptake of higher concentrations of ^{3}H-choline (10^{-4} M) is unaffected by such lesions. The medial septal nucleus and nucleus of the diagonal band contain a presumably cholinergic tract which projects to the hippocampus (Lewis and Shute, 1967). These experiments strongly suggest that the high affinity choline transport, which mediates the accumulation of low concentrations of this compound, represents accumulation into cholinergic neurons, while the low affinity uptake is mediated by some other tissue component.

B.   Studies with the Guinea Pig Ileum

The lesioning studies of Kuhar et al. (1972 a) provided strong indirect evidence that the choline uptake we had monitored in the corpus striatum was accumulated into cholinergic neurons. Unfortunately we were not in a position to "lesion" the cholinergic input to the corpus striatum to demonstrate this point directly. Accordingly, experiments were undertaken utilizing the guinea pig ileum, because it is possible to remove its cholinergic innervation simply by dissecting away the myenteric plexus.

In experiments with the ileum, strips of longitudinal muscle were incubated in Krebs-Ringer phosphate solution at 37°C without Soman for four minutes with concentrations of ^{3}H-choline ranging as low as 10^{-8} M, because there was less danger of leakage of endogenous choline into the medium than was the case for brain synaptosomes. Otherwise techniques were similar to those used with the brain.

Just as was observed in the brain, choline was accumulated by ileal strips via two distinct transport systems. A high affinity system had a Km of about 1×10^{-6} M while the low affinity system had a Km of about 9×10^{-5} M (Figure 8).

Conversion of choline to acetylcholine increased as ^{3}H-choline concentration in the medium was lowered so that at 10^{-6} and 5×10^{-7} ^{3}H-choline, about 80% of the radioactivity in the tissue was present as ^{3}H-acetylcholine (Table 4). At 10^{-4} M ^{3}H-choline, on the other hand, only 48% of tissue radioactivity was present as acetylcholine. This caused concern as to whether the apparent high affinity transport simply reflected the activity of choline acetyltransferase. Accordingly, incubations were performed at 10°C, because at this low temperature, though choline was still accumulated at 15% the rate at 37°C, only 15-20% of tissue radioactivity was acetylcholine. Under the conditions, the high affinity transport system for choline could still be demonstrated.

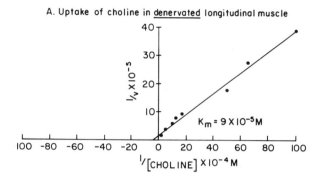

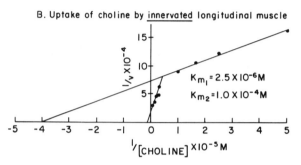

Figure 8.   Kinetics of choline uptake in innervated and denervated longitudinal intestinal muscle. Minces of longitudinal muscle obtained from guinea pig small intestine as described in Table 5 were incubated in various concentrations of ^{3}H-choline chloride for 4 minutes at 37°C in 2 ml of Krebs-phosphate medium. Uptake was stopped by the rapid addition of 8 ml of cold medium. The minced tissue was collected immediately by low pressure filtration and washed with 16 ml of Krebs medium. The filters containing the minced tissue were transferred to scintillation vials, extracted with 1 ml of 0.8 N perchloric acid and the radioactivity determined by liquid scintillation spectrometry in 20 ml of Triton X: toluene phosphor. All incubations were performed in quadruplicate.

Removal of the myenteric plexus greatly reduced the accumulation of low concentrations of ^{3}H-choline (Table 5). At 5 x 10^{-7}, 1 x 10^{-6} and 3.3 x 10^{-6} M, ^{3}H-choline, accumulated radioactivity fell about 90% after denervation. The reduction in uptake of low choline concentrations with denervation strongly suggests that the high affinity transport system is associated with the cholinergic neurons. Kinetic analysis of choline uptake revealed that with removal of the myenteric plexus, the high affinity choline uptake system vanished while the low affinity system persisted unperturbed (Figure 8).

TABLE 4

REDUCTION OF ILEAL ACETYLCHOLINE SYNTHESIS BY DENERVATION

CHOLINE METABOLISM	[CHOLINE] IN MEDIUM			
	5×10^{-7}M	1×10^{-6}M	1×10^{-5}M	1×10^{-4}M
Innervated Gut				
% Choline	19	18	28	52
% Acetylcholine	81	82	72	48
Denervated Gut				
% Choline	80	78	86	84
% Acetylcholine	20	22	14	16

Longitudinal muscle strips from guinea pigs were obtained and incubated in various concentrations of choline chloride as described in Table 5. The strips were then homogenized in 0.3 ml of acidic ethanol solution containing 0.1 mmole physostigmine sulfate, 0.3 mmole acetylcholine and 0.3 mmole choline. The choline metabolites from the supernatant fluid were analyzed by high voltage electrophoresis in a 0.2 M pyridine acetate buffer, pH 4.7, at 18 V/cm for 1 hr and visualized with iodine vapor. The paper was cut into serial 0.5 mm segments, extracted with 0.3 ml of water and counted in 10 mls of Triton-X phosphor. More than 99% of the radioactivity taken up by the tissue was recovered as choline and acetylcholine. Values did not vary more than 15%.

TABLE 5

REDUCTION OF INTESTINAL CHOLINE UPTAKE BY DENERVATION

VELOCITY OF CHOLINE UPTAKE (moles choline/ gram tissue/ 4 min x 10^{-7} M)	5×10^{-7}M	1×10^{-6}M	3.3×10^{-5}M
INNERVATED GUT	21 ± 3	33 ± 4	85 ± 5
DENERVATED GUT	2 ± 0.8	4 ± 1	16 ± 7

Male guinea pigs (500 g) were killed by a blow on the head and
their small intestines were rapidly removed from their mesenteric
attachment and placed in cold Krebs-phosphate medium (pH 7.4 at
37°C). Longitudinal muscle strips which included adherent myenteric (Auerbach's) plexus along part of their length were dissected free from the underlying circular muscle. Matched pairs
of innervated and denervated one inch muscle strips were selected
and incubated for 4 min at 37°C in 2 ml of Krebs-phosphate medium
containing various concentrations of choline chloride and 2-8 Ci
of ^{3}H-choline (17 Ci/mmole). Uptake was stopped by the rapid
addition of 8 ml cold medium and each strip was quickly transferred
with fine forceps through 5 serial washes with the medium. After
homogenization in acidic ethanol, aliquots of the supernatant
fluid were assayed for protein and radioactivity.

With denervation, conversion of choline to acetylcholine fell to about 15-20% irrespective of the concentrations of ^{3}H-choline in the medium. This may indicate that there is some non-neural synthesis of acetylcholine in the guinea pig intestine, as has been suggested by Feldberg and Lin (1950). Alternatively, it is possible that the denervation was incomplete.

In summary a variety of evidence indicates that the high affinity transport of choline reflects accumulation by cholinergic nerve terminals. Because its Km is about 1/10 that of choline acetylase, the high affinity choline transport may be rate limiting in the regulation of acetylcholine formation in vivo. It is possible that drugs which selectively inhibit this high affinity choline uptake may constitute valuable tools in the study of cholinergic nervous transmission. Moreover, this high affinity choline uptake system may furnish an heuristic approach to the labelling of cholinergic neurons in the brain and the peripheral nervous system. The "transmitter-pool" uptake of other transmitter precursors, especially the amino acid precursors, may be susceptible to experimental attack using techniques which we have found fruitful with choline.

REFERENCES

Aprison, M. and Werman, R. 1965. The distribution of glycine in cat spinal cord and roots. Life Sci. 4: 2075.
Arregui, A., Logan, W.J. and Snyder, S.H. 1972. Specific glycine accumulating synaptosomes in the spinal cord of the rat. Proc. Natl. Acad. Sci., (in press).
Askari, A. 1966. Uptake of some quaternary ammonium ions by human erythrocytes. J. Gen. Physiol. 49: 1147.
Birks, R.I. and MacIntosh, F.C. 1961. Acetylcholine metabolism of a sympathetic ganglion. Can. J. Biochem. Physiol. 39: 787.
Blasberg, R. 1968. Specificity of cerebral amino acid transport: a kinetic analysis. In: Progress in Brain Research (Eds. Lajtha, A. and Ford, D.H.) Elsevier, Amsterdam, Vol. 29, pp. 245-256.
Blasberg, R.G., Levi, G. and Lajtha, A. 1970. A comparisoin of inhibition of steady state, net transport, and exchange fluxes of amino acids in brain slices. Biochim. Biophys. Acta 203: 464.

Bloom, F.E. and Iversen, L.L. 1971. Localizing ^{3}H-GABA in nerve
    terminals of rat cerebral cortex by electron microscopic
    autoradiography. Nature 229: 629.
Browning, E.T. 1971. Free choline formation by cerebral cortical
    slices from rat brain. Biochem. Biophys. Res. Comm., 45: 1586.
Christensen, H.N. and Liang, M. 1965. An amino acid transport
    system of unassigned fraction in the Erlich ascites tumor
    cell. J. Biol. Chem. 240: 3601.
Cleland, W.W. 1967. The statistical analysis of enzyme kinetic
    data. Adv. Enzymol. 29: 1.
Coyle, J.T. and Snyder, S.H. 1969. Catecholamine uptake by
    synaptosomes in homogenates of rat brain: stereospecificity
    in different areas. J. Pharmac. Exp. Ther. 170: 221.
Curtis, D.R., Hosli, L., Johnston, G.A.R. and Johnston, I.H. 1968.
    The hyperpolarization of spinal motoneurones by glycine and
    related amino acids. Exp. Brain Res. 5: 235.
Davidoff, R.A., Graham, L.T., Shank, R.P., Werman, R. and Aprison,
    M.H. 1967. Changes in amino acid concentrations associated
    with loss of spinal interneurons. J. Neurochem. 14: 1025.
Diamond, I. and Kennedy, E.T. 1969. Carrier-mediated transport
    of choline into synaptic nerve endings. J. Biol. Chem. 244:
    3258.
Dixon, M. 1953. The determination of enzyme inhibitor constants.
    Biochem. J. 55: 170.
Feldberg, W. and Lin, R.C.Y. 1950. Synthesis of acetylcholine in
    wall of digestive tract. J. Physiol. 111: 96.
Glowinski, J. and Iversen, L.L. 1966. Regional studies of
    catecholamines in the rat brain. I. The disposition of
    [^{3}H] norepinephrine, [^{3}H] dopamine and [^{3}H] dopa in various
    regions of the brain. J. Neurochem. 13: 655.
Graham, L.T., Jr., Shank, R.P., Werman, R. and Aprison, M.H. 1967.
    Distribution of some synaptic transmitter suspects in cat
    spinal cord: glutamic acid, aspartic acid, gamma-amino-
    butyric acid, glycine and glutamine. J. Neurochem. 14: 465.
Green, A.I. and Haubrich, D.R. 1971. Accumulation of radioactivity
    after incubation of rat brain slices with H^3-choline. Trans.
    Amer. Soc. Neurochem. 2: 75.
Haga, T. 1971. Synthesis and release of (^{14}C) acetylcholine in
    synaptosomes. J. Neurochem. 18: 781.
Helbronn, E. and Carlsson, B.J. 1960. Qualitative separation of
    choline esters by means of high voltage paper electrophoresis.
    Chromatog. 4: 257.
Hemsworth, B.A., Darmer, K.I., Jr., and Bosmann, H.B. 1971.
    The incorporation of choline into isolated synaptosomal and
    synaptic vesicle fractions in the presence of quaternary
    ammonium compounds. Neuropharmacol. 10: 109.
Hökfelt, T. 1970. Electron microscopic identification of monoamine
    nerve ending particles in rat brain homogenates. Brain Res.
    22: 147.

Hökfelt, T. and Ljundahl, A. 1971. Light and electron microscope autoradiography on spinal cord slices after incubation with labelled glycine. Brain Res. 32: 189.

Johnston, G.A.R. 1968. The intraspinal distribution of some depressant amino acids. J. Neurochem. 15: 1013.

Johnston, G.A.R., DeGroat, W.C. and Curtis, D.R. 1969. Tetanus toxin and amino acid levels in cat spinal cord. J. Neurochem. 16: 797.

Johnston, G.A.R. and Iversen, L.L. 1971. Glycine uptake in rat CNS slices and homogenates: evidence for different uptake systems in spinal cord and cerebral cortex. J. Neurochem. 18: 1951.

Kuhar, M.H., Green, A.I., Snyder, S.H. and Gfeller, E. 1970. Separation of synaptosomes storing catecholamines and gamma-aminocutyric acid in rat corpus striatum. Brain Res. 21: 405.

Kuhar, M.J., Shaskan, E.G. and Snyder, S.H. 1971. The subcellular distribution of endogenous and exogenous serotonin in brain tissue: comparison of synaptosomes storing serotonin, norepinephrine and α-aminobutyric acid. J. Neurochem. 18: 333.

Kuhar, M.J., Roth, R.H. and Aghajanian, G.K. 1972. A reduction in synaptosomal uptake of serotonin in rats with midbrain raphe lesions. J. Pharmac. Exp. Ther. 181: 36.

Kuhar, M.J., Roth, R.H. and Aghajanian, G.K. 1972 a. Choline uptake into synaptosomes from the hippocampus; reduction after electrolytic destruction of the medial septal nucleus. Fed. Proc. 31: 516Abs.

Lewis, P.R. and Shute, C.C.D. 1967. The cholinergic limbic system: projections to hippocampal formation, medial cortex, nuclei of the ascending cholinergic reticular system, and the subfornical organ and supra-optic crest. Brain 90: 521.

Lineweaver, H. and Burk, D. 1934. The determination of enzyme dissociation constants. J. Amer. Chem. Soc. 56: 658.

Logan, W.J. and Snyder, S.H. 1971. Unique high affinity uptake systems for glycine, glutamic and aspartic acids in central nervous tissue of the rat. Nature 234: 297.

Logan, W.J. and Snyder, S.H. 1972. High affinity uptake systems for glycine, glutamic and aspartic acids in synaptosomes of rat central nervous tissue. Brain Res. 42: 413.

McLennan, H. 1970. Synaptic Transmission (2nd Edition), Philadelphia: W.B. Saunders Co., pp. 78-105.

Mangan, J.L. and Whittaker, V.P. 1966. The distribution of free amino acids in subcellular fractions of guinea-pig brain. Biochem. J. 98: 128.

Marchbanks, R.M. 1969. The conversion of ^{14}C-choline to ^{14}C-acetylcholine in synaptosomes in vitro. Biochem. Pharmacol. 18: 1763.

Martin, K. 1968. Concentrative accumulation of choline by human erythrocytes. J. Gen. Physiol. 51: 497.

Matus, A. and Dennison, M. 1971. Autoradiographic localization of tritiated glycine at "flat-vesicle" synapses in spinal cord. Brain Res. 32: 195.

Potter, L.T. 1968. Uptake of choline by nerve endings isolated from the rat cerebral cortex. In: The Interaction of Drug and Subcellular Components of Animal Cells (Ed. Campbell, P.N.) London: Churchill, pp. 293.

Potter, L.T., Glober, A.S. and Saelens, J.K. 1968. Choline acetyltransferase from rat brain. J. Biol. Chem. 243: 3864.

Schuberth, J., Sundwall, A., Sorbell, B. and Lindell, J.-O. 1965. Uptake of choline by mouse brain slices. J. Neurochem. 13: 347.

Schultz, S.G., Yu-Tu, L., Alvarez, O.O. and Curran, P.F. 1970. Dicarboxylic amino acid influx across brush border of rabbit ileum. Effects of amino acid charge on the sodium-amino acid interaction. J. Gen. Physiol. 56: 621.

Snyder, S.H., Logan, W.J., Bennett, J.P. and Arregui, A. 1973. Amino acids as central nervous transmitters: Biochemical studies. Neurosciences Res. (in press).

Sung, C.P. and Johnstons, R.M. 1965. Evidence for active transport of choline in rat kidney cortex slices. Can. J. Biochem. 43: 1111.

Tagliamonte, A., Tagliamonte, P., Perez-Cruet, J. and Gessa, G.L. 1971. Increase of brain tryptophan caused by drugs which stimulate serotonin synthesis. Nature 229: 125.

Werman, R., Davidoff, R.A. and Aprison, M.H. 1968. Inhibitory of glycine on spinal neurons in the cat. J. Neurophysiol. 31: 81.

Whittaker, V.P. 1965. The application of subcellular fractionation techniques to the study of brain function. Prog. Biophys. Molec. Biol. 15: 39.

Winter, C.G. and Christensen, H.N. 1965. Contrasts in neutral amino acid transport by rabbit erythrocytes and reticulocytes. J. Biol. Chem. 240: 3594.

Wofsey, A.R., Kuhar, M.J. and Snyder, S.H. 1971. A unique synaptosomal fraction which accumulates glutamic and aspartic acids in brain tissue. Proc. Natl. Acad. Sci. 68: 1102.

Wurtman, R.J. and Fernstrom, J.D. 1972. L-Tryptophan, L-tyrosine and the control of brain monoamine biosynthesis. In: Perspectives in Neuropharmacology (Ed. Snyder, S.H.), New York: Oxford Univ. Press, pp. 143.

CENTRAL NORADRENERGIC RECEPTORS: LOCALIZATION, FUNCTION AND

MOLECULAR MECHANISMS

Floyd E. Bloom, Barry J. Hoffer, and George R. Siggins

Laboratory of Neuropharmacology, Division of Special
Mental Health Research, National Institute of Mental
Health, St. Elizabeths Hospital, Washington, D.C. 20032

Fluorescence histochemical data make it eminently clear that
the catecholamine-containing neurons of the brain are restricted
to a relatively small region of the pons and mesencephalon and
yet send very discrete axonal tracts to spinal cord, diencephalon
and cortices. In order to determine the effects of norepinephrine
(NE) on postsynaptic neurons and the changes in these effects
produced by drugs which influence behavior, the location and
function of the presumed NE-mediated synapses must be determined
for each of the regions receiving these fibers. Such data has
now been accumulated in detail for the NE projection to the
cerebellum (see below) and has been partially elucidated for
several other regions. This paper will describe the methods now
being used in our laboratory to determine the localization and
function of NE-mediated synapses.

Early studies utilizing microiontophoretic drug administrations assumed that both the presence and absence of responses
were meaningful data. Quantitative assessment of the proportion
of neurons which would or would not respond to NE in a given
region might then imply the relative "importance" of noradrenergic
transmission. However, in contrast to some early studies which
indicated little or no significant actions of NE on spinal or
cortical neurons (see review, Bloom, 1968), subsequent studies
showed NE to be effective in altering the discharge patterns of
neurons in almost every region of the brain tested. This turn-
about in interpretation reflected increasing awareness of several
potential technological pitfalls: the type and depth of anesthesia, the presence of spontaneous synaptic activity versus
amino acid-induced activity, the physiological or cytological
identification of the neuronal types being tested, and the use

223

of current neutralization procedures (Salmoiraghi and Stefanis, 1967; Salmoiraghi and Weight, 1967).

There are only two possible general types of positive responses which neurons can manifest to microiontophoretic administration of NE; the cell can either fire faster or slower. Thus, depending on the cell type tested, NE can either depress discharge rates, as it does in several cortical areas, or facilitate discharge rates as has been reported for certain groups of hindbrain neurons (Bradley and Wolstencroft, 1962; Boakes et al., 1971; Couch, 1970). The presence of one type of response in one brain region need not per se mitigate against the validity of the other type of response in another brain region, although this view has been expressed (see Hebb, 1970).

However, the interpretation of responses becomes particularly boggy when separate groups working on apparently similar neurons under apparently identical conditions report opposite qualitative responses. For example, Straughan and his colleagues have emphasized excitatory responses of cortical neurons to NE (Johnson et al., 1969 a,b), while the earlier reports of Krnjevic and Phillis (1963 a,b) had indicated only a few relatively unimpressive and generally depressant effects of NE (see review, Bloom, 1968). This particular topic has recently received attention in experiments by Frederickson et al. (1971), who have shown that spontaneously active neurons are most likely to be excited by NE when the test solution is more acid than pH 4.0. At pH 4.0, most cells responded solely by depression of their spontaneous or amino acid-induced discharge. On the basis of the effects of NE on mesenteric blood vessels, Stone (1971) has suggested that excitatory effects of NE on central neurons are secondary to vascular constriction and anoxia.

DO RESPONSES IMPLY SYNAPTIC RECEPTORS

By proper regard for each of the necessary experimental controls peculiar to microiontophoresis, it has been possible to obtain reproducible effects on neuronal discharge. However, such data do not necessarily indicate the responses to be a reflection of an underlying NE-mediated input to the cells being tested. The most crucial bit of practicable data needed to corroborate this inference would be to demonstrate that selective stimulation of the afferent NE-axons reproduces the effects produced by microiontophoresis of NE. Since the cells of origin for the cortical NE projections have only recently been established (Olson and Fuxe, 1971; Ungerstedt, 1971), the next best evidence has been to establish that the cells being tested do receive NE-containing synapses. In the absence of such corroborative data, responses cannot be functionally interpreted.

LOCALIZING NOREPINEPHRINE-CONTAINING SYNAPSES

The varicosities of the axons demonstrated by fluorescence histochemistry indicate presumed sites of transmitter release. However, because of the limited resolution of the optical microscope relative to the very fine nature of the complexly inter-related cellular processes of the neuropil, electron microscopic methods are needed to determine precisely which neurons in a given region receive synaptic contact from NE-containing axons.

No single electron microscopic histochemical method has yet achieved the consistency and selectivity of localization desired for analysis of NE-transmitting synapses. Permanganate fixation methods (Hökfelt, 1967, 1968, 1972; Richardson, 1966) offer the most direct approach to the successful visualization of small granular synaptic vesicles, which seem identical morphologically and pharmacologically to the storage vesicles of NE in peripheral sympathetic nerve terminals. However, technical problems (such as poor penetration yielding small usable tissue samples) limit this method to regions with a high density of NE axons (e.g., pons, hypothalamus).

We have found most useful for our purposes a combination of two methods: autoradiographic localization of processes which accumulate tracer amounts of ^{3}H-NE in vivo (Aghajanian and Bloom, 1967) or in vitro (Lenn, 1967); and the acute degeneration which occurs in NE terminals within 8-48 hours after injection of 6-hydroxydopamine (6-OHDA) into the cerebrospinal fluid (see Bloom, 1971; Malmfors and Thoenen, 1971).

For these reasons we have attempted to apply as many of the available methods as are possible when seeking to localize NE-containing synaptic terminals, and find the most satisfactory localizations to be based upon complementary results from multiple approaches (Bloom et al., 1971). A promising future line of investigation is based upon the exploitation of axoplasmic trans-port. The distribution of a specific NE axonal pathway could be revealed by autoradiography of labeled macromolecules synthesized exclusively in the perikaryon from a restricted application of labelled precursor (Cowan et al., 1972), directly to the NE-containing neurons (Pickel, Forman and Bloom, unpublished).

By application of the combination of fluorescence histo-chemistry, autoradiography of H^3-NE and acute degeneration after 6-OHDA, NE-containing synapses have been identified as projecting to olfactory mitral cells (Dahlstrom et al., 1965; Bloom, unpub-lished results), to hypothalamic neurons of the supraoptic nucleus (Barker et al., 1971; Nicoll and Barker, 1971) and to a

portion of the neurons of the rat raphe nuclei (Loizu, 1969;
Bloom and Costa, 1971). These neurons in each region have been
tested for the actions of NE applied by microiontophoresis. In
the olfactory bulb, antidromic activation of the lateral olfactory
tract was used to identify mitral cells which showed a homogeneous
inhibitory response to NE (Bloom et al., 1964 a). Blockade of NE
responses with alpha blockers (Bloom et al., 1964 b) or longterm
depletion of NE neuronal stores (Bloom et al., 1964 b) reduced,
but did not eliminate the recurrent inhibition of mitral cells
produced by lateral olfactory tract stimuli (Salmoiraghi et al.,
1964). Supraoptic neurons, which were identified by antidromic
activation of their axons in the posterior pituitary, exhibit
uniform inhibitory responses to NE (Barker et al., 1971) but
this effect is not involved in the recurrent antidromic inhibition
(Nicoll and Barker, 1971). Neurons of the cat and rat raphe
nuclei exhibit less consistent qualitative responses: feline
median raphe cells are frequently excited (Crayton and Bloom,
1969) while only about half of the neurons in the rat dorsal
raphe (Aghajanian and Haigler, personal communication), and
pontine raphe (Couch, 1970) show this response. For the latter
nucleus, cells which were excited by 5-HT were usually depressed
by NE and vice versa (Couch, 1970).

While a physiologically significant responsiveness to NE can
be demonstrated in the three central regions just described, it
has not yet proven possible to uncover the source of these
presumed NE-synapses, nor to relate these effects of NE to the
physiology of the region. Much basic research in psychiatry has
concentrated upon the changes in catecholamine metabolism produced
by psychoactive drugs which are used to treat or induce states
of behavioral dysfunction (Schildkraut and Kety, 1967; c.f. Snyder,
1970). Since such studies require clarification of the role of NE
in cortical synaptic integration, we have begun an examination of
a specific population of cortical neurons whose function would
appear to be involved in the cortical integration of sensory
phenomena (Nelson et al., 1972). The polysensory neurons of the
squirrel monkey postarcuate cortex are characterized by their
topographical location, and by their ability to respond to photic,
auditory and somatic sensory stimuli, and hence constitute a
definable neuronal population.

The combination of histochemical and cytochemical methods,
described above, has been applied to the polysensory neurons
and has demonstrated the presence of an extensive network of
finely arborized monoamine-containing axons and terminals which
appear to establish both axosomatic and axodendritic synapses to
these cortical neurons. Based upon the density of nerve terminals
which are positively labelled by cytochemical markers before and
after chronic treatment with 6-OHDA, the NE-containing projection

would appear to be less dense than the 5-HT-containing projection. Accordingly, both of these transmitter substances, as well as a variety of other transmitter candidates have been tested on the polysensory neurons.

More than 90% of the polysensory cortical neurons respond to NE and 5-HT by depression of spontaneous or induced discharge (Nelson et al., in preparation). These responses were maximal within 5-10 seconds and exhibited very low thresholds of micro-iontophoretic currents. A few cells exhibited long latency excitatory responses to NE which generally required higher current-doses. However, the long latency excitatory responses and their thresholds were promptly converted to typical depressant responses after brief concurrent iontophoretic administrations of desmethylimipramine, even when the latter drug was given at doses which produced no obvious direct action on cell firing. The low incidence and high threshold of these responses, and their conversion to inhibition by the action of desmethylimipramine suggests that in the cortex, as in other central nervous system regions, the main cellular action of NE is inhibition.

THE NE PATHWAY TO CEREBELLAR PURKINJE CELLS

The major obstacle to the previous investigators of the presumed adrenergic synapses in the olfactory bulb, hypothalamus, pons, and cerebral cortex has been the inability to demonstrate the effects of the presumed adrenergic synaptic pathway. To obtain this evidence requires determination of the cells of origin of the distal adrenergic synapses and a description of the synaptic potentials generated in the postsynaptic cells upon selective stimulation of the NE cell bodies. Only one complete NE projection has been examined by both electrophysiology and cytochemistry, and this section will summarize our work (see Hoffer et al., 1971 a,b; Siggins et al., 1971 a-d) concerning the noradrenergic locus coeruleus (LC)-to-cerebellar Purkinje cell synapse.

Structural Basis of the Pathway and its Synapses

The norepinephrine-containing axons of the cerebellar cortex are clearly visualized in normal animals by the formaldehyde-induced fluorescence method of Falck and Hillarp (Falck et al., 1962), and are readily identified in cerebellar cortices of normal animals (Bloom et al., 1971) as well as in cerebellar slices incubated in vitro with catecholamine analogs to enhance the fluorescence (Hökfelt and Fuxe, 1969). The thin varicose fibers invade the Purkinje and molecular layers from the underlying white matter; little or no branching can be seen within the granule cell layer, but occurs frequently in the outer

cortical layers. As the axons progress toward the surface of the
folium, they course mainly along the edges of the Purkinje
dendrites (i.e., perpendicular to the outer surface) giving off
branches which tend to course mainly across the folium (i.e.,
parallel to the surface) in both frontal and sagittal planes of
sectioning. These fibers do not, therefore, correlate with any
of the classical Purkinje afferent fiber systems revealed by
silver staining or other intravital staining techniques (O'Leary
et al., 1968).

The norepinephrine-containing fibers can be located at the
electron microscopic level by autoradiography of sites taking
up H^3-norepinephrine or by the degeneration which ensues after
exposure to 6-hydroxydopamine (Bloom et al., 1971). The results
of the two ultrastructural methods indicate that the majority
of reactive nerve terminals synapse with Purkinje dendrites in
the mid-to-outer molecular layer, and occasionally contact the
Purkinje denritic surface in the inner molecular layer. Their
ultrastructural features clearly distinguish them from climbing
fibers (O'Leary et al., 1968; Larramendi, 1970) although they
do appear to climb along the Purkinje dendrite before giving off
their terminal branches.

The fluorescence of normal fibers can be somewhat enhanced
by a 15-30 minute in vitro incubation with alpha methyl norepinephrine (10^{-7} M), indicating perhaps that many of the normal
fibers are ordinarily missed due to sub-detectable levels of
amine. When animals are pretreated with reserpine there is no
enhancement of the fluorescence under these conditions (see
Hökfelt and Fuxe, 1969). Animals given 6-hydroxydopamine 1-2 weeks
before the incubation in vitro show virtually no fluorescent
catecholamine fibers, and no enhancement of the fluorescence
occurs after exposure in vitro to alpha-methyl norepinephrine.
Occasionally, fluorescent axons of the green color attributable
to catecholamines can be seen within the deeper folia of 6-
hydroxydopamine treated animals but these fibers are swollen,
show few varicosities and end bluntly (see Bloom et al., 1971).
They are apparently surviving preterminal axons trimmed of their
terminal arborizations by the toxic action of 6-hydroxydopamine;
ultrastructurally, such preterminals show large numbers of large
granular vesicles and mitochondria (Bloom, 1971).

Although statistical analyses suggest that the norepinephrine-
containing fibers constitute less than 1% of cerebellar cortical
nerve terminals (see Bloom et al., 1971), multiple varicosities
and extensive axonal branching offers the possibility of adequate
synaptic terminals to each Purkinje dendritic field.

These cytological studies indicate, therefore, that only

certain cerebellar nerve terminals will take up H^3-NE or alpha-
methyl norepinephrine and react to 6-hydroxydopamine. Each of
the cytochemical methods indicates that the endogenous norepinephrine is contained within axons which synapse with Purkinje
cell dendrites and dendritic spines.

Effects of Norepinephrine on Purkinje Cells

Effects on discharge pattern and rate: The effects of NE
have now been evaluated by microelectrophoretic testing of several
hundred rat cerebellar Purkinje cells under a variety of anesthetic conditions (Hoffer et al., 1971 a). On virtually all
cells tested, NE reduces the spontaneous discharge rate with a
delay of from 5-30 seconds after the onset of the ejection current.
When doses of NE did not produce a complete cessation of discharge,
groups of action potentials at control frequencies were interrupted
by long pauses. Larger amounts of NE were then capable of break-
ing this cyclical discharge pattern into single spikes, slowing
the cell still further, and ultimately stopping discharge altogether.

While mean rate is a convenient index to the general activity
of cells, the interspike interval histogram reveals more precise
information about discharge pattern. Study of the interspike
interval histogram indicates that NE effects are manifested on a
particular aspect of Purkinje cell discharge. Microelectro-
phoresis of NE produces no change in climbing fiber bursts.
Furthermore, during the slowing elicited by small submaximal
doses of NE, single spike discharge, as represented by the major
histogram peak, tends to occur at the same most probable interspike intervals as during the control period. It is the population of long pauses which appears markedly augmented by NE.

Mediation of the response by cyclic AMP: In many parts of
the peripheral autonomic nervous system, the cellular mechanism
of the response of sympathetically-innvervated tissues involves
the stimulation of adenyl cyclase by norepinephrine (Sutherland,
et al., 1968). This enzyme synthesizes cyclic 3',5' adenosine
monophosphate (cyclic AMP) and the cyclic nucleotide triggers
the cellular events mediated by the sympathetic innervation. In
the central nervous system, the cerebellum has one of the highest
regional levels of both cyclic AMP and adenyl cyclase and a very
low level of the cyclic AMP catabolizing enzyme, phosphodiesterase
(Sutherland et al., 1962; Weiss and Kidman, 1969). These biochemical findings prompted our original investigations into the
neuropharmacological and electrophysiological effects of cyclic
AMP in the cerebellum (Siggins et al., 1969, 1971 a,c). The
results of our experiments led us to propose that the inhibitory
effects of NE on rat cerebellar Purkinje cells are mediated by
cyclic AMP (Hoffer et al., 1971 b; Siggins et al., 1969).

In brief, this hypothesis is based upon the following points:
1) Both norepinephrine and cyclic AMP slow the discharge of
Purkinje cells by prolongation of the pauses between single spikes.
2) In many cases the response and recovery latencies with cyclic
AMP are briefer than with norepinephrine. 3) The duration and the
magnitude of the response to norepinephrine and to cyclic AMP are
increased by either parenteral or electrophoretic administration
of methyl xanthines, such as theophylline or aminophylline, or
of papaverine, compounds which are known to inhibit phosphodiesterase (see Kukovetz and Poch, 1970; Weiss and Kidman, 1969).
4) The response to norepinephrine can be completely blocked by
electrophoretic administration of MJ-1999, a beta-adrenergic
inhibitor (Lish et al., 1965), and also by nicotinate and by
prostaglandins of the E series (Siggins et al., 1971 a); all of
these substances are known to block the ability of norepinephrine
to elevate levels of cyclic AMP in peripheral tissues (Krishna
et al., 1966; Butcher and Baird, 1968). 5) Finally, the transmembrane responses to norepinephrine and to cyclic AMP both
involve a novel type of hyperpolarization, in which there is no
increase in the passive membrane conductance to ionic flow such
as occurs in the response to other inhibitory substances like
GABA (Siggins et al., 1971 c).

Moreover, since the response to norepinephrine and to cyclic
AMP and their potentiation by methyl xanthines can be seen quite
well in animals pretreated with 6-hydroxydopamine to remove the
endogenous catecholamine nerve terminals, all these results
strongly support a direct postsynaptic activation of adenyl
cyclase as one step in the molecular mechanism causing the
inhibition by norepinephrine (see Siggins et al., 1971 b).
Regardless of the biophysical mechanism (see Weight, 1971) by
which the Purkinje membrane response to NE and cyclic AMP, the
similarity of these unique hyperpolarizations accompanied by
increased membrane resistance adds significantly to the list
of common features in their actions and provides further support
for the postsynaptic mediation of NE inhibition by cyclic AMP.

Activation of the Pathway from Locus Coeruleus

Further characterization of the natural endogenous transmitter and its effect on Purkinje cells requires experimental
activation of the proposed adrenergic pathway, and identification
of the origin of the noradrenergic projection to the cerebellum
thus assumes critical importance. It has been suggested that the
nerves containing catecholamine in rat cerebellar cortex arise
largely from discrete bilateral nuclei of fluorescent cells in
the dorsal medullary brain stem (the locus coeruleus, LC)
(Hoffer et al., 1972; Olson and Fuxe, 1971; Ungerstedt, 1971).

Purkinje cells, but not cortical interneurons, showed a remarkably uniform inhibitory response to stimulation of LC with trains of pulses: ninety-four of 102 cells (twenty animals) recorded extracellularly displayed depression of spontaneous discharge rate. This summated response was greatest at relatively low stimulus frequencies (3-50/S) and was markedly diminished at faster rates. Complete cessation of discharge outlasting the stimulation period by 4-65 seconds (mean, 21 S) could be obtained with 20-100 pulses at 10 S^{-1}. At this frequency, threshold currents ranged from 0.03 to 1.2 mA (mean, 0.35 mA) (Siggins et al., 1971 d).

Although the response to a single LC stimulus often escaped detection on direct visual inspection, construction of post stimulus time histograms reproducibly revealed reduced probability of spike discharge over prolonged intervals of 60 to 470 ms (mean, 293 ms) with long latent periods of 50-290 ms (means, 148 ms). During these late inhibitions, cell discharge was often only incompletely suppressed; however, a single short burst of two to five pulses produced the inhibition.

With trains of pulses, large hyperpolarizations extending well beyond the stimulation period and averaging 14 mV (range, 2-39 mV) were recorded. An index of membrane resistance was obtained by measuring the size of climbing fiber spikes (Hoffer et al., 1971 b), or in obviously injured cells excitatory post-synaptic potentials (EPSPs), and by measuring the potential deflexions produced by hyperpolarizing currents (0.5-1 nA, 40 ms duration) passed through the recording micropipette in conjunction with a Wheatstone bridge circuit. In all cases, input resistance, as measured by these two parameters, either increased (ten cells) or did not change (two cells) during the LC evoked hyperpolarizations. In this respect, LC stimulation exactly mimics the action of exogenously applied norepinephrine and cyclic AMP, which also produce hyperpolarizations without a decrease in membrane resistance.

Although the effects of LC stimulation produce the same qualitative effect on Purkinje cells as the iontophoretic admin-istration of norepinephrine, additional studies are required to confirm the noradrenergic nature of the LC effects. If the effects of LC stimulation were due to release of norepinephrine from the nerve terminals already demonstrated to synapse with Purkinje cells, pharmacological depletion of norepinephrine should seriously impair the LC inhibitory response. Indeed, when animals are acutely pretreated with reserpine (1.5 mg/kg, IV) and alpha-methyl-tyrosine (100-200 mg/kg, IP), the loss of the LC inhibitory effects, whether to single or multiple shocks, correlates well with the regional loss of norepinephrine (Glowinski and Baldessarini, 1966), as does the subsequent recovery.

In addition, when prostaglandin E_1 or E_2 is administered to
Purkinje cells during stimulation of LC, the inhibitory effects
of LC stimulation are reproducibly and reversibly blocked. Of
all the substances tested in the rat cerebellar cortex, norepinephrine is the only substance whose response is antagonized
by prostaglandins (Siggins et al., 1971 a). Furthermore, micro-
iontophoretic administration of papaverine potentiates not only
Purkinje cells responses to NE and cyclic AMP (see above), but
also enhances the inhibition produced by LC stimulation. These
recent results strongly suggest that the LC gives rise to the
norepinephrine-cyclic AMP mediated inhibition of Purkinje cells.

Immunofluorescent Localization of Cyclic AMP in Purkinje Cells

In order to test the hypothesis that synaptically released
NE inhibits Purkinje cells by activating adenyl cyclase, we have
developed an immuno-cytochemical method (Wedner et al., 1971)
which permits the localization of intracellularly bound cyclic
AMP in unfixed frozen tissue sections. When this method is
applied to rat cerebellum, staining is dependent upon the
functional state of the tissue. Samples taken immediately
(within 30 seconds) after decapitation or from animals which are
anesthetized show positive staining in the nuclei of granule
cells and in less than 15% of the Purkinje cells. Samples taken
after post-decapitation intervals of 3-5 minutes (known to
produce elevations of cerebellar cyclic AMP (Breckenridge, 1964))
show more than 90% of Purkinje cells to exhibit positive immuno-
cytochemical staining for cyclic AMP (Bloom et al., 1972). In
preliminary studies, similar increases in cyclic AMP content of
individual Purkinje cells have been documented by this staining
technique after stimulation of locus coeruleus in normal animals,
but not in animals pretreated with 6-OHDA (unpublished results).
Topical application of NE, but not GABA, histamine, serotonin or
acetylcholine, also appear to increase Purkinje cell cyclic AMP
(unpublished results). These data, therefore, provide yet another
step in the documentation of the hypothesis that cyclic AMP mediates
the NE-induced inhibition of Purkinje cells via a synaptic pathway
from locus coeruleus.

CONCLUSIONS

The response to norepinephrine can be evaluated electro-
physiologically to determine the function of identified NE-
containing synaptic terminals on neurons in cerebral and cerebellar cortex. In these cells, NE produces an inhibitory effect.
In the cerebellum, this is caused by a hyperpolarization of the
membrane occurring by a novel membrane effect not involving an
increased membrane conductance to ions. The origin of the NE-

containing afferents has been suggested to be the locus coeruleus and stimulation of this nucleus will produce effects which emulate the cerebellar action of NE. The NE projection to the cerebellar cortex, therefore, represents a highly characterized monoamine-containing pathway of the brain, and the only central norepinephrine-containing pathway yet found susceptible to experimental manipulation by electrophysiological means. The responses and interactions of this specific synaptic system with psychoactive drugs should provide a meaningful source of interpretable data concerning the function of norepinephrine-transmitting neurons in integrated behavior.

In concluding, it might be profitable to consider how the present knowledge of the function of one particular NE-mediated system might be employed to pursue the mechanism of action of particular behaviorally active drugs. Such a problem appears simple, but is in fact relatively complex because all parts of the brain are at least indirectly connected by pathways which conduct rapidly and synapse by several unknown types of chemical transmission. When a drug is given and a response is observed by microelectrode recording of cellular discharge patterns, any delay longer than 5 msec. after the drug enters the brain allows the possibility that intervening neurons have mediated the drug response rather than the cell or cell group under electrode observation. Because all behavioral and electrophysiological changes produced by drugs must have originated from changes in the activity of certain interacting groups of cells, the interpretation of cellular actions of drugs can be partially simplified by assuming that there are 2 basic ways a drug can be causing this effect:

1. The drug may change neuronal behavior by specifically modifying one or more types of neurochemical transmission. Thus, a drug could act as an agonist at all muscarinic cholinergic synapses or by prolonging the duration of NE-receptor occupancy (e.g. by inhibiting the re-uptake of NE by presynaptic terminals).

2. A drug might act by influencing a specific group of target cells by virtue of an interaction with surface receptors which are unrelated to synaptic events and then produce an intracellular effect which is translated into an altered rate of cellular discharge. If these target cells participate in other nerve circuits which can generate or modulate behaviors, then behavior will be altered through an initial non-synaptic action. A good example of both types of reasoning with respect to the mechanisms of action of LSD appears in the recent review by Aghajanian (1972).

It is not too difficult to understand that these two theories

could be really considered as one, except that in the second case
the receptors influenced by the drug have acted upon synaptic
receptors belonging to a pathway whose transmitter has not yet
been identified. It would, therefore, seem to us that an
appropriate area for further investigation would be some means
to explore the surfaces of cells to establish the existence of
synaptic and non-synaptic receptors for those key groups of
nuclei--like the locus coeruleus, substantia nigra and raphe--
whose neurochemical circuitry is known to some extent. In such
cases, the role played by these nuclei in generating and modifying
discrete behavioral responses could then be determined. It might
then be possible to detect whether the alterations in neuronal
regulatory steps produced by drugs depend upon specific receptors
peculiar to the drug or to selective receptors characteristic
of the neurotransmitter substance at whose synapses the drug is
able to exert its effect.

REFERENCES

Aghajanian, G.K. 1972. LSD and CNS transmission. Ann. Rev.
    Pharmacol. 12: 157.
Aghajanian, G.R. and Bloom, F.E. 1967. Electron-microscopic
    localization of tritiated norepinephrine in rat brain
    effects of drugs. J. Pharmacol. Exp. Ther. 156: 407.
Barker, J.L., Crayton, J.C., and Nicoll, R.A. 1971. Supraoptic
    neurosecretory cells: Adrenergic and cholinergic sensitivity.
    Science 171: 208.
Bloom, F.E. 1968. Electrophysiological pharmacology of single
    nerve cells. In: Psychopharmacology, A 10 Year Progress
    Report (Ed. Effron, D.H.) Washington, D.C.: U.S. Govt.
    Printing Office.
Bloom, F.E. 1971. Fine structural changes in rat brain after
    intracisternal injection of 6-hydroxydopamine. In:
    6-Hydroxydopamine (Eds. Malmors, T. and Thoenen, H.)
    Amsterdam: North Holland Publishing Co., pp. 135.
Bloom, F.E. and Costa, E. 1971. The effects of drugs on seroton-
    ergic nerve terminals. In: Advances in Cytopharmacology
    (Ed. Edelson, E.) New York: Raven Press, Vol. I., pp. 379.
Bloom, F.E., von Baumgarten, R., Oliver, A.P., Costa, E. and
    Salmioraghi, G.C. 1964 a. Microelectrophoretic studies on
    adrenergic mechanisms of rabbit olfactory bulb neurons.
    Life Sci. 3: 131.
Bloom, F.E., Costa, E. and Salmoiraghi, G.C. 1964 b. Analysis
    of individual rabbit olfactory bulb neuron response to
    microelectrophoresis of acetylcholine, norepinephrine and
    serotonin synergists and antagonists. J. Pharmacol. Exp.
    Ther. 146: 16.

Bloom, F.E., Hoffer, B.J. and Siggins, G.R. 1971 Studies on
    norepinephrine-containing afferents to Purkinje cells of
    rat cerebellum: I. Localization of the fibers and their
    synapses. Brain Res. 25: 501.
Bloom, F.E., Battenberg, E., Hoffer, B.J., Siggins, G.R., Steiner,
    A.L., Parker, C.W. and Wedner, H.J. 1972. Noradrenergic
    stimulation of cyclic adenosine monophosphate in rat
    Purkinje neurons. Science (submitted for publication).
Bloom, F.E., Hoffer, B.J. and Siggins, G.R. 1972. Norepinephrine
    mediated synapses: A model system for neuropsychopharmacology.
    Biol. Psychiat. 4(2): 157.
Boakes, R.J., Bradley, P.B., Brookes, N., Candy, J.M. and Wolstencroft,
    J.H. 1971. Actions of noradrenaline, other sympathomimetic
    amines and antagonists on neurones in the brainstem of the
    cat. Brit. J. Pharmacol. 41: 262.
Bradley, P.B. and Wolstencroft, J.H. 1962. Excitation and
    inhibition of brainstem neurones by noradrenaline and
    acetylcholine. Nature 196: 840.
Breckenridge, B. 1964. The measurement of cyclic adenylate in
    tissues. Proc. Nat. Acad. Sci. 52: 1580.
Butcher, R.W. and Baird, C.E. 1968. Effects of prostaglandins
    on adenosine 3',5'-monophosphate levels in fat and other
    tissues. J. Biol. Chem. 243: 1713.
Chu, N-S. and Bloom, F.E. 1972. Single neuron activity of the
    norepinephrine-containing locus coeruleus nucleus of the
    brainstem in the cats. Fed. Proc. 31: 377.
Couch, J.R. 1970. Responses of neurons in the raphe nuclei to
    serotonin, norepinephrine and acetylcholine and their
    correlation with an excitatory synaptic input. Brain Res.
    19: 137.
Crayton, J.C. and Bloom, F.E. 1969. Responsiveness of cat raphe
    nucleus to microelectrophoresis of norepinephrine and serotonin.
    Anat. Rec. 163: 173.
Cowan, M.W., Gottlieb, D.I., Hendrickson, A.E., Price, J.L. and
    Woolsey, T.A. 1972. The autoradiographic demonstration of
    axonal connections in the central nervous system. Brain Res.
    37: 21.
Dahlström, A. and Fuxe, K. 1964. Evidence for the existence of
    monoamine-containing cell bodies. Acta. Physiol. Scand.
    62:Suppl. 232.
Dahlström, A., Fuxe, K., Olson, L. and Ungerstedt, U. 1965. On
    the distribution and possible function of monoamine nerve
    terminals in the olfactory bulb of the rabbit. Life Sci. 4: 2071.
Falck, B., Hillarp, N-A., Thieme, G. and Torp, A. 1962. Fluores-
    cence of catecholamines and related compounds condensed with
    formaldehyde. J. Histochem. Cytochem. 10: 348.
Frederickson, R.C.A., Jordan, L.M. and Phillis, J.W. 1971. The
    action of noradrenaline on cortical neurons: effect of pH.
    Brain Res. 35: 556.

Fuxe, F., Hokfelt, T. and Ungerstedt, U. 1970. Morphological and functional aspects of central monoamine neurons. Int. Rev. Neurobiol. 13: 93.

Glowinski, J. and Baldessarini, R.J. 1966. Metabolism of norepinephrine in the central nervous system. Pharmacol. Rev. 18: 1201.

Hebb, C. 1970. CNS at the cellular level: identity of transmitter agents. Ann. Rev. Physiol. 32: 165.

Hoffer, B.J., Siggins, G.R. and Bloom, F.E. 1971 a. Studies on norepinephrine-containing afferents to Purkinje cells of rat cerebellum: II. Sensitivity of Purkinje cells to norepinephrine and related substances administered by microiontophoresis. Brain Res. 25: 523.

Hoffer, B.J., Siggins, G.R., Oliver, A.P. and Bloom, F.E. 1971 b. Cyclic AMP mediation of norepinephrine inhibition in rat cerebellar cortex: A unique class of synaptic responses. Ann. N.Y. Acad. Sci. 185: 531.

Hoffer, B.J., Chu, N-s., and Oliver, A.P. 1972. Cytochemical and electrophysiological studies on central catecholamine-containing neurons. Proc. Vth Intl. Congress Pharmacol., pp. 103.

Hökfelt, T. 1967. Electron microscopic studies on brain slices from regions rich in catecholamine terminals. Acta. Physiol. Scand. 69: 119.

Hökfelt, T. 1968. In vitro studies on central and peripheral monoamine neurons at the ultrastructural level. Z. Zellforsch. 91: 1.

Hökfelt, T. 1972. Ultrastructural localization of intra-neuronal monoamines - some aspects on methodology. Prog. Brain Res. 34: 213.

Hökfelt, T. and Fuxe, K. 1969. Cerebellar monoamine nerve terminals, a new type of afferent fiber to the cortex cerebelli. Exp. Brain Res. 9: 63.

Iversen, L.L. 1967. The Uptake and Storage of Noradrenaline in Sympathetic Nerves, Cambridge University Press.

Iversen, L.L. and Uretsky, N.J. 1971. Biochemical effects of 6-hydroxydopamine on catecholamine-containing neurons in the rat central nervous system. In: 6-Hydroxydopamine. (Eds. Malmfors, T. and Thoenen, H.) Amsterdam: North Holland Publishing Co., pp. 171.

Johnson, E.S., Roberts, M.H.T., Sobieszek, A. and Straughan, D.W. 1969 a. Noradrenaline sensitive cells in cat cerebral cortex. Int. J. Neuropharmacol. 8: 549.

Johnson, E.S., Roberts, M.H.T. and Straughan, D.W. 1969 b. The responses of cortical neurones to monoamines under differing anaesthetic conditions. J. Physiol (Lond) 203: 261.

Jones, B.E., Bobillier, P. and Jouvet, M. 1969. Effects de la destruction des neurones contenant des catecholamines du mesencephale sur le cycle veille sommeils du chat. C.R. Soc. Biol. Paris 163: 176.

Jouvet, M. 1969. Biogenic amines and the state of sleep. Science 163: 32.

Kakiuchi, S. and Rall, T.W. 1968. The influence of chemical agents on the accumulation of adenosine 3',5'-phosphate in slices of rabbit cerebellum. Molec. Pharmacol. 4: 367.

Krishna, G., Weiss, B.W., Davies, J.L. and Hynie, S. 1966. Mechanism of nicotinic acid inhibition of hormone-induced lipolysis. Fed. Proc. 25: 719.

Krnjevic, K. and Phillis, J.W. 1963 a. Actions of certain amines on cerebral cortical neurones. Brit. J. Pharmacol. 20: 471.

Krnjevic, K. and Phillis, J.W. 1963 b. Iontophoretic studies of cortical neurones in the mammalian cerebral cortex. J. Physiol. (Lond) 165: 274.

Kukovetz, W.R. and Poch, G. 1970. Cardiostimulatory effects of cyclic 3',5'-adenosine monophosphate and its acylated derivatives. Naunyn-Schmiedeberg Arch. Pharmak. 266: 236.

Larramendi, L.M.H. 1969. Analysis of synaptogenesis in the cerebellum of the mouse. In: Neurobiology of Cerebellar Evolution and Development. (Ed. Llinas, R.) Chicago: Amer. Med. Ass. Press, pp. 803.

Lenn, N.J. 1967. Localization of uptake of tritiated norepinephrine by rat brain in vivo and in vitro using electron microscopy. Amer. J. Anat. 120: 377.

Lish, P.M., Weikel, J.H. and Dugan, K.W. 1965. Pharmacological and toxicological properties of two new β-adrenergic receptor antagonists. J. Pharmacol. Exp. Ther. 149: 161.

Loizou, L.A. 1969. Projections of the nucleus locus coeruleus in the albino rat. Brain Res. 15: 563.

Malmfors, T. and Thoenen, H. (Eds.) 1971. 6-Hydroxydopamine and Catecholamine Neurons. Amsterdam: North Holland Publishing Co., pp. 368.

Nelson, C.N., Hoffer, B.J., and Bloom, F.E. 1972. Evidence for monoamine inputs to frontal polysensory cortex in the squirrel monkey. Fed. Proc. 31: 270.

Nelson, J., Sheu, Y-s. and Bloom, F.E. 1972. A chronic micro-electrode advancer (in preparation).

Nicoll, R.A. and Barker, J.L. 1971. The pharmacology of recurrent inhibition in the supraoptic neurosecretory system. Brain Res. 35: 501.

O'Leary, J.L., Petty, J., Smith, J.M., O'Leary, M. and Inukai, J. 1968. Cerebellar cortex of rat and other animals. A structural and ultrastructural study. J. Comp. Neurol. 134: 401.

Olson, L. and Fuxe, K. 1971. On the projections from the locus coeruleus noradrenaline neurons. Brain Res. 28: 165.

Richardson, K.C. 1966. Electron microscopic identification of autonomic nerve fibers. Nature 210: 756.

Salmoiraghi, G.C. and Bloom, F.E. 1964. The pharmacology of individual neurons. Science 144: 493.

Salmoiraghi, G.C. and Stefanis, C. 1967. A critique of iontophoretic studies of central nervous system neurons. Int. Rev. Neurobiol. 10: 1.

Salmoiraghi, G.C. and Weight, F.F. 1967. Micromethods in neuro-pharmacology: An approach to the study of anesthetics. Anesthesiology 28: 54.

Salmoiraghi, G.C., Bloom, F.E. and Costa, E. 1964. Adrenergic mechanisms in rabbit olfactory bulb. Am. J. Physiol. 207: 1417.

Siggins, G.R., Hoffer, B.J. and Bloom, F.E. 1969. Cyclic adenosine monophosphate: Possible mediator for norepinephrine effects on cerebellar Purkinje cells. Science 165: 1018.

Siggins, G.R., Hoffer, B.J. and Bloom, F.E. 1971 a. Studies on norepinephrine-containing afferents to Purkinje cells of rat cerebellum. III. Evidence for mediation of norepinephrine effects by cyclic 3'5'-adenosine monophosphate. Brain Res. 25: 535.

Siggins, G.R., Hoffer, B.J. and Bloom, F.E. 1971 b. Prostaglandin-norepinephrine interactions in brain: Microelectrophoretic and histochemical correlates. Ann. N.Y. Acad. Sci. 180: 302.

Siggins, G.R., Oliver, A.P., Hoffer, B.J. and Bloom, F.E. 1971 c. Cyclic adenosine monophosphate and norepinephrine: Effects on transmembrane properties of Purkinje cells. Science 171: 192.

Siggins, G.R., Hoffer, B.J., Oliver, A.P. and Bloom, F.E. 1971 d. Activation of a central noradrenergic projection to cerebellum. Nature 233: 481.

Snyder, S.H., Taylor, K.M., Coyle, J.T. and Meyerhoff, J.L. 1970. The role of brain dopamine in behavioral regulation and the actions of psychotropic drugs. Amer. J. Psychiat. 127: 117.

Stone, T.W. 1971. Are noradrenaline excitations artifacts? Nature 234: 145.

Sutherland, E.W., Rall, T.W. and Menon, T. 1962. Adenyl cyclase. I. Distribution, preparation and properties. J. Biol. Chem. 237: 1220.

Sutherland, E.W., Robinson, G.A. and Butcher, R. 1968. Some aspects of the biological role of adenosine 3',5'-monophosphate. Circulation 3: 279.

Ungerstedt, U. 1971. Stereotaxic mapping of the monoamine pathways in the rat brain. Acta. Physiol. Scand. Suppl. 367.

Wedner, H.J., Hoffer, B.J., Battenberg, E., Steiner, A.L., Parker, C.W. and Bloom, F.E. 1972. A method for detecting intracellular cyclic adenosine monophosphate by immunofluorescence. J. Histochem. Cytochem. (in press).

Weight, F.F. 1971. Mechanisms of synaptic transmission. Neuro-sciences Res. 4: 1.

Weiss, B. and Kidman, A'D. 1969. Neurobiological significance of cyclic 3'5'-adeonsine monophosphate. In: Advances in Biochemical Psychopharmacology (Eds. Costa, E. and Greengard, P.) New York: Raven Press, Vol. 1, pp. 131.

REGULATION OF 5-HT SYNTHESIS IN CENTRAL SEROTONINERGIC NEURONS

Jacques Glowinski, Michel Hamon and Francis Héry

Groupe NB, Laboratoire de Biologie Moléculaire
Collège de France, 11 place Marcelin Berthelot
Paris 5e - France

INTRODUCTION

The first step of synthesis of 5-hydroxytryptamine (5-HT) in central serotoninergic neurons plays a major role in the regulation of the transmitter formation similar to that observed in catecholaminergic neurons. But, during the past few years it has been generally assumed that the regulation of 5-HT synthesis differed in at least two ways from that of catecholamines (CA) in noradrenergic or dopaminergic neurons. The concentrations of tryptophan normally present in the mammalian brain are below the Michaelis constant (Km) of tryptophan hydroxylase (Jéquier et al., 1967; Peters et al., 1968), while the concentrations of tyrosine are not below the Michaelis constant of tyrosine hydroxylase (McGeer et al., 1967). The intraneuronal concentrations of tryptophan may not be sufficient to saturate the enzyme and small variations in the availability of the amino acid may rapidly affect the rate of 5-HT synthesis. This does not seem to be the case for tyrosine in catecholaminergic neurons. Consequently, much effort has been made to study the role of tryptophan in the regulation of the transmitter synthesis. Central 5-HT levels increase much more markedly after MAO inhibition than those of CA, and as shown in in vitro studies, 5-HT did not apparently inhibit tryptophan hydroxylase activity (McGeer and Peters, 1969, Grahame-Smith, 1964; Jéquier et al., 1969) whereas tyrosine hydroxylase activity was inhibited by increased CA levels (Udenfriend et al., 1965). These earlier observations, and a more recent one which will be discussed extensively, have led various workers (Lin et al., 1969; Millard and Gal, 1971; Meek and Fuxe, 1971) to suggest that 5-HT synthesis was not regulated by end-product like the synthesis of norepinephrine (Lin et al., 1969) or dopamine (Javoy et al., 1972) in central

239

catecholaminergic neurons.   Information concerning both the role
of tryptophan and 5-HT in the regulation of 5-HT synthesis, have
been obtained in our laboratory.   We would like to discuss and
illustrate by experimental results these two important aspects of
5-HT metabolism.

ROLE OF TRYPTOPHAN IN THE REGULATION OF 5-HT SYNTHESIS

Experimental manipulations of tryptophan availability, such
as feeding rats with diets containing little (Gal and Drewes, 1962) or
large amounts of tryptophan (Wang et al., 1962; Green et al., 1962),
or more directly injections of large doses of the amino acid
(Ashcroft et al., 1965; Consolo et al., 1965; Fernstrom and Wurtman,
1971) respectively depress or elevate the brain concentrations of
5-HT.   On the other hand, it has recently been shown that changes
in the turnover or in the synthesis rate of 5-HT in central serotoninergic neurons induced by various pharmacological treatments
were associated with pronounced elevation of brain tryptophan
levels.   For instance, amphetamine (Reid, 1970), reserpine (Tozer
et al., 1966) or lithium (Perez-Cruet et al., 1970; Sheard and
Aghajanian, 1970), drugs which are able to activate the synthesis
of 5-HT induced marked increase in central levels of tryptophan
and 5-hydroxyindoleacetic acid (5-HIAA) (Tagliamonte et al., 1971).
These effects were associated in most cases with an increase in
plasma levels of tryptophan when the body temperature rose above
40°C.   In fact, the exposure of rats to high temperature environment stimulated the synthesis of 5-HT.   This was suggested by the
rise in central 5-HIAA levels, and the increase in brain and plasma
tryptophan levels (Tagliamonte et al., 1971 b).   In contrast,
parachlorophenylalanine, the inhibitor of 5-HT synthesis (Koe and
Weissman, 1966), decreased the levels of tryptophan both in brain
and plasma (Tagliamonte et al., 1971 b).   In their very interesting
study, Tagliamonte et al. (1971 b) also reported that other psychotropic drugs were able to increase the levels of tryptophan and in
most cases those of 5-HIAA.   According to these authors, the
estimation in the brain of the precursor and of the metabolite of
5-HT can give valuable indications about the variations of central
5-HT synthesis.   In fact, we also observed in a few cases, that
treatments which increased 5-HT synthesis, coincidentally raised the
levels of tryptophan in the brain.   This was seen particularly in
various structures of the rat brain 15 or 120 minutes after progesterone treatment (10 mg/rat), and in the mouse brain shortly after
slight ether anaesthesia or 10 minutes after LSD (500 µg/kg)
administration (Table 1).   A similar observation was made by Diaz
and Huttunen (1971)--the persistent increase in serotonin turnover
seen in brain of rats chronically injected with LSD was associated
with a moderate but significant increase in tryptophan concentration.
MAO inhibitors and probenecid have been largely used as pharmacological tools for the estimation of the rate of 5-HT synthesis

TABLE 1

Effect of Various Pharmacological Treatments on
Tryptophan, 5-HT and 5-HIAA Levels in the Mouse and Rat Brain

DETERMINATION	TRY (µg/g)		5-HT (µg/g)		5-HIAA (µg/g)	
Treatment	Control	Treated	Control	Treated	Control	Treated
ETHER	4.25 ± 0.20	5.23 ± 0.19*	0.67 ± 0.02	0.67 ± 0.03	0.50 ± 0.02	0.50 ± 0.02
PROBENECID	4.18 ± 0.20	5.85 ± 0.40*	0.76 ± 0.02	0.80 ± 0.03	0.36 ± 0.03	0.56 ± 0.01*
LSD	4.88 ± 0.30	6.62 ± 0.38*	0.64 ± 0.01	0.70 ± 0.01*	0.48 ± 0.03	0.54 ± 0.03
PARGYLINE	4.18 ± 0.20	5.11 ± 0.30*	0.74 ± 0.03	0.89 ± 0.02*	0.30 ± 0.02	0.27 ± 0.01
PROGESTERONE	3.53 ± 0.11	5.87 ± 0.34*	0.59 ± 0.02	0.72 ± 0.06	0.54 ± 0.02	0.96 ± 0.09*

The effect of ether was estimated 3 min after the beginning of the light anesthesia. The effects of probenecid (200 mg/kg, i.p.), LSD (500 µg/kg i.p.) and pargyline (75 mg/kg i.p.) were estimated respectively 30, 10 and 10 min after the drugs administration. All these experiments were made on the mouse brain. The effect of progesterone (10 mg/animal) was estimated on the brainstem of spayed female rat two hours after the treatment. Results are the mean ± S.E.M. of groups of eight animals. * $p < .05$

(Costa and Neff, 1970). We were surprised to see that endogenous levels of tryptophan were increased in mouse brain 30 minutes after the administration of probenecid (200 mg/kg) and only for a short time (less than 15 minutes) after the intraperitoneal injection of pargyline (75 mg/kg) (Table 1). Similar observations have been made by Tagliamonte et al. (1971 b) in rat brain two hours after the intraperitoneal injection of probenecid (300 mg/kg) or of the MAO inhibitor, phenelzine (100 mg/kg). These results suggest a direct action of these drugs on the synthesis of 5-HT and should limit their use for the estimation of the turnover rate of this transmitter.

The estimation of endogenous levels of tryptophan in tissues may not be always the most valuable approach to appreciate the role of the amino acid in the regulation of 5-HT synthesis. The amino acid is very likely localized in various pools in tissues exhibiting different turnover rates. In fact, recently Shields and Eccleston (1972) have suggested the coexistence of two pools of tryptophan in serotoninergic neurons. They also mentioned that tryptophan newly taken up may play a major role in serotonin synthesis. This is in agreement with our own observations about the role of tyrosine newly taken up in the synthesis of dopamine in striatal dopaminergic terminals (Besson et al., 1971) and with a recent report of Costa et al. (1972) in which it was calculated that the specific activity of tyrosine was much higher in the nor-adrenergic terminals of the heart than in tissues shortly after the pulse injection of labelled tyrosine.

Very early in our effort to understand some of the changes in the activity of serotoninergic neurons occurring in sleep processes, we observed, using isotopic methods, that the increase of 5-HT synthesis was associated with marked changes in the tissue accumulation of newly taken up tryptophan. The stimulated formation of ^{3}H-5-HT and of its metabolite, ^{3}H-5-HIAA was generally related to the enhanced accumulation of ^{3}H-tryptophan in tissues (Héry et al., 1970). Since these first experiments, this observation has been made in numerous situations after the intravenous or intracisternal injection of ^{3}H-tryptophan, and the most interesting, in slices of brain tissues incubated with the labelled amino acid. A rapid survey of the various results obtained may help to clarify the respective role of plasma tryptophan and of its transport into nervous tissues in the regulation of 5-HT synthesis. First, as already mentioned, the synthesis of 5-HT is rapidly activated after the onset of light ether anaesthesia (Bourgoin et al., 1972) or after the intraperitoneal administration of LSD (500 µg/kg) (Hamon et al., 1972) to mice. These effects were demonstrated by measuring the initial accumulation of ^{3}H-5-HT and of ^{3}H-5-HIAA in brain 10 minutes after the intravenous injection of labelled tryptophan (Table II) The increase in the initial accumulations of the newly synthesized

TABLE II

Effect of Various Treatments on ^{3}H-tryptophan Initial Accumulation
and ^{3}H-5-HT Synthesis in the Mouse and Rat Brain

DETERMINATION		^{3}H-TRY nCi/g		^{3}H-5-HT nCi/g		^{3}H-5-HIAA	
Treatment	Injection	Control	Treated	Control	Treated	Control	Treated
ETHER	IV	104.7 ± 8.6	147.8 ± 11.5*	3.46 ± 0.21	5.61 ± 0.37*	1.28 ± 0.09	2.12 ± 0.15*
LSD	IV	140.0 ± 10.0	185.8 ± 14.8*	4.16 ± 9.30	4.82 ± 0.42	1.54 ± 0.07	1.93 ± 0.1*
PROGESTERONE	IC	8834. ± 1030.	14231. ± 1375.*	177. ± 21.	298. ± 21.*	nd	nd
FOOD DEPRIVATION	IC	747. ± 77.	913. ± 64.	32.9 ± 2.5	43.0 ± 2.9*	nd	nd

^{3}H-tryptophan (30 μCi) was injected intravenously just before the ether anesthesia which lasted 3 min,
mice were killed 10 min after the ^{3}H precursor injection. The ^{3}H-amino-acid was injected (i.v., 30 μCi)
5 min after LSD injection (500 μg/kg, i.p.) and mice were sacrificed 10 min later. ^{3}H-tryptophan,
^{3}H-5-HT and ^{3}H-5-HIAA were estimated in the whole brain. In experiments made on rat, ^{3}H-tryptophan was
injected intracisternally, four hours after progesterone treatment (10 mg/kg per animal) (53 μCi) or
four days after food deprivation (25 μCi), animals were sacrificed respectively 15 or 45 min after the
^{3}H-amino-acid injection and ^{3}H-tryptophan and ^{3}H-5-HT were estimated in the hypothalamus of the spayed
female rats (progesterone) or in the whole brain of male rats (food deprivation). Results are the
mean ± S.E.M. of groups of eight animals. *p <.05 when compared with control rats.

transmitter and of its acid metabolite were associated with parallel
increases of ^{3}H-tryptophan levels in tissues. The acute injection of
LSD induces a biphasic effect on 5-HT synthesis (Hamon et al., 1972),
the hallucinogen inhibited 5-HT synthesis one hour after its administration; various authors have already observed this long-term effect
of LSD on 5-HT synthesis (Andén et al., 1968; Lin et al., 1969;
Schubert et al., 1970). In our own experiments, levels of labelled
5-HT and 5-HIAA were markedly reduced at that time when compared
with control animals, and the enhanced accumulation of ^{3}H-tryptophan
seen 10 minutes after LSD injection was no more detectable. Secondly,
the estimation of synthesis of 5-HT can also be made by injecting
^{3}H-tryptophan intracisternally, although this method does not allow
an homogeneous labelling of central serotoninergic neurons. Nevertheless the intracisternal route offers some advantages: (1) changes
in transmitter synthesis can be seen in discrete areas of the
brain; (2) difficulties which may be raised by modifications of the
peripheral metabolism of tryptophan or by variations in plasma
tryptophan concentrations can be mostly avoided; (3) the delivery of
labelled tryptophan to nervous tissues seems to last longer than
with the acute intravenous injection of the amino acid. Using this
method, an increased accumulation of newly synthesized ^{3}H-5-HT
was seen in discrete structures or in the whole brain of rats two
hours after progesterone treatment (10 mg/rat) or after food deprivation for four days (Table II). These changes in the transmitter
formation appeared to be directly related to a parallel increase
in the accumulation of ^{3}H-tryptophan in tissues. The selective
deprivation for 91 hours of paradoxical sleep (P.S.) in rat,
stimulates the synthesis and utilization of 5-HT in various parts
of the brain (Héry et al., 1970). Forty-five minutes after the
intracisternal injection of ^{3}H-tryptophan, the levels of ^{3}H-5-HT
were about 150% those of controls in the telencephalon-diencephalon
and in the brainstem-mesencephalon. They even reached 265% control
values in the spinal cord. These effects appeared again to be
completely linked to changes in the accumulation of ^{3}H-tryptophan
in tissues in the two first structures, but only partly in the last
one, since the ^{3}H-precursor levels reached 150% control values in
the various structures. No changes in the accumulation of the
labelled precursor or ^{3}H-5-HT could be seen when ^{3}H-5-hydroxy-
tryptophan was substituted for ^{3}H-tryptophan in these experiments
in vivo. This strongly suggested that the increased synthesis of
5-HT observed in P.S. deprived rats, could be related to specific
modifications of tryptophan transport. Further confirmation of
the importance of newly taken up tryptophan to the regulation of
5-HT synthesis were obtained in recent experiments undertaken to
study the diurnal variations of serotoninergic neuronal activity
(Héry et al., 1972). In rats placed in constant temperature and
noise environment and submitted to regular alternative cycles of
light and darkness (12h - 12h) for at least three weeks, an activation of 5-HT synthesis could be demonstrated in various structures

of the brain at different times of the light period. In contrast,
the synthesis was depressed during darkness when the locomotor
activity of the animals was maximal. While the "light-off" appeared
to trigger the important changes in 5-HT synthesis seen in the cortex
and in the brainstem, this was less apparent in the hypothalamus.
Nevertheless, the total accumulation of ^{3}H-5-HT and of its metabolite
^{3}H-5-HIAA estimated 7 minutes after the intracisternal injection
of ^{3}H-tryptophan was significantly higher at 15 hours during the
light period than at 21 hours during darkness in the hypothalamus
and in brainstem (Figure 1, Figure 2). These changes in the
formation of 5-HT were, as in previous experiments, associated with
parallel modifications of the accumulation of ^{3}H-tryptophan in
tissues (Figure 1, Figure 2). As indicated by the estimation of
tryptophan specific activity in tissues, the changes in 5-HT
synthesis were not related to modifications in the rate of conversion of tryptophan into 5-HT, but were only dependent on those
of the initial accumulation of ^{3}H-tryptophan. In fact, endogenous
levels of tryptophan were similar at 15 and 21 hours in both structures and slightly but significantly higher in plasma during darkness
than during the light period suggesting that 5-HT synthesis is not
always dependent on the levels of tryptophan in plasma as proposed
by some authors (Fernstrom and Wurtman, 1971).

Further evidence of the correlation between the increased
synthesis of 5-HT and the activation of the initial accumulation of
tryptophan in nervous tissues was provided by complementary experiments carried out in vitro on slices of isolated structures of the
rat brain. Tagliamonte et al. (1971 a) have reported that dibutyryl-
cyclic AMP increased the endogenous levels of tryptophan and 5-HIAA
in the rat brain 120 minutes after its intraventricular injection
(100 µg/rat). These authors were able to demonstrate a parallel
increase in the accumulation of labelled tryptophan and in the
formation of ^{3}H-5-HT and its metabolite in brainstem slices of rats
incubated with dibutyryl-cyclic AMP. These results were confirmed
in our laboratory using striatal slices of the rat brain (Hamon
et al., 1972). Similar findings could be made with slices of discrete
structures of animals sacrificed during various states of activity
of central serotoninergic neurons. The daily variations of 5-HT
synthesis described previously could also be visualized in vitro
by measuring the synthesis of 5-HT in hypothalamic and brainstem
slices of rats killed respectively at 15 and 21 hours during light
and darkness. The total formation of ^{3}H-5-HT and its main metabolite ^{3}H-5-HIAA, estimated at the end of a 20 minute incubation
of slices in presence of ^{3}H-tryptophan, was significantly higher
during light than during darkness in both structures (Figure 2).
Similar changes were seen concerning the accumulation of ^{3}H-
tryptophan in tissues (Héry et al., 1972) (Figure 1, Figure 2).

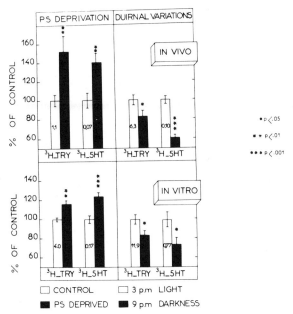

Figure 1. Effect of paradoxical sleep (PS) deprivation and diurnal variations on ^{3}H-5-HT formation from ^{3}H-tryptophan in the rat brainstem.

^{3}H-5-HT formation from ^{3}H(G)-tryptophan (5.4 Ci/mmole) was estimated in vivo (upper part) and in vitro (bottom part). In the experiments on PS deprivation (I)(left part), rats were deprived of PS for
91 hours by putting them on small supports surrounded by water, and
^{3}H-5-HT formation was estimated just at the end of the PS deprivation
period in the brainstem-mesencephalon. In the experiments on 5-HT
diurnal variations (II)(right part), rats were subjected to alternate
cycles of 12 hours of light and darkness (light from 7 a.m. to 7 p.m.
and darkness from 7 p.m. to 7 a.m.) for three weeks, and ^{3}H-5-HT
formation in the brainstem was estimated in the middle of two successive light and dark periods. In the experiments (I) control and PS-
deprived rats were injected intracisternally with 25 µCi of ^{3}H-trypto-
phan under light ether anaesthesia and killed 45 min later. Brainstem-
mesencephalon slices of control and PS-deprived rats were incubated
for 30 min with 10 µCi of ^{3}H-tryptophan. Endogenous levels of 5-HT
and tryptophan were unchanged at the time of estimation of ^{3}H-5-HT
formation. In the experiments (II) rats kept in light or darkness
were injected with 50 µCi of ^{3}H-tryptophan under light ether anaesthesia and killed 15 min later. Brainstem slices were incubated for
30 min with 25 µCi of ^{3}H-tryptophan. Endogenous levels of 5-HT and
tryptophan were respectively 0.64 µg/g, 4.19 µg/g and 0.53 µg/g,
3.71 µg/g in the brainstem of rats kept in light and darkness. ^{3}H-5-
HT and ^{3}H-tryptophan were estimated in tissues in in vivo as well as
in vitro studies. Results, expressed as per cent of respective controls (I) or of values obtained in animals kept in light (II), are the
mean + S.E.M. of groups of 8 to 10 animals. Numbers correspond to the
absolute values of ^{3}H-tryptophan and ^{3}H-5-HT (expressed in µCi/g) in
control animals. (From Héry et al., 1970 and 1972).

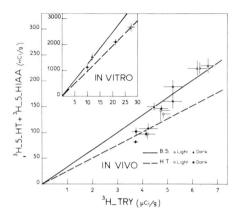

Figure 2. Correlations between ^{3}H-tryptophan initial accumulation
and the total formation of ^{3}H-5-HT and ^{3}H-5-HIAA in experiments
on diurnal variations of central 5-HT metabolism.

    Rats were kept for three weeks under a regular cycle of light
and dark periods of 12 hours each as described in Figure 1 (experiment II). Total ^{3}H-5-HT and ^{3}H-5-HIAA formation from ^{3}H-tryptophan
was estimated in the hypothalamus (HT) and the brainstem (BS).
In the experiment made in vivo, ^{3}H-tryptophan, ^{3}H-5-HT and ^{3}H-5-
HIAA levels were estimated at various successive times of the light
(13, 15 and 17 hours) and of the dark (19, 21, 23 and 1 hour)
periods 7 minutes after the intracisternal injection of ^{3}H-trypto-
phan (50 µCi). In the experiment performed in vitro, hypothalamic
and brainstem slices of rats killed at 15 or 21 hours were incubated
for 30 minutes with ^{3}H-tryptophan (25 µCi/5 ml) total ^{3}H-5-HT and
^{3}H-5-HIAA levels were estimated both in slices and their incubating
medium. ^{3}H-tryptophan was estimated in slices. The correlation
coefficients were calculated for each structure on the basis of
individual data and were respectively: R = 0.54 (p <.01) and
R = 0.87 (p <.01) for the hypothalamus and the brainstem in the
experiments in vitro (from Héry et al., 1972).

Therefore, a good correlation between the changes in the formation of
5-HT and in the initial accumulation of ^{3}H-tryptophan in tissues
was found in vitro as well as in vivo (Figure 2). Recent experiments
in which ^{3}H-tryptophan was estimated in slices 4 minutes after the
beginning of the incubation revealed that the changes in the accumulation of ^{3}H-tryptophan in slices were related to modifications of the
initial transport of the amino acid (Héry and Rouer, unpublished
observations). It should also be pointed out, that changes in 5-HT
synthesis induced by P.S. deprivation could also be demonstrated
in vitro; parallel increases in the accumulation of ^{3}H-tryptophan
and in the total formation of ^{3}H-5-HT were seen in brainstem slices
(Héry et al., 1970) (Figure 1).

These various results clearly indicate that changes in 5-HT synthesis in central serotoninergic neurons are not always related to tryptophan levels in plasma. Furthermore, variations in the rate of 5-HT synthesis induced by stimulation of neuronal activity or by psychotropic drugs seem also not to be necessarily dependent on the acceleration of tryptophan conversion into 5-HT. In most cases the changes in 5-HT synthesis observed appear to be linked to modifications of the availability of intraneuronal tryptophan to the pool implicated in 5-HT synthesis. The turnover rate of tryptophan in this intraneuronal pool may be markedly accelerated when synthesis of 5-HT is activated; this may be related to mechanisms which still have to be elucidated with the pronounced changes in the initial accumulation or transport of exogenous tryptophan in tissues. It should be emphasized that the mechanism implicated in the rapid variations of tryptophan metabolism is still operating in vitro after the in vivo activation of serotoninergic neurons. Such changes in the regulation of tryptophan metabolism in serotoninergic neurons could be induced by the acceleration of 5-HT utilization as observed for the conversion of tyrosine into dopa in catecholaminergic neurons (Weiner, 1970). However, our experiments with the daily variations of 5-HT synthesis suggest that this may not always be the case--a desynchronization between synthesis and release processes could be detected. The rate of synthesis of 5-HT in serotoninergic neurons was depressed during the dark period when compared with the light period although the utilization and release processes of the transmitter were activated at this time (Héry et al., 1972).

FEEDBACK REGULATION OF 5-HT SYNTHESIS

Evidence for the existence of a mechanism of negative feedback which controls the synthesis of 5-HT in serotoninergic neurons has been obtained in our laboratory in experiments performed in vivo as well as in vitro; they have been described in detail in various articles (Macon et al., 1971; Hamon et al., 1972 a,b) and reviews (Glowinski et al., 1972; Glowinski, 1972). Therefore, we would like just to summarize the most important facts and avoid the full description of the experimental conditions used in these studies.

A marked increase in the intraneuronal levels of 5-HT, induced by MAO inhibitors or by uptake of exogenous 5-HT in tissues, depresses the synthesis of ^{3}H-5-HT from its precursor ^{3}H-tryptophan. The effects of MAO inhibitors were seen in vivo by measuring the rate of conversion of ^{3}H-tryptophan into ^{3}H-5-HT at various times after the acute injection of pargyline (75 mg/kg) or pheniprazine (10 mg/kg) or after the chronic administration of pheniprazine (10 mg/kg, 48, 24 and 3 hours before the sacrifice of the animals) (Macon et al., 1971). They were also demonstrated in vitro by measuring the rate of conversion of tryptophan into 5-HT in striatal slices of rats pretreated for three hours with pargyline or pheniprazine.

As newly synthesized 5-HT is localized in a pool exhibiting a very rapid turnover rate (the half-life of 5-HT in this pool is less than 10 minutes), the measurement of the initial accumulation in tissues of ^{3}H-5-HT alone underestimates the total formation of the transmitter. A better index of 5-HT synthesis can be obtained by measuring the initial formation of both ^{3}H-5-HT and its metabolite ^{3}H-5-HIAA. This was done in vitro using brain slices of normal and MAOI pretreated rats by measuring the total accumulation of ^{3}H-5-HT and its main metabolite both in the tissue and their incubating medium at the end of a 30 minute incubation in presence of labelled tryptophan. In the experiments in vivo, this difficulty was avoided by comparing the accumulation of ^{3}H-5-HT synthesized in the 15 minutes which followed the intracisternal administration of ^{3}H-tryptophan at shorter time (20 minutes) or at longer time (180 minutes) after the intraperitoneal injection of the drugs. In both cases the activity of MAO was completely inhibited. In these conditions, the formation of ^{3}H-5-HT from labelled tryptophan was decreased by about 35% in the brainstem of rats at a later time (180 minutes) when compared to a shorter time (20 minutes) with both inhibitors. This effect appears related to the changes in intraneuronal levels of 5-HT since the amine levels were about three times those of controls and much higher than those observed 20 minutes after the drug administration. The inhibition of ^{3}H-5-HT synthesis was even more pronounced after the chronic injection of pheniprazine and a good inverse correlation could be seen between the increase in 5-HT levels and the extent of synthesis inhibition. Those results strongly suggested an inhibition of the conversion of tryptophan into 5-HT by intracellular levels of the transmitter since no changes in the endogenous levels of tryptophan could be seen at the times used in this study. The mechanism involved seems to operate at the first step of 5-HT synthesis, since no inhibition of the ^{3}H-5-HT formation was seen when ^{3}H-5-hydroxytryptophan was substituted to ^{3}H-tryptophan. The inhibiting effects of long treatments with both inhibitors (180 minutes) on ^{3}H-5-HT synthesis from ^{3}H-tryptophan could be confirmed in vitro in striatal slices rich in serotoninergic terminals (Hamon et al., 1972 a,b). In this case, the total formation of ^{3}H-5-HT and its metabolite was reduced by about 30 to 35% in MAOI pretreated rats (180 minutes) when compared to controls. Thus, MAO inhibitors rapidly induce a sustained reduction in 5-HT synthesis still detectable in vitro. This very likely excludes a possible interference of peripheral effects of MAOI, or other possible actions than MAO inhibition, in their effects on 5-HT synthesis. Other evidence for the inhibiting effect on 5-HT synthesis of enhanced intraneuronal levels of 5-HT induced by MAO inhibitors, have been recently obtained by Carlsson et al. (1972). These authors observed a reduced accumulation of 5-hydroxytryptophan after the injection of a potent decarboxylase inhibitor in brains of mice pretreated with nialamide or pargyline. Thus, they confirmed the inhibitory

end-product regulation acting at the first step of the 5-HT biosynthetic process induced by MAO pretreatment. However, Carlsson
and his colleagues (1972) did not exclude an indirect effect of
5-HT (i.e. on postsynaptic receptors) to explain the reduction of
5-HT synthesis. This process, as well as the existence of an
intraneuronal negative feedback mechanism could be related to the
decrease in the rate of firing of midbrain raphe units seen after
various treatments with MAO inhibitors as suggested by Aghajanian
et al. (1970).

Intraneuronal levels of 5-HT in serotoninergic neurons can
be raised rapidly by incubating slices with exogenous 5-HT. We
have used this procedure to study more precisely the regulation of
5-HT synthesis by the end product of the biosynthetic pathway. 5-HT
levels in striatal slices reached about six times control values at
the end of a 40 minute incubation in presence of 3.10^{-6} M of 5-HT.
When ^{3}H-tryptophan was added 10 minutes after the exogenous amine,
the total accumulation of ^{3}H-5-HT and its metabolite, both in slices
and their incubating medium, was reduced by about 40% at the end
of the incubation. This effect is undoubtedly related to changes
in intraneuronal levels of 5-HT since chlorimipramine ($1.5 \ 10^{-6}$ M)
reduced significantly the inhibitory effect of exogenous 5-HT on
5-HT synthesis. This drug, as expected, partially inhibited the
accumulation of exogenous 5-HT in slices (22%) and efficiently
blocked the reuptake of the newly synthesized transmitter as indicated by the marked rise in ^{3}H-5-HT levels in medium.

It should be noticed that in this experiment, as well as in
those made with MAO inhibitors, care was made to measure ^{3}H-5-HT
and ^{3}H-5-HIAA in the incubating medium. For example, the exogenous
5-HT displaced very efficiently the newly synthesized transmitter
which is released and rapidly inactivated. Furthermore, we have
also taken in account in our estimation of 5-HT synthesis that small
quantities of ^{3}H-tryptamine are formed from ^{3}H-tryptophan and
rapidly converted into ^{3}H-indoleacetic acid in striatal slices.
The direct inhibitory effect of exogenous 5-HT on 5-HT synthesis
has also been recently shown by Karobath (1972) in synaptosomal preparations of the rat brain. However, the effect appeared less pronounced than in striatal slices. The demonstration in vitro of a
feedback regulation of 5-HT synthesis after loading of serotoninergic
terminals or synaptosomes with 5-HT revealed that the regulation of
5-HT synthesis cannot be attributed solely to an interneuronal feedback process, a mechanism which could not be excluded in the various
experiments made in vivo by us and other workers.

The inhibitory effect of exogenous 5-HT on its own synthesis in
slices provides an interesting working model to further explore
the mechanisms involved in the inhibitory process of 5-HT synthesis

(Hamon et al., 1972 b). Catechols have been shown to inhibit
tryptophan hydroxylase activity in slices (Goldstein and Frenkel,
1971; Héry and Rouer, unpublished observations), however, the
possible interference of released dopamine in the action of exogenous
5-HT in the conversion of tryptophan into 5-HT seems to be excluded.
Exogenous 5-HT was still able to inhibit 5-HT synthesis in striatal
slices containing low levels of DA. Similar inhibitions of the
transmitter synthesis were seen in slices of control rats and in
those of animals in which dopaminergic neurons had been destroyed
by an intraventricular injection of 6-hydroxydopamine or in which DA
levels had been reduced by injections of α-methyl-para-tyrosine,
the inhibitor of CA synthesis.

The inhibitory action of exogenous 5-HT on 5-HT synthesis
could be related to changes in the availability of newly taken up
tryptophan. However, we failed to see changes in the long-term
accumulation (30 minutes) of tracer concentrations of labelled
tryptophan in striatal slices incubated with exogenous 5-HT or
in those of MAOI pretreated rats. The initial uptake of ^{3}H-
tryptophan in slices was also not affected by exogenous 5-HT.
This is in agreement with similar experiments made on synaptosomes
(Grahame-Smith and Parfitt, 1970; Karobath, 1972). On the other
hand, the inhibitory effect of exogenous 5-HT on 5-HT synthesis
could still be seen in striatal slices incubated with dibutyryl-
cyclic AMP which activates both the transport of tryptophan and
the formation of 5-HT (Hamon et al., 1972 b) (Figure 3). However,
changes in tryptophan transport or in tryptophan turnover in the
5-HT synthesizing pool of serotoninergic neurons have still to be
considered to explain the negative feedback regulation process.
Unfortunately, the overall estimation of ^{3}H-tryptophan accumulation in slices or even in synaptosomal preparations may mask specific
events occurring at the level of serotoninergic terminals or
varicosities.

From earlier experiments, it can be said at the present time
that the negative feedback regulation of 5-HT synthesis, operating
before the decarboxylation of 5-hydroxytryptophan, is not the result
of an end product inhibition of tryptophan hydroxylase activity.
Exogenous 5-HT has not been shown to inhibit tryptophan hydroxylase
activity in homogenates of rat brain (McGeer and Peters, 1969), in
those of dog and rabbit brainstem (Grahame-Smith, 1964) nor in
partially purified enzymatic preparations of rat brainstem (Jéquier
et al., 1969). We could confirm these results--10^{-4} M 5-HT did
not inhibit tryptophan hydroxylase activity recovered in a soluble
form after purification of the enzyme from the pig and rat brain
(Youdim, Hamon and Bourgoin, unpublished observations). In some
cases, but not constantly, 5-HT even appeared to stimulate the
enzyme activity. However, final conclusions about this problem
should not be made too rapidly, two forms of tryptophan hydroxylase

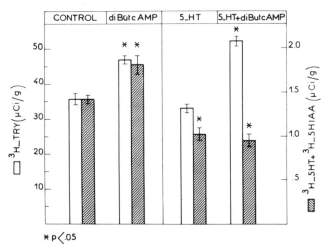

* p < .05

Figure 3. Effect of exogenous 5-HT and dibutyryl-cyclic AMP on serotonin synthesis in striatal slices of the rat.

Slices were preincubated for 5 min with 5-HT (2.10^{-6} M) or dibutyryl-cyclic AMP (dibut-c AMP) (10^{-3} M) or both, ^{3}H-tryptophan (G, 2 Ci/mmole) 22 μCi/5 ml) was then added for 30 min and total formation of ^{3}H-5-HT and ^{3}H-5-HIAA in slices and their incubating medium was estimated at the end of the incubation period. ^{3}H-tryptophan was estimated in slices; results are the mean ± S.E.M. of experiments made with 9 striata. p <0.5 when compared with respective ^{3}H-tryptophan and ^{3}H-5-HT + ^{3}H-5-HIAA of control values.

have been found in brain tissues (Ichiyama et al., 1970; Peters, 1972) and the characteristics of the enzyme are still not well established. Furthermore, if tryptophan hydroxylase is partly bound to membrane intraneuronally, an hypothesis which presently cannot be excluded, its properties in its normal cellular environment may be quite different from those detected in isotropic conditions. Indeed it has been recently shown, that purified enzymes fixed to artificial protein membranes exhibit different Km and Vmax characteristics than those observed in solutions (Thomas et al., 1972).

CONCLUSIONS

Further experiments are still required to fully elucidate the mechanisms involved at a molecular level in the control of 5-HT synthesis. However, the various results described and discussed strongly suggest that tryptophan transport or its distribution in the pool of 5-HT synthesis in serotoninergic neurons play a major role in the regulation of the amine synthesis. It is worthwhile to recall that the inhibitors of tryptophan hydroxylase which act both on the activity of the enzyme and on tryptophan transport are the most potent to decrease serotonin synthesis in vivo (Peters, 1972). On the other hand, we have seen that the effects of dibutyryl-cyclic AMP on 5-HT synthesis are related to its action on the initial accumulation of tryptophan. This is particularly interesting and suggests a stimulating working hypothesis. Changes in cyclic AMP occurring in glial cells could also contribute to the control of tryptophan delivery to serotoninergic neurons and consequently to the regulation of 5-HT synthesis. Various observations support this hypothesis. Increased levels of cyclic AMP have already been detected in pharmacological (Cramer et al., 1972) or physical situations (Hamadah et al., 1972) which stimulate 5-HT synthesis. 5-HT has also been shown to inhibit adenyl cyclase activity in the pineal gland (Weiss and Costa, 1968). Finally, a very important increase in cyclic AMP has been found in glial cells incubated with NE. Modulation of cyclic AMP levels in surrounding glial cells of serotoninergic neurons induced by NE, drugs or other factors may contribute to the changes in 5-HT synthesis and to the inter-neuronal regulation of serotoninergic neurons (Figure 4).

There is now little doubt that 5-HT synthesis is regulated at least in some pharmacological situations or experimental conditions which activate serotoninergic neurons activity by the intraneuronal levels of the transmitter. In fact, it was shown in earlier experiments that the synthesis of 5-HT could be stimulated by the previous depletion of amine stores induced by reserpine (Tozer et al., 1966). 5-HT synthesis is also much more accelerated by external physical stimuli, such as stress (Thierry et al., 1968; Rosecrans

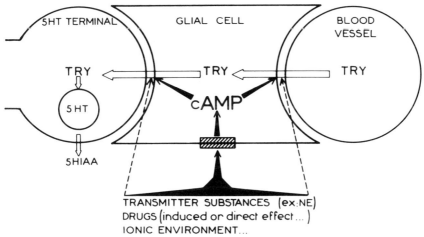

Figure 4. A hypothetical model for the control of the delivery of tryptophan to serotoninergic neurons by cyclic AMP.

As discussed in the text, tryptophan transport to serotoninergic neurons may partly be regulated by modifications of cyclic AMP levels in surrounding glial cells induced by various factors.

and Sheard, 1969), when 5-HT levels have been previously reduced
by parachlorophenylalanine. The results obtained with MAO
inhibitors or with the uptake of exogenous 5-HT in serotoninergic
neurons reveal that an important rise in 5-HT levels can rapidly
depress the transmitter synthesis. This process appears, at
least in part, to be dependent on intraneuronal regulatory mechanisms.
The role of tryptophan transport in the regulation of 5-HT synthesis
could be demonstrated in physiological situations, however little
is yet known about the regulatory functions of the intraneuronal
levels of 5-HT in the natural dynamic states of serotoninergic
neurons.

ACKNOWLEDGEMENTS

     This research was mainly supported by grants of l'Institut
National de la Santé et de la Recherche Médicale (INSERM), and also
la Direction de la Recherche et Moyens d'Essais (DRME), le Centre
National de la Recherche Scientifique (CNRS), la Fondation pour la
Recherche Médicale Francaise, and la Société Chimique des Usines
Rhône-Poulenc.

REFERENCES

Aghajanian, G.K., Graham, A.W. and Sheard, M.H. 1970. Serotonin
     containing neurons in brain. Depression of firing by mono-
     amine oxidayse inhibitors. Science 169: 1100-1102.
Andén, N.-E., Corrodi, H., Fuxe, K. and Hökfelt, T. 1968. Evidence
     for a central 5-hydroxytryptamine receptor stimulation by
     lysergic acid diethylamide. British J. of Pharm. 34: 1-7.
Ashcroft, G.W., Eccleston, D. and Crawford, T.B.B. 1965. 5-
     Hydroxyindole metabolism in rat brain. A study of intermediate
     metabolism using the technique of tryptophan loading. J.
     Neurochem. 12: 483-492.
Besson, M.J., Cheramy, A. and Glowinski, J. 1971. Effects of
     some psychotropic drugs on dopamine synthesis in the rat
     striatum. J. of Pharmacol. 177: 196-205.
Bourgoin, S., Morot-Gaudry, Y., Hamon, M. and Glowinski, J. 1972.
     Limitations of ether anaesthesia in biochemical studies on
     5-HT metabolism, (in preparation).
Carlsson, A., Bedard, P., Lindqvist, M. and Magnusson, T. 1972.
     Physiological control of 5-HT synthesis and turnover in the
     brain. Fifth International Congress on Pharmacology 256-
     257. (Abstracts of invited presentations).
Consolo, S., Garattini, S., Ghielmetti, R., Morselli, P. and
     Valzelli, L. 1965. The hydroxylation of tryptophan in vivo
     by brain. Life Sciences 4: 625-630.
Costa, E., Green, A.R., Koslow, S.H., Lefevre, H.J., Revuelta, A.V.
     and Wang, C. 1972. Dopamine and norepinephrine in nor-

adrenergic axons: an in vivo study of their precursor product
relationship by mass fragmentography and radiochemistry.
Pharmac. Rev., (in press).
Costa, E. and Neff, N.H. 1970. Estimation of turnover rates to
study the metabolic regulation of the steady-state level of
neuronal monoamines. In: Handbook of Neurochemistry
(Ed. Lajtha,) New York: Plenum Press, Vol. IV, pp. 45-90.
Cramer, H., Ng, L.K.Y. and Chase, T.N. 1972. Effect of probenecid
on levels of cyclic AMP in human cerebrospinal fluid. J.
Neurochem. 19: 1601-1602.
Diaz, J.L. and Huttunen, M.O. 1971. Persistent increase in brain
serotonin turnover after chronic administration of LSD in the
rat. Science 174: 62-64.
Fernstrom, J.D. and Wurtman, R.J. 1971. Brain serotonin content.
Physiological dependence on plasma tryptophan levels. Science
173: 149-152.
Gal, E.M. and Drewes, P.A. 1962. Studies on the metabolism of
5-HT (II) Effect of tryptophan deficiency in rats (27520).
Proc. Soc. for Exp. Biol. and Med., vol. 110, pp. 369-371.
Glowinski, J. 1972. Some new facts about synthesis, storage and
release processes of monoamines in the central nervous system.
In: Perspectives in Neuropharmacology (Ed. Snyder, S.H.)
Oxford Univ. Press, Inc., pp. 349-404.
Glowinski, J., Hamon, M., Javoy, F. and Morot-Gaudry, Y. 1972.
Rapid effects of MAO inhibitors on synthesis and release of
central monoamines. In: Advances in Psychopharmacology
(Ed. Sandler and Costa), 5: 423-439.
Grahame-Smith, D.G. 1964. Tryptophan hydroxylation in brain.
Biochem. and Biophys. Res. Comm. 16(6): 586-592.
Grahame-Smith, D.G. and Parfitt, A.G. 1970. Tryptophan trans-
port across the synaptosomal membrane. J. Neurochem. 17:
1339-1353.
Green, H., Greenberg, S.M., Erickson, R.W., Sawyer, J.L. and
Ellizon, T. 1962. Effect of dietary phenylalanine and
tryptophan upon rat brain amine levels. J. Pharmacol. Exp.
Ther. 136: 174-178.
Hamadah, K., Holmes, H., Barker, G., Hartman, G.C. and Parke, D.V.
1972. The effect of electro-convulsive therapy on the urinary
excretion of adenosine 3',5'-cyclic monophosphate. Proc.
of the Biochemical Soc. (Cambridge), pp. 15. 529th Mtg. July, 1972.
Hamon, M. Bourgoin, S., Morot-Gaudry, Y. and Glowinski, J. 1972.
Biphasic effects of acute LSD treatment on central synthesis
and release of 5-HT. (In preparation).
Hamon, M. Bourgoin, S. and Glowinski, J. 1972. Feedback regulation
of serotonin synthesis in the rat striatum. J. Neurochem.
(in press).
Hamon, M., Bourgoin, S., Morot-Gaudry, Y. and Glowinski, J. 1972.
End product inhibition of serotonin synthesis in the rat
striatum. Nature (New Biology) 237: 184-187.

Héry, F., Pujol, J.F., Lopez, M., Macon, J. and Glowinski, J. 1970. Increased synthesis and utilization of serotonin in the central nervous system of the rat during paradoxical sleep deprivation. Brain Res. 21: 391-403.

Héry, F., Rouer, E. and Glowinski, J. 1972. Daily variations of serotonin metabolism in the rat brain. Brain Res. 43: 445-465.

Ichiyama, A., Nakamura, S., Nishizuka, Y. and Hayaishi, O. 1970. Enzymic studies on the biosynthesis of serotonin in mammalian brain. J. Biol. Chem. 245: 1699-1709.

Javoy, F., Agid, Y., Bouvet, D. and Glowinski, J. 1972. Feedback control of dopamine synthesis in dopaminergic terminals of the rat striatum. J. Pharmacol. (in press).

Jéquier, E., Robinson, D.S., Lovenberg, W. and Sjoerdsma, A. 1969. Further studies on tryptophan hydroxylase in rat brainstem and beef pineal. Biochem. Pharmac. 18: 1071-1081.

Karobath, M. 1972. Serotonin synthesis with rat brain synaptosomes. Effects of serotonin and monoamine oxidase inhibitors. Biochem. Pharmacol. 21: 1253-1263.

Goldstein, M. and Frenkel, R. 1971. Inhibition of serotonin synthesis by dopa and other catechols. Nature (New Biology) 233: 179-180.

Koe, B.K. and Weissman, A. 1966. p-chlorophenylalanine - a specific depletor of brain serotonin. J. Pharmacol. Exp. Ther. 154: 499-516.

Lin, R.C., Neff, N.H., Ngai, S.H. and Costa, E. 1969. Turnover rates of serotonin and norepinephrine in brain of normal and pargyline treated rats. Life Sciences B: 1077-1084.

Lin, R.C., Ngai, S.H. and Costa, E. 1969. Lysergic acid diethylamide: role in conversion of plasma tryptophan to brain serotonin (5-hydroxytryptamine). Science, N. Y., 166: 237.

McGeer, E.G. and Peters, D.A.V. 1969. In vitro screen of inhibitors of rat brain serotonin synthesis. Can. J. Biochem. 47(5): 501-506.

McGeer, E.G., Gibson, S. and McGeer, P.L. 1967. Some characteristics of brain tyrosine hydroxylase. Can. J. Biochem. 45: 1557-1563.

Macon, J.B., Sokoloff, L. and Glowinski, J. 1971. Feedback control of rat brain 5-hydroxytryptamine synthesis. J. Neurochem. 18: 323-331.

Meek, J.L. and Fuxe, K. 1971. Serotonin accumulation after monoamine oxidase inhibition. Biochem. Pharm. 20: 693-706.

Millard, S.A. and Gal, E.M. 1971. The contribution of 5-hydroxyindole pyruvic acid to cerebral 5-hydroxyindole metabolism. Intern. J. Neuroscience 1: 211-218.

Perez-Cruet, J. Tagliamonte, A., Tagliamonte, P. and Gessa, G.L. 1970. Stimulation of brain serotonin turnover by lithium. Pharmacologist 12: 257.

Peters, D.A.V. 1972. Inhibition of brain tryptophan-5-hydroxylase by amino acids. The role of L-tryptophan uptake inhibition. Biochemical Pharmac. 21: 1051-1053.

Peters, D.A.V., McGeer, P.L. and McGeer, E.G. 1968. The distribu-
    tion of tryptophan hydroxylase in cat brain. J. Neurochem.
    15: 1431-1435.
Reid, W.D. 1970. Turnover rate of brain 5-hydroxytryptamine
    increased by d-amphetamine. British J. Pharm. 40: 483-491.
Rosecrans, J.A. and Sheard, M.H. 1969. Effects of an acute stress
    on forebrain 5-hydroxytryptamine (5-HT) metabolism in CNS
    lesioned and drug pretreated rats. Eur. J. Pharm. 6: 197-199.
Schubert, J., Nyback, H. and Sedvall, G. 1970. Accumulation
    and disappearance of ^{3}H-5-hydroxytryptamine formed from ^{3}H-
    tryptophan in mouse brain; effect of LSD-25. Eur. J. Pharm.
    10: 215-224.
Sheard, M.H. and Aghajanian, G.K. 1970. Neuronally activated
    metabolism of brain serotonin: effect of lithium. Life Sciences
    9: 285-290.
Shields, P.J. and Eccleston, D. 1972. Effects of electrical
    stimulation of rat midbrain on 5-hydroxytryptamine synthesis
    as determined by a sensitive radioisotope method. J. Neurochem.
    19(2): 265-272.
Tagliamonte, A., Tagliamonte, P., Forn, J., Perez-Cruet, J., Krishna,
    G. and Gessa, G.L. 1971 a. Stimulation of brain serotonin
    synthesis by dibutyryl-cyclic AMP in rats. J. Neurochem.
    18: 1191-1196.
Tagliamonte, A., Tagliamonte, P., Perez-Cruet, J., Stern, S. and
    Gessa, G.L. 1971 b. Effect of psychotropic drugs on trypto-
    phan concentration in the rat brain. J. Pharm. Exp. Ther.
    177: 475-480.
Thierry, A.M., Fekete, M. and Glowinski, J. 1968. Effects of stress
    on the metabolism of noradrenaline, dopamine and serotonin
    (5-HT) in the central nervous system of the rat (II). Modifi-
    cations of serotonin metabolism. Eur. J. Pharm. 4: 384-389.
Thomas, D., Broun, G. and Selegny, E. 1972. Monoenzymatic model
    membranes: diffusion-reaction kinetics and phenomena. Biochimie
    54: 229-244.
Tozer, T.N., Neff, N.H. and Brodie, B.B. 1966. Application of
    steady-state kinetics to the synthesis rate and turnover time
    of serotonin in the brain of normal and reserpine-treated rats.
    J. Pharmacol. Exp. Ther. 153: 177-182.
Udenfriend, S., Zaltman-Nirenberg, P. and Nagatsu, T. 1965.
    Inhibitors of purified beef adrenal tyrosine hydroxylase.
    Biochem. Pharmacol. 14: 837-845.
Wang, H.L., Harwalkar, V.H., Waisman, H.A. 1962. Effect of dietary
    phenylalanine and tryptophan on brain serotonin. Arch. Biochem.
    Biophys. 97: 181-184.
Weiner, N. 1970. Regulation of norepinephrine biosynthesis. Ann.
    Rev. Pharm. 10: 273-285.
Weiss, B. and Costa, E. 1968. Selective stimulation of adenyl cy-
    clase of rat pineal gland by pharmacologicall active catechol-
    amines. J. Pharmacol. Exp. Ther. 161: 310-319.

REDUNDANT MACROMOLECULAR MECHANISMS IN CENTRAL SYNAPTIC REGULATION

Arnold J. Mandell

Department of Psychiatry
University of California at San Diego
La Jolla, California   92037

Viewing in retrospect the evolution of our understanding of central biogenic amine mechanisms, we seem to have arrived at a third generation of neuropharmacological explanation. In the earliest correlations between drug action, behavioral effects, and neurochemical parameters, the level of measurable biogenic amine was the major dependent variable in relation to action and behavior. For example, comparisons were made between the behavioral and biochemical effects of reserpine and monoamine oxidase inhibitors. Reserpine depleted the brain stores of measurable amines (serotonin, dopamine, norepinephrine) and depressed behavior in animals and mood in humans. Monoamine oxidase inhibitors, intruding on a major metabolic route of aminic degradation, resulted in increased brain amines, increased spontaneous exploratory behavior in animals and elevation of mood in humans. This chemical hydrodynamic model represented the conclusion that motor activity and psychic energy rose and fell with the level of the biogenic amines in the brain.

With the emergence of new drugs explanations became more complicated. Acute and chronic administration of tricyclic antidepressants did not alter gross aminic levels, yet they obviously altered behavior in humans and in animals. Indirect measurement of synthesis, conversion, release, and degradation developed with the use of isotopic neurotransmitters or their precursors. The new logic of turnover suggested that functional level of neurotransmitter was more significant than total level. Most psychotropic drugs were found either to alter nerve ending release or uptake of putative amine neurotransmitters, or to alter their access to receptors. Transmitter synthesis was thought to be regulated by product feedback inhibition of the rate-limiting biosynthetic enzyme. For example, it was believed that competition for the pteridine cofactor by either dopamine or norepinephrine could explain the increases in catecholamine synthesis resulting from drug-facilitated release of the neurotransmitter at nerve endings. Tricyclic antidepressants blocked reuptake of neuro-transmitters, prolonging the probability of neurotransmitter-receptor interaction. Phenothiazines were thought to block the receptor. Cocaine and amphetamine were thought to release and block reuptake of neurotransmitter. Morphine was thought to block pain-activated receptors. This thinking represented the second generation of neuropharmacological explanation.

Recent work with pulse-labeled, neurally-activated adrenergic structures has shifted research emphasis. Rate of synthesis now emerges as a determinant of the level of functional neurotransmit-ter at the synapse. Many studies indicate that a neurally active amine system releases newly-synthesized neurotransmitter preferen-tially over that from a stored pool (Kopin et al. 1968). Other dimensions of central amine synapses have now been involved. In-vestigators studying drugs of abuse that interfere with pre-synaptic and post-synaptic neurotransmitter relationships have found potential regulatory participants in receptors and alterations in receptor sensitivity. Reports of functional recovery following central sympathectomy with 6-hydroxydopamine have directed our attention to receptors (Laverty and Taylor 1970). Emphasis now rests on secondary and tertiary alterations (with various latency) in the neurotransmitter biosynthetic apparatus and in the respon-siveness of receptors (Mandell et al. 1972a).

In animals and in humans, the more complicated psychotropic drugs, such as tricyclic antidepressants and phenothiazines, take weeks, or even months, to manifest all their actions, and atten-tion is directed toward the longer-term effects of addictive drugs, tolerance and withdrawal, as outcomes of chronic administration. Much current study was born of difficulties in understanding the latency to action of major psychotropic drugs and the long-term effects of chronic drug administration. Focusing on responses to drug administration made by adaptive mechanisms in the neuro-transmitter system, we see a constellation of neural processes. Five mechanisms appear to act in concert to regulate these responses to acute and chronic administration of drugs in the brain. Their relative importance, their circumstances of activation, and their quantitative significance remain mysteries. However, using this model of multiple, redundant if you will, adaptive synaptic mechanisms, we have been able to predict rather systematically the neurochemical alterations likely to be induced by drugs.

MACROMOLECULAR MECHANISMS INVOLVED
IN THE REGULATION OF
NEUROTRANSMITTER SYNTHESIS AND EFFICACY

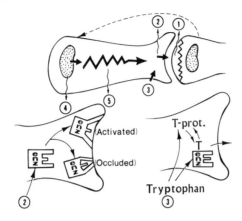

Figure 1. (1) The receptor area is postulated to increase or decrease in sensitivity to infused neurotransmitter. (2) Enzymes in the nerve ending may be inhibited by occlusion or activated by alterations in physical conformation resulting in increased Km or Vmax. (3) Uptake is thought to involve a drug-sensitive mechanism, a storage pool, and a direct conversion pathway. (4) Nuclear enzyme synthesis or degradation is probably affected by intra- or inter-neuronal feedback communication. (5) Axoplasmic flow is thought to affect the latency of enzymatic increase or decrease in the nerve ending.

(1) ALTERATIONS IN RECEPTOR FUNCTION

Diaphragmatic muscle when denervated is supersensitive to cholinergic transmitter compounds, and its stereo-specificity to activating compounds is altered. Peripheral sympathetic structures also are known to respond with supersensitivity to denervation. Similar mechanisms have been speculated to occur in brain and to explain tolerance and withdrawal. However, little direct evidence is extant. Segal and Geyer have evolved models in which receptor sensitivity can be induced and studied. By slowly infusing small volumes of putative neurotransmitter (dopamine, norepinephrine,

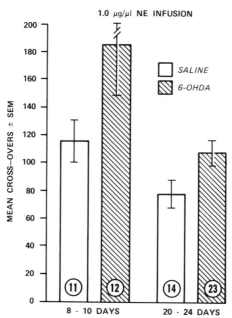

Figure 2. The effect of intraventricular norepinephrine on spontaneous motor activity at two intervals following intraventricular administration of 6-hydroxydopamine. Following the destruction of catecholamine nerve endings by 6-hydroxydopamine, receptor function registers heightened sensitivity.

serotonin) into the ventricles of freely moving rats, they have demonstrated a relationship between drug action, drug effects, and later responsiveness to infused neurotransmitter. Three weeks after intraventricular infusion of 6-hydroxydopamine, which is incorporated by catecholamine nerve endings and destroys them, tyrosine hydroxylase activity in the midbrain and striatum was reduced by more than 75%. Following a short period of retarded behavior and apparent physical illness, the animals had returned gradually to grossly normal behavior. At that time low volumes of norepinephrine were infused chronically to the ventricles of the animals. Figure 2 charts the augmented response to infused norepinephrine reflected by increased spontaneous exploratory behavior and probably due to functional supersensitivity of the catecholamine receptors. On the other hand, the pre-synaptic nerve apparatus which removes some active neurotransmitter via reuptake was destroyed by the 6-hydroxydopamine. Consequently, the behavioral potentiation might be explained by this loss of neurotransmitter

inactivation. Drs. Segal and Geyer are gathering data which may
rule out this alternative (Geyer and Segal 1973). For example,
alpha-methyltyrosine (aMT) inhibits biosynthesis of dopamine and
norepinephrine probably by blocking tyrosine uptake into the nerve
ending and by inhibiting tyrosine hydroxylase. Figure 3 illustrates
that catecholamine infusions in the brain following chronic treatment with aMT potentiate later responses to intraventricular catecholamines. Chronic administration of reserpine does the same
thing. When central biogenic amine synapses are impaired by drugs
and normal neurotransmitter-receptor interaction is decreased, the
receptor function appears capable of compensatory alterations in
sensitivity.

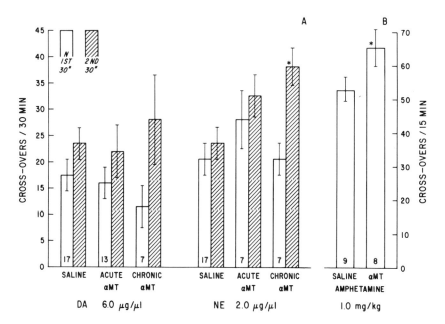

Figure 3 A. Effects of acute and chronic alpha-methyltyrosine
(aMT) on NE- and DA-induced behavioral activity. Rats were tested
3 hours after a single injection of 125 mg/kg of aMT or saline and
again 3 hours after the last of 8 daily doses of aMT or saline.
Chronic aMT treatment significantly increased response to NE infusion. Behavioral activity during DA infusion was not significantly
altered. 3B. Animals injected with amphetamine 24 hours after
the last injection of aMT were significantly more active than
controls (p<.05).

TABLE 1

The Effects of Methadrine on Choline Acetyltransferase
Activity in Chick Optic Lobe

Drug	Administration	nmole/mg protein/hr
Saline	Chronic	130.6 $\pm$ 6.6 (SEM)
Methadrine	Acute	155.5 $\pm$ 6.7
Methadrine	Chronic	165.4 $\pm$ 5.1*

Six animals in each group received either 10 mg/kg i.p. of
methadrine or 1 ml/kg of saline. Acute administration: One
injection 6 hr before assay. Chronic administration: one
injection every 12 hr for 5 days. * p<0.01.

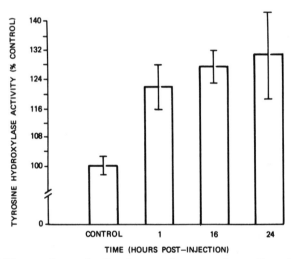

Figure 4. Effect of a single dose of reserpine, 5 mg/kg i.p., on
striatal tyrosine hydroxylase activity at various times after drug
administration. There was a significant increase in enzyme activity
at 1 hr which lasted at least 24 hr. p<0.05. N = 6 per group.

(2) ALTERATIONS IN ENZYME CONFORMATION AND ACTIVITY

By maintaining to some degree the integrity of the nerve
ending fraction during brain tissue homogenization, it is possible
to study the rate of conversion of substrate to neurotransmitter
after acute drug administration as a function of the physical
state of the enzyme. Some drug-induced alterations in neurotransmitter biosynthetic enzyme (NBE) activity in nerve ending regions
manifest very short latency. In contrast, alterations in amount
of NBE require hours to days to reach the nerve ending. Table 1
compares the effects of acute and chronic administration of amphetamine on bird striatal choline acetylase activity. Figure 4 depicts
synaptosomal tyrosine hydroxylase activity in rat striatum after
acute administration of reserpine. We have studied short latency
changes in nerve ending enzyme activity (Mandell et al. 1972b)
as follows. One to 15 mg/kg of amphetamine were administered to
rats, and the animals were sacrificed at 5 min to 1 hour. Subcellular fractions were prepared according to the method of Gray
and Whittaker (1962). We found an amphetamine-induced, progressive
shift of enzyme activity from the soluble to the particulate
fraction at doses up to 5 mg/kg. (Figure 5) The observable

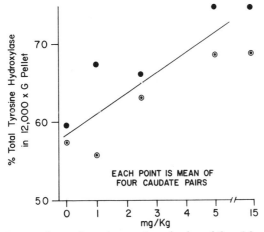

Figure 5. Effect of methamphetamine hydrochloride on percent of
total measurable striatal tyrosine hydroxylase in post-spin (11,000
g) pellet studied 1 hr after drug administration. Each point represents the mean (+ SEM) for 8 caudate pairs (8 animals). Saline-
injected controls did not change significantly over non-injected
controls. The increase achieved significance at 2.5 mg/kg (p<0.05).
High variance of response at 1 mg/kg may indicate a response threshold. Fifteen mg/kg did not produce greater effect than 5 mg/kg
produced.

duration of the effect was also dose-dependent, lasting 4 hours
at 1 mg/kg and 8 hours at 5 mg/kg. Apparently the physical state
of tyrosine hydroxylase can be altered by drugs, suggesting that
the bound state versus the free state might be regulatory of the
enzyme's activity.

Kuczenski has shown that a specific sulfated mucopolysaccharide
(heparin) can alter the conformation of tyrosine hydroxylase,
thereby decreasing its Km for the pteridine cofactor and increasing its Vmax (Kuczenski and Mandell 1972a, 1972b). This conformational change could partially mimic the effect of membrane binding
on the kinetic properties of the soluble enzyme. The top part of
Figure 6 shows what happened when the sulfated mucopolysaccharide
was added to an assay and kinetics were determined for $DMPH_4$ binding; there was marked increase in the affinity of tyrosine hydroxylase for the $DMPH_4$ cofactor. In contrast, the lower part of the
figure indicates that bound enzyme was not activated when the
sulfated mucopolysaccharide was added (activation had already
taken place). We do not know whether this binding-activation is
regulatory or whether it is the normal end state in a process by

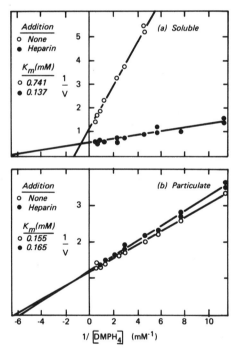

Figure 6. Lineweaver-Burke plot of the activity of caudate (a)
soluble tyrosine hydroxylase and (b) particulate tyrosine hydroxylase as a function of $DMPH_4$ concentration in the presence and
absence of 0.0286 mg/ml of heparin.

which the soluble, less active, NBE is transported down the axon
to the nerve ending membrane where it is activated for use. It is
tempting to relate a drug-inducable shift in the enzyme's physical
state to an increase or decrease in enzyme activity. By varying
the ionic composition in media containing soluble enzyme and nerve
ending membrane components we have shown a decrease in tyrosine
hydroxylase activity. That is, it appears that membrane binding
can occlude tyrosine hydroxylase as well as activate it. (Table 2).
We have elucidated similar acute alterations in tryptophan hydroxylase activity following reserpine (Figure 7). In short, we feel
that physical-state alteration of NBE activity may be significant
in the regulation of neurotransmitter biosynthesis.

TABLE 2

The Effect of Ionic Medium on Subcellular Distribution
And Specific Activity of Caudate Tyrosine Hydroxylase

	Subcellular Distribution (% total activity)		Specific Activity (ionic assay = 100%)	
	.32 M Sucrose	.001 M Na_2PO_4	Ionic Assay	Non-ionic Assay
Supernatant	48%	78%	100%	53 $\pm$ 4%
Pellet	52%	22%	100%	24 $\pm$ 2%

Sucrose homogenization yielded approximately 50-50 distribution of
tyrosine hydroxylase activity between supernatant and pellet after
17,000 x g centrifugation. Hypotonic homogenization yielded more
solubilized enzyme. Fractions were assayed in standard assay
("ionic") and in an assay that optimized binding (0.32 M sucrose
with 0.001 M histidine buffer, pH 6.2). Sucrose-induced reduction:
47%; binding-induced reduction: 76%.

---

(3) ALTERATIONS IN SUBSTRATE UPTAKE PROCESSES

We have found that morphine inhibits intrasynaptosomal tryptophan hydroxylase activity without altering the rate of substrate
uptake. However, a number of other drugs and treatments do alter
tryptophan uptake into nerve endings. The uptake mechanism
appears to be energy-dependent, stereo-specific, and drug-sensitive
(Knapp and Mandell 1973a). Figure 8 summarizes the kinetics of
tryptophan uptake into septal synaptosomes. A low affinity and a
high affinity uptake system are manifest. The low affinity system
has a Km of 6.6×10^{-3} M, and the high affinity system has a Km of
5×10^{-5} M. We have found that the high affinity system is more

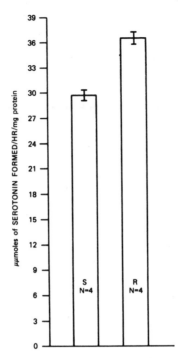

Figure 7. Activity of septal synaptosomal tryptophan hydroxylase 24 hours after a single dose of reserpine, 1.5 mg/kg, or saline.

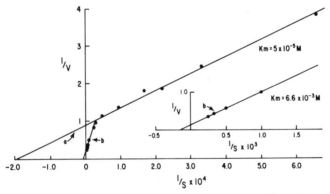

Figure 8. Kinetics of the uptake of tryptophan into septal synaptosomes, showing both high and low affinity systems.

drug-sensitive. For example, lithium appears to increase serotonin
biosynthesis in septal and striatal synaptosomes by stimulating
the high affinity uptake mechanism for tryptophan without altering
the low affinity uptake system (Knapp and Mandell 1973b). Cocaine
inhibits the high affinity uptake system for tryptophan without
altering the low affinity system (Figure 9). In Figure 10, soluble
enzyme activity, synaptosomal conversion of tryptophan to serotonin,
and nerve ending uptake of tryptophan are compared in vitro at
various concentrations of cocaine. Cocaine reduces the rate of
conversion of tryptophan to serotonin indirectly by affecting the
tryptophan uptake mechanism (Knapp and Mandell 1972a).

The relationship between substrate uptake and conversion to
neurotransmitter in the serotonin system is not precisely explica-
ted. After 15 minutes of incubation in substrate followed by disruption of the synaptosomes and chromatography almost 90% of
radioactive tryptophan remained unconverted. This suggests that
there is an intrasynaptosomal storage pool of substrate. On the
other hand, there was immediate conversion of some radioactive
tryptophan to serotonin. We are thinking that there may be a

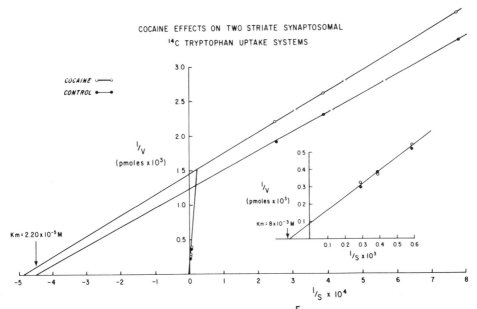

Figure 9. The effect of cocaine (1×10^{-5} M) on two tryptophan
uptake systems. The drug inhibits the uptake of the high affinity
system without altering the low affinity system.

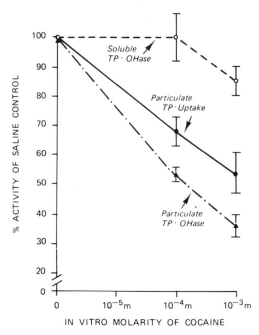

Figure 10. The effects of three concentrations of cocaine hydrochloride on hydroxylation and uptake of tryptophan by particulate
and hydroxylation by soluble enzyme. Each point represents the
mean ± SEM for six experiments. Cocaine does not inhibit soluble
enzyme significantly; it appears to inhibit particulate uptake and
thereby to affect hydroxylation by particulate enzyme.

tryptophan-binding protein in synaptosomes for storage of substrate
like the one that has been demonstrated in bacteria (Wiley 1970).
All this implies a complicated regulatory scheme in the nerve
ending, including a drug-sensitive uptake mechanism, a storage pool,
and a direct uptake-to-conversion pathway.

(4) LONG-LATENCY ALTERATIONS IN NBE AMOUNT OR ACTIVITY

Several workers have demonstrated that adrenergic drugs given
chronically produce a trans-synaptic increase in adrenal and sympathetic nerve ending tyrosine hydroxylase, dopamine-beta-hydroxylase, and phenylethanolamine-N-methyltransferase (Thoenen et al.
1969; Molinoff et al. 1970). Using ganglionic blockers and inhibitors of protein synthesis, they concluded that it is possible to
produce trans-synaptic induction of NBEs at the periphery, whence
feedback activates a compensatory increase in NBE activity. Like-

wise, working in the central nervous system, we have shown that
chronic reserpine administration increases tyrosine hydroxylase
activity in various areas in rat brain (Segal et al. 1971). Figure
11 records the results of daily administration of .5 mg/kg of
reserpine for several days. By the ninth day there was an increase
in the enzyme activity comparable to that reported in the peripheral sympathetic system by Thoenen et al. (1969). Figure 12
demonstrates a similar, drug-induced increase in the rate-limiting
serotonergic enzyme, tryptophan hydroxylase (Knapp and Mandell
1972a). Morphine pellets implanted under the skins of rats allowed
chronic administration of the opiate over 5 days. Morphine, taken
into the synaptosomes, inhibits tryptophan hydroxylase. This
requires a 10^{-4} M concentration of morphine in vitro, generally
thought to be too high to achieve in vivo, but Scrafani et al.
(1969) have demonstrated synaptosomal concentration of morphine
which could eliminate that discrepancy. Immediately upon inhibition of nerve ending serotonin biosynthesis there appears to be an
increase in cell body enzyme activity which is later seen at the
nerve ending. With time, there appears to be a compensatory
increase in tryptophan hydroxylase activity. Data from similar
experiments indicate that amphetamine and monoamine oxidase inhibitors, chronically administered, decrease midbrain tyrosine hydroxylase activity. A similar compensatory change has been observed over

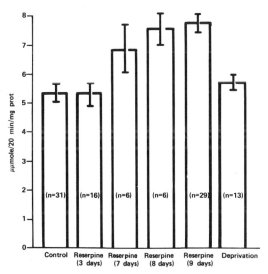

Figure 11. The effects of reserpine treatment on midbrain tyrosine
hydroxylase activity in rats. Each bar represents the mean + SEM
of the indicated number of observations. Nine days of chronic
reserpine treatment induced a significant increase in activity. p<0.05.

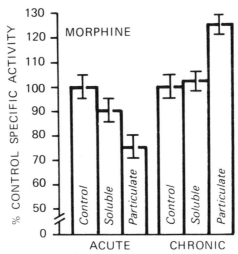

Figure 12. The effects of acute and chronic morphine treatment on two measurable forms of regional brain tryptophan hydroxylase in the rat graphed as percent of control specific activity. Particulate enzyme activity is significantly reduced and increased with acute or chronic administration respectively. p<0.05.

chronic administration of lithium. Lithium augments tryptophan uptake into synaptosomes and conversion of tryptophan into serotonin at nerve endings (Knapp and Mandell 1973b). This is associated with an almost immediate decrease in midbrain enzyme activity, which decrease arrives at serotonergic nerve endings two weeks later.

In general, then, we have come to believe that the reflexive alterations in NBE levels may be a consistent adaptation to chronic administration of drugs that alter synaptic function. Induced changes in neurotransmitter dynamics at the nerve ending may alter NBE activity, probably by modifications in the rate of NBE synthesis prompted by intra- or inter-neuronal communication. The cell body region of the biogenic amine system is first to manifest the adaptive changes. Enzyme amount seems to be involved because alterations induced in the cell body region are seen several days later at the nerve ending.

(5) AXOPLASMIC FLOW OF NEUROTRANSMITTER BIOSYNTHETIC ENZYMES

The consistent latency that we have observed between alterations in NBE activity in cell body and nerve ending regions
suggests that alteration to the nerve ending moves with axoplasmic
flow of either increased or decreased NBE. Previous work on axoplasmic flow rate suggests that particulate enzyme moves with
"fast flow," and soluble enzyme moves with "slow flow." In an
effort to describe the flow rate of an NBE we have inhibited
tryptophan hydroxylase with parachlorphenylalanine (PCPA) and
followed the defective enzyme activity as it moves from the midbrain to the septum (Figure 13; Knapp and Mandell 1972b). After a
single injection of PCPA, tryptophan hydroxylase activity was observed in the midbrain soluble cell body fraction and in the septal
synaptosomal fraction. Irreversible, nondialyzable inhibition of
midbrain tryptophan hydroxylase activity peaked at two days and
gradually disappeared. In the septal synaptosomes during the first
few hours there was an apparent inhibition of conversion of tryptophan to serotonin which we have since attributed to competitive
inhibition of tryptophan uptake by PCPA. More importantly, defective tryptophan hydroxylase was seen to arrive at the septal nerve
ending beginning with day 13 and extending at least through day 22.

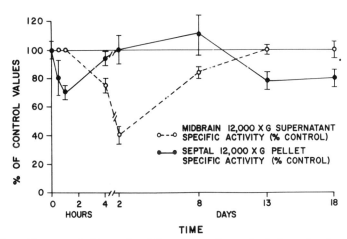

Figure 13. The activity of midbrain and septal tryptophan hydroxylase after acute administration of 300 mg/kg PCPA. Initial reversible decrease in septal enzyme activity was followed by return to
control levels and then delayed decrease. Midbrain activity decreased more slowly and more profoundly, and return to control levels
was delayed.

It appeared to leave the midbrain and arrive at the septum in appropriate temporal sequence. This axoplasmic flow rate can be calculated, from the distance between midbrain and septum in the rat, as 1 to 2 mm per day, or "slow flow." We wonder if the latency to action of some psychotropic drugs and the time required for the development of tolerance and withdrawal to chronic addictive drugs might be functions of this inevitable delay. Fibiger et al. (1972) have identified a similar flow of tyrosine hydroxylase from the midbrain to the corpus striatum. Their rate was a bit faster, 5 to 10 mm per day, but probably within the "slow flow" range.

DISCUSSION

Having reviewed five central biogenic amine neurotransmitter mechanisms found to be drug-sensitive and of short or long latency, we construe as adaptive the delayed (by axoplasmic flow) changes in NBE at nerve endings following impairment of synaptic processes. Alterations in receptor sensitivity in opposition to acute drug intervention also seem adaptive. The "purpose" of changes in substrate uptake processes and acute changes in physical conformation of NBEs are not as clear.

The relative quantitative importance of these mechanisms in response to various agents and manipulations is not yet known. We are intrigued with the possibility that similar responses are inducible by environmental stimuli (or lack of them)(Segal et al. 1973). Figure 14 graphs the effects of extended sensory isolation on the activity of tyrosine hydroxylase and tryptophan hydroxylase in the rat midbrain, striatum, and septum, i.e., progressive increase in midbrain tyrosine hydroxylase activity, delayed increase of that activity in striatum or nerve endings, and decrease in septal tryptophan hydroxylase activity. We are trying to discover whether immediate decrease in septal tryptophan hydroxylase activity following isolation is due to alterations in tryptophan uptake processes or in tryptophan-to-serotonin conversion.

Increased sensitivity to shock, startle, and amphetamine is known to be caused by sensory isolation. Assuming the catecholamines are activating, the biosynthetic substrate for excitability would increase with progressive isolation. Assuming serotonin is sedating, reduced activity of the serotonin biosynthetic unit would lead to neural excitation. Both increases in catecholamines and reductions in serotonin would produce a more excited animal. In any case, it is becoming clear that biogenic amine mechanisms are sensitive to environment as well as to drugs.

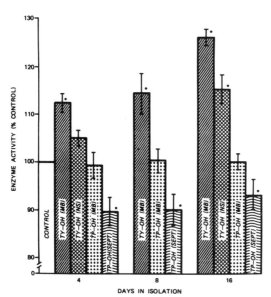

Figure 14. Brain enzyme activity expressed as mean percent of that
of control (grouped) animals in rats isolated for intervals of 4,
8, and 16 days. Midbrain (MB) and neostriatal (NS) tyrosine
hydroxylase (TY-OH) levels increased significantly in 16 days of
isolation. Septal (SEPT) tryptophan hydroxylase (TP-OH) decreased.
Midbrain TP-OH remained unchanged for the intervals of isolation
tested. p<0.05.

Simple statements concerning primary psychotropic drug action
may not be sufficient at the frontier of neuropharmacological
exploration, and the brain's macromolecular adaptive changes
(particularly in response to chronic drug administration) may be
more informative than earlier models involving only subcellular
mobility.

REFERENCES

Fibiger, H.C., Pudritz, R.E., McGeer, P.L., and McGeer, E.G. 1972.
    Axonal transport in nigrostriatal and nigrothalamic neurons;
    effects of medial forebrain bundle lesions and 6-hydroxydopa-
    mine. J. Neurochem. 19: 1697.
Geyer, M., and Segal, D. 1973 Differential effects of reserpine and
    alpha-methyl-p-tyrosine on norepinephrine and dopamine induced
    behavioral activity. Psychopharmacologia (in press)

Gray, E.G. and Whittaker, V.P. 1962. The isolation of nerve endings from brain: an electron-microscopic study of cell fragments derived by homogenization and centrifugation. J. Anat. 96: 79.

Knapp, S. and Mandell, A.J. 1972a. The effects of narcotic drugs on the brain's serotonin biosynthetic systems. Science 177: 1209.

Knapp, S. and Mandell, A.J. 1972b. Parachlorophenylalanine: its three phase sequence of interactions with the two forms of brain tryptophan hydroxylase. Life Sciences 2(16): 761.

Knapp, S. and Mandell, A.J. 1973a. Some drug effects on the functions of the two physical forms of tryptophan-5-hydroxylase; influence on hydroxylation and uptake of substrate. in Serotonin and Behavior, edited by J. Barchus and E. Usdin. Academic Press (in press).

Knapp, S. and Mandell, A.J. 1973b. Long-term lithium administration: effects on the brain's serotonergic biosynthetic systems. (submitted to Science)

Kopin, I.J., Breese, G.R., Krauss, K.R., and Weise, V.K. 1968. Selective release of newly synthesized norepinephrine from the cat spleen during sympathetic nerve stimulation. J. Pharm. Exp. Ther. 161: 271.

Kuczenski, R.T. and Mandell, A.J. 1972a. Allosteric activation of hypothalamic tyrosine hydroxylase by ions and sulfated mucopolysaccharides. J. Neurochem. 19: 131.

Kuczenski, R.T. and Mandell, A.J. 1972b. Regulatory properties of soluble and particulate rat brain tyrosine hydroxylase. J. Biol. Chem. 247: 3114.

Laverty, R. and Taylor, K.M. 1970. Effects of intraventricular 2,4,5-trihydroxyphenylethylamine (6-hydroxydopamine) on rat behavior and brain catecholamine metabolism. Br. J. Pharmacol. 40: 836.

Mandell, A.J., Segal, D.S., Kuczenski, R.T., and Knapp, S. 1972a. Some macromolecular mechanisms in CNS neurotransmitter pharmacology and their psychobiological organization. in The Chemistry of Mood, Motivation, and Memory, edited by J. McGaugh. Plenum Press pp. 105-148.

Mandell, A.J., Knapp, S., Kuczenski, R.T., and Segal, D.S. 1972b. A methamphetamine induced shift in the physical state of rat caudate tyrosine hydroxylase. Biochem. Pharmacol. 21: 2737.

Molinoff, P.B., Brimijoin, W.S., Weinshilboum, R. and Axelrod, J. 1970. Nerually mediated increase in dopamine-beta-hydroxylase activity. Proc. Nat. Acad. Sci. U.S.A. 66: 453.

Scrafani, J.T., Williams, N., and Clouet, D.N. 1969. Binding of dihydromorphine to subcellular fractions of rat brain. The Pharmacologist 11: 256.

Segal, D.S., Sullivan, J.L., Kuczenski, R.T., and Mandell, A.J.
    1971. Effects of long-term reserpine treatment on brain
    tyrosine hydroxylase and behavioral activity. Science 173:
    847.
Segal, D.S., Knapp, S., Kuczenski, R.T., and Mandell, A.J. 1973.
    The effect of environmental isolation on regional rat brain
    tyrosine and tryptophan hydroxylase activity. Behavior. Biol.
    1: 1.
Thoenen, H., Mueller, R.A., and Axelrod, J. 1969. Trans-synaptic
    induction of adrenal tyrosine hydroxylase. J. Pharmacol. Exp.
    Ther. 169: 249.
Wiley, W.R. 1970. Tryptophan transport in neurospora crassa:
    a tryptophan-binding protein released by cold osmotic shock.
    J. Bacteriol. 103: 656.

RELATION OF BRAIN SEROTONIN TO THE INHIBITION AND ENHANCEMENT

OF MORPHINE TOLERANCE AND PHYSICAL DEPENDENCE

E. Leong Way, Ing K. Ho and Horace H. Loh

Department of Pharmacology, School of Medicine,
University of California, San Francisco, California
and The Langley Porter Neuropsychiatric Institute
San Francisco, California

Studies in our laboratory on the mechanisms of morphine
tolerance and physical dependence suggest that cerebral macromolecules may play an important role. The protein synthesis
inhibitor, cycloheximide, was found to prevent the development of
tolerance to and physical dependence on morphine (Way, Loh and
Shen, 1968; Loh, Shen and Way, 1969). A logical extension of this
work was to consider those reactions or enzymes associated with
the putative neurotransmitters. We suggested that one of the
proteins involved may be associated with serotonin (5-HT) synthesis on the basis that brain turnover of 5-HT during the morphine
tolerant-dependent state was greater than under normal conditions
and that tolerance and dependence could be reduced by p-chlorophenylalanine (PCPA) (Shen, Loh and Way, 1970), a relatively
specific inhibitor of 5-HT synthesis (Koe and Weissman, 1966).
Unfortunately, various laboratories have not been able to confirm
certain aspects of our work. We propose to analyze these
discrepancies and present additional data which support our original findings.

Effect of PCPA on morphine tolerance: We use mice or rats
rendered highly tolerant to morphine within three days by the
subcutaneous implantation of a specially formulated morphine
pellet (Way, Loh and Shen, 1969). On occasions we may use
repeated injections of morphine and more recently serial implantation of two pellets for six days. Tolerance to morphine is noted
by the increase in amount of the drug necessary to produce
analgesia. The prolongation in tail-flick reaction time to
thermal stimulus is used for a quantal assay to determine the
median analgetic dose (AD50) of morphine.

279

We have repeated our experiments and confirmed our previous finding that PCPA reduced tolerance development. In two separate experiments on mice, the several fold increase in the morphine AD50 that results after pellet implantation was found to be reduced by approximately one-half with PCPA treatment (Ho et al., 1972). The results are consistent with those by Maruyama et al. (1971) who reported that PCPA reduced development of tolerance to morphine analgesia by the writhing test but are not in agreement with the negative findings with the hot-plate procedure by Cheney and Goldstein (1971). Not only have we been able to repeat our previous findings in the mouse, but we were also able to substantiate the results in the rat.

In the rat, three days after initiating the serial implantation of two morphine pellets 36 hours apart, the morphine AD50 increased from 4 mg/kg to 16 mg/kg (Figure 1). The injection of

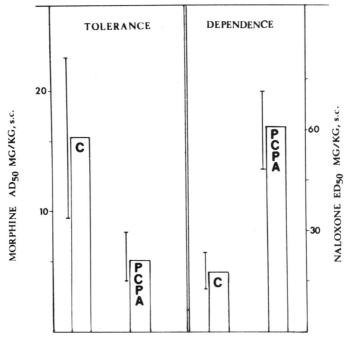

Figure 1. PCPA inhibition of morphine tolerance and physical dependence development in the rat. The animals were rendered tolerant and dependent by morphine pellet implantation. The left panel indicates the s.c. morphine AD50 and 95% confidence limits for animals treated either with PCPA or its vehicle (C). The right panel indicates the s.c. naloxone ED50 for precipitating withdrawal jumping with and without PCPA treatment (Ho et al., 1972).

PCPA during the implantation period yielded an AD50 (6.2 mg/kg) which was not significantly different from that obtained in animals prior to pellet implantation. PCPA alone also did not alter the AD50. We conclude from the data that PCPA inhibits the development of tolerance to morphine in the rat as well as in the mouse.

Additional findings to support an associated role for 5-HT in morphine tolerance were obtained in experiments with tryptophan. Recent studies indicate that the regulation of brain 5-HT synthesis may depend upon the availability of its amino acid precursor (Fernstrom and Wurtman, 1971). As a consequence, we decided to investigate the influence of tryptophan on morphine tolerance and physical dependence development.

Tryptophan was found to accelerate the development of tolerance. In paired experiments on mice implanted with a morphine pellet for three days, a control group receiving saline prior to and once daily during the period of implantation developed a 15-fold tolerance; the morphine AD50 increased from 4.9 to 72 mg/kg. In the test group receiving injections of tryptophan, 75 mg/kg, i.p., daily during the period of implant instead of saline, the AD50 increased almost 50-fold from 7.4 to 350 mg/kg. On the other hand, no significant change in the morphine AD50 was noted between vehicle and tryptophan injected mice receiving a placebo implant. Thus as judged by the relative increase in the AD50, tryptophan treated animals became nearly five times as tolerant as the vehicle treated group. Similar experiments in the rat also resulted in enhancement of tolerance development to morphine by tryptophan.

PCPA prevented the accelerating effect of tryptophan on tolerance development. As shown in Figure 2, in mice rendered tolerant by pellet implantation, those mice receiving repeated injections of tryptophan exhibited a morphine AD50 about three times higher than that of the control group receiving the vehicle. In contrast, in animals given PCPA together with repeated injections of tryptophan, the AD50 of morphine was about the same as that of the control group receiving the vehicle (Ho, Loh and Way, 1972).

Effect of PCPA on morphine dependence: The degree of dependence in dependent mice with and without PCPA treatment was assessed by precipitated withdrawal and by abrupt withdrawal. The procedure for rendering mice dependent on morphine was the same as that in the tolerant study since mice rendered tolerant to morphine by double pellet implantation are also highly dependent on morphine. Precipitated withdrawal was induced by naloxone, the most characteristic sign being stereotyped jumping. The degree of dependence is inversely related

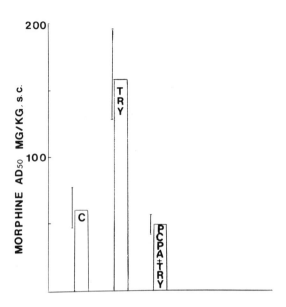

Figure 2. PCPA inhibition of tryptophan acceleration of morphine
tolerance development in mice rendered tolerant by morphine
pellet implantation (Ho, Loh and Way, 1972).

to the dose of naloxone required to elicit the behavior; hence,
the naloxone ED50 provides an index of dependence intensity (Way,
Loh and Shen, 1969). The degree of dependence after abrupt withdrawal was assessed by weighing the animals at fixed intervals
after removing the morphine pellet. Loss in body weight during
abstinence was reported to be a reliable index of morphine
dependence in the rat (Hosoya, 1959; Akera and Brody, 1968) and
the mouse (Shuster, Hannum and Boyle, 1963). Dependent animals
exhibit considerable weight loss 12 to 24 hours after pellet
removal.

     Our additional experiments with PCPA substantiate our
original studies (Way, Loh and Shen, 1968; Shen, Loh and Way,
1970) with respect to its ability to reduce physical dependence
development on morphine. Confirmatory evidence was noted in the
rat as well as the mouse.

     In the mouse, by prolonging the state of physical dependence
on morphine, it was possible to demonstrate by naloxone precipitated withdrawal that PCPA pretreatment could reduce dependence
development. More protracted dependence was obtained by implant-
ing a second morphine pellet in dependent animals and allowing
another three days for further dependence development. In such
animals, the amount of naloxone needed to precipitate withdrawal

jumping was roughly three times greater in the PCPA group than in the control group.

Attenuation of morphine dependence development by PCPA was also demonstrated by its effect on weight loss after abrupt withdrawal. As shown in Figure 3, the weight loss, occurring after removal of the implanted pellets from dependent mice, was reduced by PCPA pretreatment. These results are not in agreement with those reported by Marshall and Grahame-Smith (1971).

Several explanations can be offered for the inability of various laboratories to obtain results with PCPA on dependence development consistent with ours. None of the groups claiming inability to support our findings attempted to repeat our experiments in detail. In our original tests (Shen, Loh and Way, 1970), we rendered mice dependent on morphine by repeated injections for

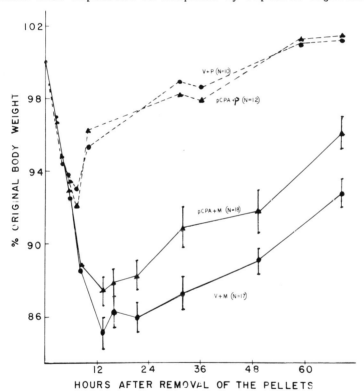

Figure 3. PCPA inhibition of body weight loss after abrupt withdrawal in mice rendered dependent by morphine pellet implantation. results in animals implanted with morphine (M) pellets are shown by the solid lines and in those receiving placebo (P) pellets by broken lines. V denotes the vehicle (Ho et al., 1972).

5 to 14 days and subjected our animals to repeated naloxone
challenge and supplementary doses of PCPA until a difference was
obtained between the control and the test group. We reported also
that in short-term experiments when mice were made dependent on
morphine by a single pellet implantation, PCPA did not block
withdrawal jumping precipitated by a single challenge by naloxone.
Instead of contradicting our findings, therefore, the four
laboratories claiming results inconsistent with ours (Maruyama
et al., 1971; Cheney and Goldstein, 1971; Marshall and Grahame-
Smith, 1971; Collier, Francis and Schneider, 1972) appear to have
confirmed our short-term tests. Moreover, our tests were performed on a much larger series of animals, and we used a quantal
response to provide a quantitative indication of the degree of
dependence inhibition by PCPA. Marshall and Grahame-Smith (1971)
used a graded response in a smaller number of mice which apparently
were not highly dependent since the animals were injected with
morphine for only a few days. While Collier, Francis and
Schneider (1972) indicated that PCPA acutely inhibits naloxone
precipitated withdrawal jumping, in our more recent experiments
our tests with naloxone were performed 54-72 hours after the last
PCPA dose.

The findings with respect to PCPA reduction of morphine
dependence in the mouse are supported by additional experiments
in the rat. As shown on the right of Figure 1 in rats rendered
dependent on morphine by double pellet implantation, PCPA reduced
dependence development as evidenced by the increase in the naloxone
ED50 to precipitate withdrawal jumping. These findings are not in
agreement with those reported by Schwartz and Eidelberg (1970) and
Algeri and Costa (1971) who were unable to demonstrate an effect
of PCPA on dependence. It should be pointed out that these
investigators carried out short-term experiments in a relatively
small series of animals and did not provide a quantitative measure
of the degree of morphine dependence. Moreover, in precipitating
abstinence with nalorphine, they studied the effects of only one
dose which, if supramaximal, could easily have masked any effect
PCPA might have on dependence development.

The involvement of 5-HT in the development of physical
dependence on morphine was also supported by additional studies
with tryptophan in mice. In addition to enhancing tolerance
development, the repeated injection of tryptophan enhanced the
development of physical dependence. Enhanced dependence was
indicated by the decrease in the amount of naloxone needed to
induce precipitated withdrawal jumping in mice treated with
tryptophan before and daily during implantation. As shown in
Figure 4, although the naloxone ED50 of the control group was not
modified by acute treatment with tryptophan, the naloxone ED50 of
the group treated with tryptophan before and during dependence

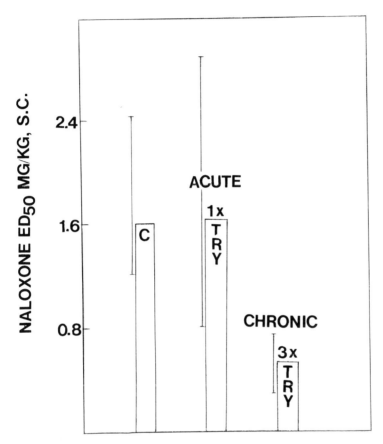

Figure 4. Tryptophan acceleration of morphine dependence development in mice rendered dependent by pellet implantation. The degree
of dependence is inversely related to the naloxone ED50. Tryptophan acutely was administered after dependence had developed,
chronically before and during pellet implantation (Ho, Loh and
Way, 1972).

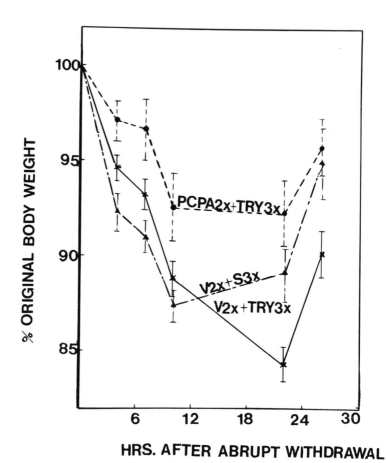

Figure 5.   PCPA inhibition of tryptophan enhancement of morphine physical dependence development.   The degree of dependence is reflected by the mean (+ S.E.) loss in body weight after abrupt withdrawal.   V = PCPA vehicle; S = tryptophan vehicle.   PCPA and tryptophan (TRY) were administered before and during the development of dependence (Ho, Loh and Way, 1972).

development was approximately one-fourth that of the control group.
In the rat, similar naloxone precipitated withdrawal experiments
also indicated a four-fold reduction in the naloxone ED50 by
tryptophan. Furthermore, the tryptophan treated animals lost
more weight than the controls when abrupt withdrawal was initiated
by pellet removal. Likewise, tryptophan also increased the weight
loss after abrupt withdrawal in the mouse. The increased weight
loss effected by tryptophan in dependent mice was largely antagonized by PCPA. As shown in Figure 5 the weight loss 20 hours after
pellet removal was considerably greater in tryptophan treated
animals than that in the control group receiving the PCPA and
tryptophan vehicles; the concomitant administration of PCPA
prevented the tryptophan effect. Thus, PCPA not only reduces
the development of physical dependence on morphine but it also
blocks the accelerating effects of tryptophan on the process.

While it was not established that the effect produced by
PCPA was related to an inhibition of 5-HT synthesis, this appears
to be a reasonable conclusion. The fact that PCPA does not
inhibit dependence development on morphine in short-term experiments raises some questions. An explanation may reside in the
inability of PCPA to deplete completely brain 5-HT and this
residual 5-HT may have a role. Perhaps, also, the effects of
PCPA are apparent only after tryptophan hydroxylase levels become
sufficiently elevated by prolonged morphine administration. The
recent findings by Knapp and Mandell (1972 a,b) may have immediate
relevance.

According to these two investigators, tryptophan hydroxylase
appears to be influenced by PCPA in a linked series of three
temporally related events, namely, competition with substrate
for entry into the nerve ending, reversible competitive inhibition
of the enzyme for substrate, and irreversible inhibition by incorporation into the enzyme during new protein synthesis in the cell
body. The defective enzyme formed in the latter event is then
transported by axoplasmic flow to nerve endings of the septal area
at the rate of about 1 to 2 mm/day. Hence, in utilizing PCPA to
elucidate biochemical mechanisms underlying behavioral and
pharmacologic phenomena, the temporal sequence of all three
mechanisms for decreasing brain 5-HT should be considered. It
is likely that some of the reported discrepancies concerning PCPA
effects on morphine tolerance and dependence are explainable in
terms of these varying mechanisms by which PCPA acts.

Brain 5-HT synthesis in morphine tolerant-dependent state:
There is general agreement that steady state levels of brain 5-HT
are not altered by repeated morphine administration. On the other
hand, the evidence concerning increased brain 5-HT turnover in
morphine tolerant-dependent state is controversial.

We first reported that the synthesis of brain 5-HT was elevated in the mouse rendered tolerant to and dependent on morphine (Way, Loh and Shen, 1968; Shen, Loh and Way, 1970). We noted, additionally, that the increased rate of 5-HT turnover resulting from chronic morphine administration was blocked by cycloheximide, an inhibitor of protein synthesis (Loh, Shen and Way, 1969) and that when morphine tolerance and dependence development was prevented by the concomitant injection of a narcotic antagonist, naloxone, daily with morphine, the increase in brain 5-HT was prevented (Shen, Loh and Way, 1970). Our findings have been corroborated and refuted. The discrepancies appear in part to be due to differences in sensitivity in analytical technic applied to a given strain or species.

We used the pargyline method (Tozer, Neff and Brodie, 1966) which involves blocking the conversion of 5-HT to 5-HIAA with the MAO inhibitor pargyline, and, on the assumption that brain 5-HT is converted solely to 5-HIAA, the rate of 5-HT synthesis may be calculated from the rate of accumulation of 5-HT. We also used the probenecid procedure of Neff, Tozer and Brodie (1967) in a limited number of studies to measure the rise in 5-HIAA when the transport of 5-HIAA from the cerebral spinal fluid to blood was blocked.

Our findings with respect to morphine enhancement of brain 5-HT in the tolerant-dependent state have been contradicted by several laboratories. Cheney et al. (1971) measured 5-HT turnover in mouse brain by following the conversion of ^{3}H-tryptophan into 5-HT (Neff et al., 1971) and reported no significant difference between morphine tolerant and non-tolerant mice. However, their conclusions appear to have been refuted (Hitzemann, Ho and Loh, 1972). Marshall and Grahame-Smith (1971) reported no change in brain serotonin turnover in morphine-dependent mice after monoamine oxidase inhibition with tranylcypromine. Although both laboratories did not use the pargyline procedure to estimate 5-HT turnover, Schecter, Lovenberg and Sjoerdsma (1972) did and failed to support our results. Also, in the rat, Algeri and Costa (1971) were unable to demonstrate an increase in serotonin turnover in morphine dependent animals by the ^{3}H-tryptophan procedure and in our own laboratory, we have not noted any increase in brain serotonin turnover in five brain regions of dependent rats (Bhargava, Friedler and Way, unpublished).

The above findings appear to be strong evidence arguing against an associated role (direct or indirect) for 5-HT in morphine tolerance and dependence. And yet, there is sufficient evidence to warrant a more optimistic viewpoint and continuation in the efforts to implicate 5-HT in morphine tolerance and dependence.

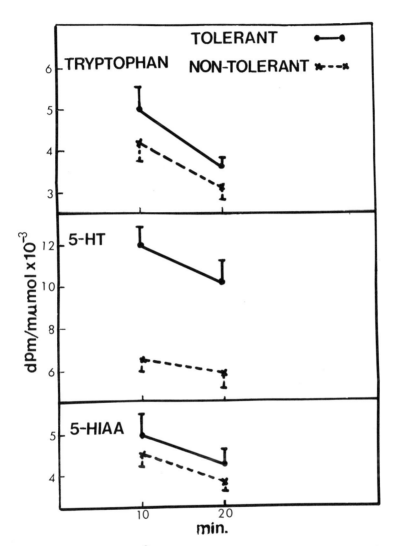

Figure 6. Conversion of ^{3}H-tryptophan into radiolabelled 5-HT and 5-HIAA in morphine tolerant and non-tolerant mice (Loh et al., unpublished).

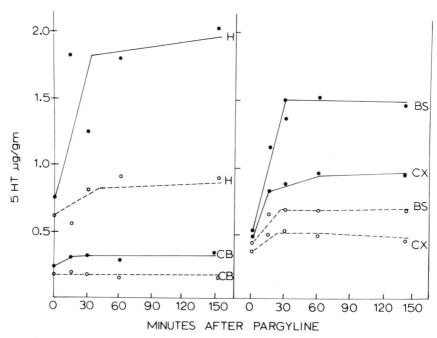

Figure 7. 5-HT levels in various brain regions of morphine tolerant (solid lines) and non-tolerant (broken lines) mice after
pargyline. H = hypothalamus; CB = cerebellum; BS = brain stem;
CX = cortex (Ho et al., 1972).

On the positive side, our observations in the tolerant-
dependent mouse that increased brain serotonin turnover occurs
has been amply confirmed (Maruyama et al., 1971). Furthermore,
these investigators studied three strains of mice and found that,
while there were quantitative differences in the response to
morphine, all three strains exhibited increased brain 5-HT turnover after development of morphine dependence. Methadone also
appears to increase brain 5-HT turnover (Bowers and Kleber, 1971).
Also, Haubrich and Blake (1969) using the probenecid procedure to
measure brain 5-HT turnover in the rat, noted that the rate of
accumulation of 5-HIAA in animals rendered tolerant to morphine by
pellet implantation was considerably greater than that in non-
tolerant controls. More recently, we have compared the brain 5-HT
turnover of morphine tolerant-dependent mice and non-tolerant ones
by the ^{3}H-tryptophan procedure (Loh et al., unpublished) and,
contrary to the results reported by Cheney et al. (1971), we have
noted a higher rate of conversion of tryptophan into 5-HT in the
tolerant-dependent state. As can be seen in Figure 6 a study of
the uptake of labelled tryptophan in brain showed higher specific
activities for tryptophan and 5-HT in morphine tolerant-dependent
mice.

We have also compared the 5-HT turnover of morphine tolerant-
dependent and non-tolerant-dependent mice in five brain regions
by the pargyline method. As can be seen in Figure 7, the turnover
is higher in the former animals, particularly in the hypothalamic
region and brain stem (Ho et al., 1972). And while our findings
in the rat in this regard were negative, results by other workers
suggest that we may not have separated the brain areas sufficiently.

Two laboratories reported independently that the rate-
limiting enzyme involved in serotonin synthesis is increased in
the morphine-dependent animal. Azmitia et al. (1970) noted an
increase in tryptophan hydroxylase activity in the midbrain
areas of rats given repeated injections of morphine and a pronounced elevation was noted in the synaptosomes of the septal
areas (Knapp and Mandell, 1972 a). These findings are of considerable import since Schecter, Lovenberg and Sjoerdsma (1972), using
a DMPH$_4$-dependent fraction prepared from whole mouse brain, were
unable to find any difference in total brain tryptophan hydroxylase
activity between tolerant and non-tolerant mice. Knapp and
Mandell (1972 a) point out the negative data can be explained on
the basis that there are two forms of tryptophan hydroxylase, a
soluble and particulate form. They mention that only the soluble
enzyme could be dependent on exogenous DMPH$_4$ since nerve endings
do not take up this cofactor and morphine did not affect the soluble
form of tryptophan hydroxylase but only the particulate form
(vide infra). Finally, our more recent experiments indicate that

5-HT turnover is higher in tolerant-dependent mice than in non-tolerant ones following a tryptophan load. In morphine pellet implanted mice pretreated with tryptophan to enhance tolerance and dependence development, the 5-HT turnover was found to be augmented.

CONCLUSIONS

The results suggest that 5-HT is involved in the processes concerned with development of tolerance to and dependence on morphine. A causal role has not been established nor has it been determined whether the association is direct or indirect. However, the fact that the 5-HT precursor, tryptophan, enhances tolerance and dependence development and the fact that PCPA blocks the effect argue strongly that more than just a remote relationship is involved. To our knowledge, the acceleration of tolerance and physical dependence has not been previously reported. More recently, we have been interested in the compound, 5,6-dihydroxy-tryptamine which has been reported to destroy serotonergic amine pathways (Baumgarten et al., 1972). Our preliminary results indicate that this compound like PCPA, inhibits the development of morphine tolerance and dependence.

While the precise mechanism by which morphine and 5-HT may interact has not been established, their relationship has been made somewhat clearer by the recent studies in Mandell's laboratory. Knapp and Mandell (1972 b) have reported that there are two types of tryptophan hydroxylase in the brain, a soluble form present primarily in serotonergic cell bodies and a particulate form at serotonergic nerve endings. An energy transport mechanism for tryptophan uptake was noted in the particulate form and they suggested that this mechanism may play an important role in the regulation of 5-HT synthesis. While the soluble form enzyme was not materially affected either by acute or chronic morphine administration, morphine acutely inhibited the synaptosomal tryptophan hydroxylase but with continued administration, an adaptive increase in the particulate nerve ending enzyme activity resulted in the septal and caudate regions.

The finding in the latter area may be highly significant inasmuch as the thalamus has been identified as a sensitive site for morphine precipitated withdrawal effects (Wei, Loh and Way, 1972) and one of the main projections of the medical thalamic nuclei is to the globus and striatum. However, since cholinergic pathways predominate in this system, the involvement of acetyl-choline in morphine action must also be considered.

It is of interest to mention, also, that an interaction has been reported to occur between 5-HT and adenosine 3',5'-monophosphate (c-AMP). It has been reported that dibutyryl c-AMP stimulates

5-HT turnover in the brain (Tagliamonte et al., 1971). Recently, we have obtained evidence that c-AMP, like tryptophan, can antagonize morphine effects (Loh et al., 1971) and accelerate the development of tolerance and physical dependence (Ho et al., 1971). These findings provide incentive to seek a possible relationship between morphine, 5-HT and c-AMP. There is increasing evidence that c-AMP has a role in the induction of enzymes in the liver (Wicks, 1971) and it is within reason to expect that it might similarly alter brain tryptophan hydroxylase.

ACKNOWLEDGEMENTS

This study was supported by NIMH grants MH-17017 and MH-19768, and NIH grant GM-01839.

REFERENCES

Akera, T. and Brody, T.M. 1968. The addiction cycle to narcotics in the rat and its relation to catecholamine. Biochem. Pharmacol. 17: 675-688.

Algeri, S. and Costa, E. 1971. Physical dependence on morphine fails to increase serotonin turnover rate in rat brain. Biochem. Pharmacol. 20: 877-884.

Azmitia, E.C., Hess, P. and Reis, D. 1970. Tryptophan hydroxylase changes in midbrain of rat after chronic morphine administration. Life Sci. 9: 633-637.

Baumgarten, H.G., Bjorklund, A., Lachenmayer, L., Nobin, A. and Stenevi, U. 1972. Long-lasting selective depletion of brain serotonin by 5,6-dihydroxytryptamine. Acta Physiol. Scand. Supplementum 373, 1972.

Bowers, M.B. and Kleber, H.L. 1971. Methadone increases mouse brain 5-hydroxyindoleacetic acid. Nature 229: 134-135.

Cheney, D.L. and Goldstein, A. 1971. The effect of p-chlorophenylalanine on opiate-induced running, analgesia, tolerance and physical dependence in mice. J. Pharmacol. Exp. Ther. 177: 309-315.

Cheney, D.L., Goldstein, A., Algeri, S. and Costa, E. 1971. Narcotic tolerance and dependence: lack of relationship with brain serotonin turnover. Science 171: 1169-1171.

Collier, H.O.G., Francis, D.L. and Schneider, C. 1972. Modification of morphine withdrawal by drugs interacting with humoral mechanisms: some contradictions and their interpretation. Nature 237: 220-223.

Fernstrom, J.D. and Wurtman, R.J. 1971. Brain serotonin content: Physiological dependence on plasma tryptophan levels. Science 173: 149-152.

Haubrich, D.R. and Blake, D.E. 1969. Effect of acute and chronic administration of morphine on the metabolism of brain serotonin in rats. Fed. Proc. 28: 793.

Hitzemann, R.J., Ho, I.K. and Loh, H.H. 1972. Narcotic tolerance,
    dependence and serotonin turnover. Science (in press).
Ho, I.K., Loh, H.H. and Way, E.L. 1972. Influence of L-tryptophan
    on morphine analgesia, tolerance and physical dependence.
    Reports of the NAS-NRC Committee on Problems of Drug
    Dependence. U.S. Govt. Printing Office (in press).
Ho, I.K., Lu, S.E., Loh, H.H. and Way, E.L. 1971. Effects of
    c-AMP on morphine tolerant and physically dependent mice.
    Pharmacologist 13: 314.
Ho, I.K., Lu, S.E., Stolman, S., Loh, H.H. and Way, E.L. 1972.
    Influence of p-chlorophenylalanine on morphine tolerance and
    physical dependence and regional brain serotonin turnover
    studies in morphine tolerant-dependent mice. J. Pharmacol.
    Exp. Ther. 182: 155-165.
Hosoya, E. 1959. Some withdrawal symptoms of rats to morphine.
    Pharmacologist 1: 77.
Koe, B.K. and Weissman, A. 1966. p-Chlorophenylalanine: A
    specific depletor of brain serotonin. J. Pharmacol. Exp.
    Ther. 154: 499-516.
Knapp, S. and Mandell, A.J. 1972a. Some drug effects on the func-
    tions of the two physical forms of tryptophan-5-hydroxylase;
    influence on hydroxylation and uptake of substrate. In:
    Serotonin and Behavior (Ed. Barchus, J.), U.S. Govt. Printing
    Office (in press).
Knapp, S. and Mandell, A.J. 1972b. Parachlorophenylalanine--Its
    three phase sequence of interactions with the two forms of
    brain tryptophan hydroxylase. Life Sci. 2(16): 761-771.
Loh, H.H., Cho, T.M., Ho, I.K. and Way, E. 1972. Regulation of
    brain serotonin biosynthesis in morphine tolerant mice,
    (in preparation).
Loh, H.H., Ho, I.K., Lu, S.E. and Way, E.L. 1971. Effect of c-AMP
    on morphine analgesia. Pharmacologist 13: 313.
Loh, H.H., Shen, F. and Way, E.L. 1969. Inhibition of morphine
    tolerance and physical dependence development and brain
    serotonin synthesis by cycloheximide. Biochem. Pharmacol.
    18: 2711-2721.
Mandell, A.J., Segal, D.S., Kuczenski, R.T. and Knapp, S. 1972. Some
    macromolecular mechanisms in CNS neurotransmitter pharmacology
    and their psychobiological organization. In: Chemistry of
    Mood, Motivation and Memory (Ed. McGaugh, J.L.), pp. 105-143.
Marshall, I. and Grahame-Smith, D.G. 1971. Evidence against a role
    of brain 5-hydroxytryptamine in the development of physical
    dependence upon morphine in mice. J. Pharmacol. Exp. Ther.
    179: 634-641.
Maruyama, Y., Hayashi, G., Smits, S.E. and Takemori, A.E. 1971.
    Studies on the relationship between 5-hydroxytryptamine
    turnover in brain and tolerance and physical dependence
    in mice. J. Pharmacol. Exp. Ther. 178: 20-29.

Neff, N.H., Tozer, T.N. and Brodie, B.B. 1967. Application of steady-state kinetics to studies of the transfer of 5-hydroxyindoleacetic acid from brain to plasma. J. Pharmacol. Exp. Ther. 158 : 214-218.

Neff, N.H., Spano, P.F., Gropetti, A., Wang, C.T. and Costa, E. 1971. A simple procedure for calculating the synthesis rate of norepinephrine, dopamine and serotonin in rat brain. J. Pharmacol. Exp. Ther. 176: 701-710.

Schecter, P.J., Lovenberg, W. and Sjoerdsma, A. 1972. Dissociation of morphine tolerance and dependence from brain serotonin synthesis rate in mice. Biochem. Pharmacol. 21: 751-753.

Schwartz, A.S. and Eidelberg, E. 1970. Role of biogenic amines in morphine dependence. Life Sciences 9(1): 613-624.

Shen, F.H., Loh, H. and Way, E.L. 1970. Brain serotonin turnover in morphine tolerant-dependent mice. J. Pharmacol. Exp. Ther. 175: 427-434.

Shuster, L., Hannam, R.V. and Boyle, W.E., Jr. 1963. A simple method for producing tolerance to dihydromorphinone in mice. J. Pharmacol. Exp. Ther. 140: 149-154.

Tagliamonte, A., Tagliamonte, P., Forn, J., Perez-Cruet, J., Krishna, G. and Gessa, G.L. 1971. Stimulation of brain serotonin synthesis by dibutyryl-cyclic AMP in rats. J. Neurochem. 18: 1191-1196.

Tozer, T.N., Neff, N.H. and Brodie, B.B. 1966. Application of steady state kinetics to the synthesis rate and turnover time of serotonin in the brain of normal and reserpine-treated rats. J. Pharmacol. Exp. Ther. 153: 177-182.

Way, E.L., Loh, H.H. and Shen, F.H. 1968. Morphine tolerance, physical dependence and synthesis of brain 5-hydroxytryptamine. Science 162: 1290-1292.

Way, E.L., Loh, H.H. and Shen, F.H. 1969. Simultaneous quantitative assessment of morphine tolerance and physical dependence. J. Pharmacol. Exp. Ther. 167: 1-8.

Wei, E.T., Loh, H.H. and Way, E.L. 1972. Neuroanatomical correlates of morphine dependence. Science (in press).

Wicks, W.D. 1971. Regulation of hepatic enzyme synthesis by cyclic AMP. Ann. N.Y. Acad. Sci. 185: 152-164.

RECENT STUDIES ON THE BINDING OF OPIATE NARCOTICS TO POSSIBLE RECEPTOR SITES

Avram Goldstein

Addiction Research Laboratory, Department of

Pharmacology, Stanford University, Stanford, CA 94305

It is not known yet if the theme of this conference, Neurotransmitter Regulation, is relevant to the problem of narcotic tolerance and dependence. In 1961, Dr. Dora B. Goldstein and I (1961) proposed a unitary theory of tolerance and dependence, based upon the Jacob-Monod (1961) concepts of repression and derepression of protein synthesis as fundamental mechanisms of biochemical regulation. In the same year, Shuster (1961) advanced virtually the same idea independently. Collier (1965) later advanced a somewhat different but related theory. And subsequently, our ideas were further refined and generalized (Goldstein and Goldstein, 1968).

The essential feature of the enzyme (receptor) expansion theory is depicted in Figure 1. It is supposed that the receptor upon which the narcotic drugs act is subject to regulation in the central nervous system, i.e., that the brain maintains a constant steady-state level of free (functional) receptor. If the receptor is an enzyme, then the regulatory control would respond, according to the classical model, to the concentration of enzyme product. But the receptor could also be a presynaptic or postsynaptic membrane protein, the amount of which (in the free functional form) would be kept constant, perhaps by a transsynaptic feedback such as described in this symposium. The normal amount of free receptor is represented at upper left of Figure 1. The acute narcotic effect, which occurs immediately, is due to occupancy of the receptor by an opiate drug, as indicated at upper right. In consequence, the amount of total receptor is expanded (either by increased rate of synthesis or by decreased rate of degradation), until the _free_ receptor has been restored to its normal amount, despite the continued presence of the narcotic. This is

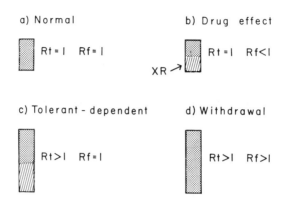

Figure 1. Receptor expansion theory of tolerance and physical
dependence. Rt: Total receptor. Rf: Free receptor. XR: Drug-
receptor complex. a) The normal state, all receptors free.
b) 50 per cent occupancy of receptor by drug causes drug effect
because free receptor is reduced in amount. c) Regulatory
processes have restored normal amount of free receptor. Function
is normal. Total receptor doubled. d) On withdrawal of drug,
excess receptor becomes free, withdrawal effects ensue, opposite
to initial drug effects. Subsequently, regulatory processes
reduce free receptor to normal amount.

shown at lower left of Figure 1. If we suppose the acute narcotic
effect to have been manifested at 50 per cent occupancy of the
receptors, then the total receptor pool will have to be doubled,
so that the free receptor can again be present in the normal
amount, and the receptor occupancy, in the presence of the same
concentration of narcotic, will still be 50 per cent. This follows
directly from the mass law, for according to classical Michaelis-
Menten kinetics (i.e., when most of the ligand molecules are free
at equilibrium), the fractional occupancy depends only upon the
free ligand concentration, not upon the receptor concentration or
amount.

We now have the well-known pharmacologic state of tolerance,
because despite the presence of a concentration of drug that
previously caused narcotic effects, there are now no such effects,
since there is no abnormality in the amount of free receptor. In
order to elicit narcotic effects again (e.g., to produce 50 per
cent occupancy of the free receptors), a total occupancy greater
than before will be required, and thus a higher drug concentration
will be needed. In the example proposed, 75 per cent total
occupancy will be needed.

The same model explains dependence. The apparently normal
state in the presence of a previously effective drug concentration
conceals a latent abnormality--the total receptor pool is excessive,
with the excess masked by bound drug molecules. Removal of the drug,
by simple withdrawal or by use of a narcotic antagonist, will expose
the receptor excess, leading to rapid onset of physiologic disturbances opposite to those produced by the narcotic initially, as
shown at lower right of Figure 1. Then the regulatory mechanism
will again come into play, synthesis will be shut off or degradation will increase, until eventually the normal state is restored
again.

This general model fits quite well with what we know about
tolerance and dependence. It predicts that these states should
be prevented by inhibitors of protein synthesis, and this has
been found to be true (Way et al., 1968). It predicts that signs
of withdrawal should be generally opposite to signs of narcotic
intoxication, and this is true on the whole (Jaffe, 1970). It
predicts that in contrast to the fast rates of onset of drug
effects and of withdrawal effects, the development and disappearance of tolerance and dependence should be relatively slower, on
a time scale compatible with known turnover rates of proteins in
the brain (hours to days), and this is also true. It predicts
that tolerance and dependence should co-vary, and that both should
behave as reversible steady-state processes, predictions borne out
experimentally (Way et al., 1969; Goldstein and Sheehan, 1969;
Cheney and Goldstein, 1971).

Unfortunately, even after ten years, no direct evidence
verifying or falsifying this theory has emerged. The problem
is, of course, that with no knowledge about the receptor, it is
impossible to measure its changes in tolerance and dependence. It
has seemed likely to us, therefore, that identification, isolation,
and characterization of the receptor are prerequisites to any real
understanding of narcotic action or of narcotic tolerance and
dependence.

Our approach to the problem has been based upon the known
pharmacologic stereospecificity of narcotic effects. Only the
D(-) isomers are active. The L(+) enantiomers are neither agonists
nor antagonists, at concentrations up to 100 times greater than the
corresponding D(-) compounds. We deduce from this fact that the
"wrong" isomers do not gain access to the receptor sites at all,
or that their affinities for the sites are very much lower. Stereospecific binding (SSB) should be indicative of narcotic receptor
binding. Such binding could be expected to comprise only a very
small fraction of the total apparent binding of narcotic molecules
to macromolecular or membrane fractions of brain, for two reasons.
First, nonspecific ionic interactions are bound to occur, since
the narcotics are cations at physiologic pH by virtue of their

protonated nitrogen atom; thus, they should interact with many
anionic components such as acidic proteins, nucleic acids,
mucopolysaccharides, and lipids. Second, like virtually all
psychoactive drugs, the narcotics are highly lipophilic--else
they could not pass the blood-brain barrier--and therefore simple
solution in lipid membranes and hydrophobic interaction with
lipophilic regions of proteins may be expected. Our basic method,
therefore, is not to look for binding per se, but rather for the
difference in binding of a radioactive narcotic, D(-)-levorphanol,
under two conditions. In condition B, a tracer amount of ^{3}H- or
^{14}C-levorphanol is introduced in vitro into a particulate suspension from brain that has been preincubated with nonradioactive
dextrorphan, the L(+) enantiomer of levorphanol. In condition C,
nonradioactive levorphanol is used for the preincubation. Since
the total narcotic concentration is identical in the two conditions,
the binding of the radioactive drug should be the same if there is
no stereospecific binding, for all the sites will be available to
both isomers. Any difference in binding (B minus C) should
measure SSB.

The absolute configuration of D(-)-levorphanol is seen in
Figure 2, which shows the molecule rotated in 90 degree steps
about an axis running from top to bottom in the plane of the paper.
The nitrogen atom, which in its protonated form presumably estab-
lishes an ionic bond to an anionic group in the receptor, is
placed in a completely lipophilic flat surface. The phenolic
oxygen, equally essential to narcotic action, and which presumably participates in a hydrogen bond to an appropriate residue of
the receptor, is situated at the end of another lipophilic region.
It is easy to imagine a stereospecific pocket that would accomodate
the D(-) isomers and exclude (or react only poorly with) the
L(+) isomers.

We have confirmed the pharmacologic stereospecificity of.
levorphanol in our laboratory. In mice, as shown in Figure 3,
levorphanol produces both analgesia and running activity (ED50
approximately 3 mg/kg, concentration in brain water about 10^{-7} M),
whereas dextrorphan is without effect up to lethality. The lethal
action is not stereospecific; its mechanism is unknown. In the
myenteric plexus-longitudinal muscle preparation from guinea pig
ileum (Kosterlitz et al., 1970), as shown in Figure 4, the ED50
for levorphanol is about 10^{-7} M, while dextrorphan, at 10-fold
greater concentration (and even at 100-fold, not shown) is
neither an agonist nor an antagonist.

Since a large part of the total nonspecific interaction of
radioactive levorphanol with mouse brain tissue appeared to be
due to simple solution of the lipophilic drug molecules in membranes, we explored the possibility of using a more hydrophilic

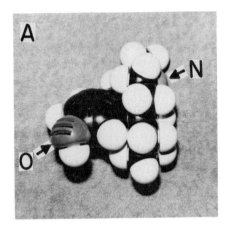
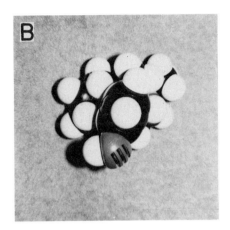
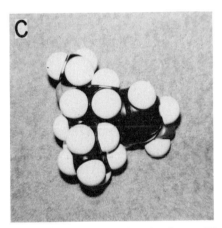
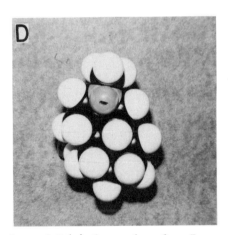

Figure 2. Stereochemical configuration of D(−)-levorphanol. In panel A, arrows show phenolic hydroxyl group at lower left, nitrogen atom embedded in surface facing to the reader's right. Panels B, C, and D depict successive 90 degree rotations of the molecule about an axis running from top to bottom in the plane of the paper. In Panel B, the phenolic hydroxyl group has been rotated toward the reader. Panel D shows most clearly the position of the nitrogen atom (not protonated here) in a flat lipophilic surface.

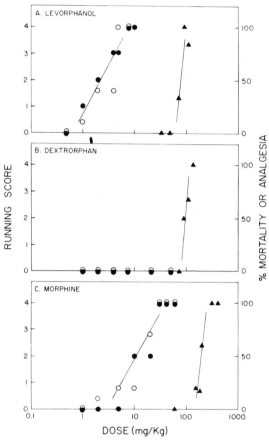

Figure 3. Stereospecificity of narcotic action in the mouse. Solid
circles: running activity. Open circles: analgesia. Triangles:
lethality. Dextrorphan is L(+) enantiomer of levorphanol. See
text for description. (Reproduced from Goldstein and Sheehan,
1969, Figure 3).

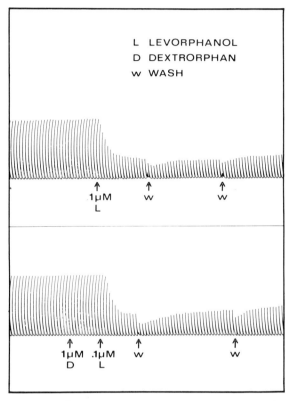

Figure 4. Stereospecificity of narcotic action on the guinea pig ileum longitudinal muscle strip with attached myenteric plexus. Isometric contractions induced by field stimulation, maximum response voltage, duration 0.5 msec. square waves, 0.1 Hz, tension approx. 0.5 g. Upper panel: normal response to levorphanol (L). Delayed recovery of tension on washing (W) is typical of levorphanol, in contrast to morphine. Lower panel: dextrorphan, at 10 times levorphanol concentration, has neither agonistic nor antagonistic action.

narcotic. Published reports (Sasajima, 1970; Hosoya and Oka, 1970)
indicated that morphine 3-glucuronide had analgesic effect when
injected intracerebrally, suggesting that this hydrophilic derivative was inactive by systemic administration only because it could
not gain access to brain tissue across the blood-brain barrier.
If true that the glucuronides of the narcotics could combine with
opiate receptors when brought into contact with them, this would
provide a means for circumventing much of the nonspecific binding,
and thereby simplifying the identification of the small amount of
SSB. As published elsewhere (Schulz and Goldstein, 1972), however,
this proved an illusory hope. In the longitudinal muscle strip
from guinea-pig ileum, with neurons of the myenteric plexus in
direct contact with the aqueous medium, morphine and levorphanol
glucuronides were inert. Moreover, we showed by means of doubly
labelled levorphanol glucuronide, that the analgesia produced on
intracerebral injection can be accounted for fully by the rapid
hydrolysis of the glucuronide that occurs in the brain tissue after
intracerebral injection.

As we reported elsewhere (Goldstein et al., 1971; Pal et al.,
1971), less than 2 per cent of the total binding of levorphanol
in mouse brain homogenate is SSB. This is almost entirely in a
membrane fraction, and it (together with a great deal of nonspecific binding material) is extractable into chloroform-
methanol (2:1). Fractionation of such extracts on Sephadex LH-20
indicated binding to a variety of lipid components, most of which
is not stereospecific. Figure 5 illustrates the competition of
nonradioactive dextrorphan for such sites, with apparent dissociation constant 1.2×10^{-3} M. Here the entire range of dextrorphan
concentrations was explored, with different concentrations of
radioactive levorphanol, from 10^{-7} M to more than 10^{-2} M. Assuming
that the binding constants for levorphanol and dextrorphan are
identical ($K_L = K_D = 1.2 \times 10^{-3}$ M) i.e., that the binding is not
stereospecific, theoretical curves can be constructed, according
to the equation

$$f = \cfrac{1}{1 + \cfrac{(D)}{K_L + (L)}}$$

which is derived from the mass law, where f is the fraction of the
binding obtained with L alone, and (D) and (L) are the concentrations of free dextrorphan and levorphanol, respectively. These
experiments were carried out by the phase partition method of
Weber et al. (1971), and the free concentrations are those measured
in the aqueous phase. A single curve is obtained as long as the
radioactive levorphanol concentration is well below K_L, i.e., at
low fractional occupanices. The curve shifts to the right at
levorphanol concentrations that produce significant fractional

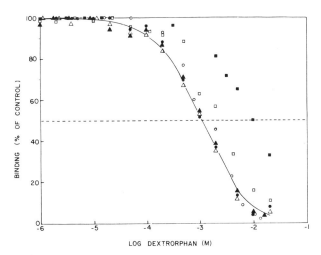

LOG DEXTRORPHAN (M)

Figure 5. Dextrorphan competition for levorphanol binding sites in chloroform-methanol extract of mouse brain. Phase distribution between chloroform-methanol (2:1) extract and citrate buffer, pH 6.0. Varied concentrations of dextrorphan, preincubated 5 min before addition of fixed concentration of ^{14}C-levorphanol. Radioactivity assayed in each phase after equilibration. Binding computed from increased apparent partition coefficient compared with no-extract control. Levorphanol concentrations in aqueous phase (M): o - o, 1.2×10^{-7}; • - •, 1.5×10^{-6}; Δ - Δ, 1.0×10^{-5}; ▲ - ▲, 1.1×10^{-4}; □ - □, 1.2×10^{-3}; ■ - ■, 1.9×10^{-2}. In each case the binding in the absence of dextrorphan is designated 100%. The log of the molar concentration of dextrorphan in the aqueous phase is shown on the x-axis.

occupancy. The experimental points are entirely in accord with the theoretical assumption that the sites are preponderantly non-stereospecific. However, a few per cent SSB could not be detected by this procedure.

A precipitate forms in the chloroform-methanol extract of mouse brain upon addition of certain alkaloids, including the opiate narcotics. The total amount of levorphanol precipitated in this way is equivalent to about 2500 nmoles per brain (400 mg wet weight, 40 mg protein), as shown in Figure 6. Throughout the range of partial precipitation, about nine molecules of levorphanol remained free for each molecule in the precipitate. This indicated a loosely bound reversible complex, a conclusion that was confirmed by sequential washes of the precipitate with chloroform-methanol, as shown in Figure 7. Of the total 2500 nmoles, about 9 nmoles is seen to be tightly bound. Of this, 3 nmoles proved to be stereo-specifically bound (shown elsewhere, Goldstein, 1972), in that it

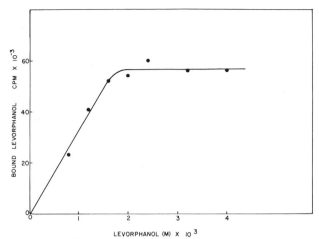

LEVORPHANOL (M) X 10^3

Figure 6. Precipitation of material from mouse brain by levorphanol. An amount of chloroform-methanol (2:1) extract equivalent
to 1/5 brain was precipitated with ^{14}C-levorphanol at various
concentrations in total volume 2 ml. The material was passed
through glass filters. Levorphanol complexed in precipitate was
calculated from difference of counts in filtrate between runs with
and without brain extract. Maximum precipitate represents 2500
nmoles bound levorphanol.

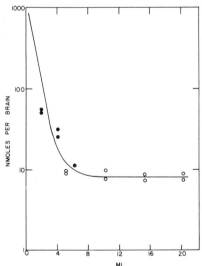

Figure 7. Tightly complexed levorphanol in precipitates from
chloroform-methanol extracts of mouse brain. Each tube contained
1/10 brain equivalent and was precipitated with 2×10^{-3} M ^{14}C-
levorphanol, then centrifuged. Solid circles represent 2 ml washes,
open circles 5 ml washes. Total wash volume is given on x-axis.
Successive washes reduce original 2500 nmoles per brain to about
9 nmoles per brain tightly complexed material.

could not be blocked by dextrorphan concentrations as high as 10^{-2} M. It is interesting that a Scatchard plot of SSB with whole homogenate of mouse brain also revealed a high-affinity binding with a capacity of 3 nmoles per brain.

Let me summarize our quantitative results. We found that the total binding of levorphanol to mouse brain homogenate followed a nonsaturable curve with increasing drug concentration. A Scatchard plot of the total binding revealed at least two components, the one of highest affinity having an apparent capacity of about 6000 nmoles per brain. A Scatchard plot of total binding in the chloroform-methanol extract (by the phase partition method) yielded a total capacity of 8000 nmoles per brain for the high-affinity component. The precipitation method gave 2500 nmoles for the corresponding total binding. On the other hand, when high-affinity SSB was examined by similar methods, a capacity of only about 3 nmoles per brain was found, both in whole homogenate and by the precipitation method. At pharmacologic concentrations, as shown previously (Goldstein et al., 1970), SSB was about 1 nmole per brain. The total binding is greatly in excess of the 50 nmoles of proteolipid protein per brain in the chloroform-methanol extract but it could represent a mole for mole combination with any of several kinds of lipids such as phospholipids (25,000 nmoles), galactolipids (3,000 nmoles), plasmalogens (5,600 nmoles) or gangliosides (1,000 nmoles) (Lapetina et al., 1968). SSB, on the other hand, could be accounted for by a small fraction of the proteolipid protein. The question whether even a few nmoles per brain is too much material to represent narcotic receptors, as suggested by Dole (1970), must be left unanswered for the moment. If the pharmacologic actions of the most potent narcotics can be triggered by a conformational change in a small fraction of the total receptors (Stephenson, 1956; Paton, 1961), our estimate may not be unreasonable.

I am grateful to Louise I. Lowney and Dr. Rudiger Schulz, whose experimental results are included here. Hoffman-LaRoche, Inc., generously supplied levorphanol and dextrorphan. The work was supported by grant 13963 from the National Institute of Mental Health.

REFERENCES

Cheney, D.L. and Goldstein, A. 1971. Tolerance to opioid narcotics, III. Time course and reversibility of physical dependence in mice. Nature 232: 477.
Collier, H.O.J. 1965. A general theory of the genesis of drug dependence by induction of receptors. Nature 205: 181.
Dole. V.P. 1970. Biochemistry of addiction. Ann.Rev.Biochem. 39: 821.
Goldstein, A. and Goldstein, D.B. 1968. Enzyme expansion theory of drug tolerance and physical dependence. Proc. Assoc. Res. Nerv. Ment. Dis. 46: 265.

Goldstein, D.B. and Goldstein, A. 1961. Possible role of enzyme
    inhibition and repression in drug tolerance and addiction.
    Presented at First International Pharmacological Meeting,
    Stockholm. Biochem. Pharmacol. 8: 48.
Goldstein, A. and Goldstein, D.B. 1968. Enzyme expansion theory
    of drug tolerance and physical dependence. Proc. Assoc.
    Res. Nerv. Ment. Dis. 46: 265.
Goldstein, A., Lowney, L.I. and Pal, B.K. 1971 Stereospecific and
    nonspecific interactions of the morphine congener levor-
    phanol in subcellular fractions of mouse brain. Proc. Nat.
    Acad. Sci. USA 68: 1742.
Goldstein, A. and Sheehan, P. 1969. Tolerance to opioid narcotics.
    I. Tolerance to the "running fit" caused by levorphanol in
    the mouse. J. Pharmacol. Exp. Ther. 169: 175.
Hosoya, E. and Oka, T. 1970. Studies on morphine glucuronide.
    Med. Center J. Univ. of Mich. 36(4): 241.
Jacob, F. and Monod, J. 1961. Genetic regulatory mechanisms in
    the synthesis of proteins. J. Mol. Biol. 3: 318.
Jaffe, J.H. 1970. Drug addiction and drug abuse. In: The
    Pharmacological Basis of Therapeutics (Eds. Goodman, L.S.
    and Gilman, A.), New York: The Macmillan Company, Chapter 16,
    pp. 276.
Kosterlitz, H.W., Lydon, R.J. and Watt, A.J. 1970. The effect
    of adrenaline, noradrenaline and isoprenaline on inhibitory
    α- and β-adrenoceptors in the longitudinal muscle of the
    guinea-pig ileum. Brit. J. Pharmacol. 39: 398.
Lapetina, E.G., Soto, E.F. and DeRobertis, E. 1968. Lipids and
    proteolipids in isolated subcellular membranes of rat brain
    cortex. J. Neurochemistry 15: 437.
Pal, B.K., Lowney, L.I. and Goldstein, A. 1971. Further studies
    on the stereospecific binding of levorphanol by a membrane
    fraction from mouse brain. Proc. Symposium on Agonist and
    Antagonist Actions of Narcotic Analgesic Drugs, Aberdeen,
    Scotland. Brit. J. Pharmacol. (in press).
Paton, W.D.M. 1961. A theory of drug action based on the rate
    of drug-receptor combination. Proc. Roy. Soc. Ser. B. 154: 21.
Sasajima, M. 1970. Analgesic effect of morphine-3-monoglucuronide.
    Keio Igaku 47: 421.
Schulz, R. and Goldstein, A. 1972. Inactivity of narcotic glucur-
    onides as analgesics and on guinea pig ileum. J. Pharmacol.
    Exp. Ther. (in press).
Shuster, L. 1961. Repression and de-repression of enzyme synthesis
    as a possible explanation of some aspects of drug action. Nature
    189: 314.
Stephenson, R.P. 1956. A modification of receptor theory. Brit.
    J. Pharmacol. 11: 379.
Way, E.L., Loh, H.H. and Shen, F.-H. 1968. Morphine tolerance,
    physical dependence, and synthesis of brain 5-hydroxytryptamine.
    Science 162: 1290.

Way, E.L., Loh, H.H. and Shen, F.-H. 1969. Simultaneous quantita-
   tive assessment of morphine tolerance and physical dependence.
   J. Pharmacol. Exp. Ther. 167: 1.
Weber, G., Borris, D.P., DeRobertis, E., Barrantes, F.J., LaTorre,
   J.L. and DeCarlin, M. 1971. The use of a cholinergic
   fluorescent probe for the study of the receptor proteolipid.
   Molec. Pharmacol. 7: 530.

INDEX